THE PHYSIOLOGY OF THE JOINTS

Seventh edition

A.I. KAPANDJI

Honorary Member of the French Society of Orthopaedics and Traumatology
Honorary Member and President (1987-1988) of the French Society of Hand Surgeons
Member of the American Society for Surgery of the Hand and of the Italian Society for Surgery of the Hand
Corresponding Foreign Member of the Argentine Society of Orthopaedics and Traumatology

THE PHYSIOLOGY OF THE JOINTS

Foreword by Professor Thierry Judet

2

Seventh edition

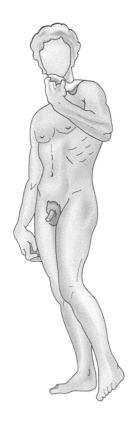

1. The Hip
2. The Knee
3. The Ankle
4. The Foot
5. The Plantar Vault
6. Walking

843 original drawings by the author
Translated by Dr Louis Honoré

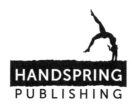

HANDSPRING
PUBLISHING

Handspring Publishing
Carmelite House
50 Victoria Embankment
London EC4Y 0DZ
www.handspringpublishing.com

Seventh edition first published in 2018 in French by Éditions Maloine under the title
Anatomie fonctionnelle: 2. Membre supérieur by A.I. Kapandji.
Copyright © Éditions Maloine 2018 – ISBN: 978-2-224-03495-5

Seventh edition first published in 2019 in English in the United Kingdom by Handspring Publishing (an imprint of Jessica Kingsley
Publishers, an imprint of Hodder & Stoughton Ltd, an Hachette UK Company) by arrangement with Éditions Maloine.

ISBN 978-1-912085-60-6

British Library Cataloguing in Publication Data

A catalogue record for this book is available from the British Library

Library of Congress Cataloguing in Publication Data

A catalogue record for this book is available from the Library of Congress

Notice
Neither the Publisher nor the Author assume any responsibility for any loss or injury and/or damage to persons or property arising out
of or relating to any use of the material contained in this book. It is the responsibility of the treating practitioner, relying on independent
expertise and knowledge of the patient, to determine the best treatment and method of application for the patient.

Cover painting: A.I. Kapandji

Printed in France

To my wife
To my mother, the artist
To my father, the surgeon
To my maternal grandfather, the mechanic

Foreword

'Look it up in Kapandji; you'll understand it then'.
Which of us, in my own generation or those that followed, having personally spent long hours reading Kapandji, has never said those words to a younger colleague? The knowledge of anatomy and biomechanics gleaned from *The Physiology of the Joints* is at the heart of our profession, whether we seek to understand a symptom, a clinical diagnostic procedure or an operative manoeuvre. Following in the footsteps of the great anatomists, who are inescapable and sometimes forbidding, Adalbert Kapandji knew from the very start how to bring a new dimension to the understanding and especially to the teaching of functional anatomy; everything becomes clear and simple, and the reader finds himself feeling a little more intelligent!

Thank you, Kap: anything can seem easy when genius is behind the scenes. And the genius here is certainly the product of an encyclopaedic knowledge. This volume follows those on the upper limb and the spinal column. It is genius based on a perfection of movement, be it in the stroke of a pen or in the elegance and efficiency of a surgical operation.
It is genius nourished by a rich imagination, applied equally to surgery and to the explanation of the 'why' and 'how' of functional anatomy. Finally, it is the genius of an impeccable teaching approach, which has never wavered over time.

The new edition bears witness to this genius. Expanded and enriched even more than the preceding editions, it deserves pride of place on the shelves of all those who are interested in movement: students and established practitioners, surgeons, rheumatologists and rehabilitation specialists as well as all physiotherapists.

Professor Thierry Judet

Preface to the sixth edition

In the sixth edition of this work on functional anatomy, the three volumes published on this subject have been re-cast and updated. With computer assistance, the author has undertaken the demanding task of re-issuing all the illustrations in colour, thus making them all the more illuminating and helpful. We can properly call this a metamorphosis, and it has been accompanied by a complete re-writing of the text. The new edition also contains many additions and improvements, not only in the original chapters, but also in the shape of a new chapter entitled 'Walking' and of an Appendix with a 'Synoptic Table of the Nerves of the Lower Limb'. Finally, faithful to the idea of three-dimensional diagrams, the author has supplied, at the end of the book, mechanical models for the reader to construct, offering real practical experience in biomechanics. Some have been omitted or simplified; some new ones have been introduced.

Preface to the seventh edition

This new edition is a carefully corrected and improved version of the original text and also contains eight new pages dealing with the elasticity of the Achilles tendon, the barycentre of the pregnant woman, additional information on the half step, the swinging of the upper limbs and the different types of walking, simple or military, and jumps. This new book should have a renewed interest for the reader.

Contents

Chapter 1

THE HIP

The hip joint (coxofemoral joint)

When quadrupeds evolved into bipeds, the hip joint, which was the proximal joint of the posterior limb, became the joint at the root of the lower limb, while the proximal joint of the anterior limb (the shoulder) became the joint at the root of the upper limb. The **upper limb** has lost its supportive and locomotor function to become a *free-hanging* limb providing logistical support to the **prehensile** hand.

Concurrently, the **lower limb** has retained its locomotor function, thus becoming the only limb responsible for **body support and locomotion.** As a result, the hip has become the only joint able to support the body at rest and during locomotion. This new role has led to profound changes in its structure.

Whereas the shoulder is a multi-articular complex functionally, the **hip**, as a single joint, ensures both the **orientation and support** of the lower limb and therefore enjoys a wide range of movements (partly offset by the lumbar spine), as well as a greater degree of stability (it is the most difficult joint to dislocate in the whole body). These features reflect its role both in body support and in locomotion.

Artificial replacement of the hip ushered in the era of *joint prostheses*, which have revolutionized orthopaedics. It is seemingly the easiest joint to model mechanically because its articular surfaces closely resemble those of a sphere, but there are still many outstanding problems, i.e. the proper size of the prosthetic head, the fraction coefficient of the surfaces in contact, their resistance to wear and tear and the potential toxicity of wear debris. More important however, is the problem of the *mode of linkage of the prosthesis to the living bone*, i.e. whether cemented or not, particularly since some prostheses can become secondarily fused as their surfaces become coated with living cells. Prosthesis research is most advanced for the hip, which also enjoys the largest number of proposed models.

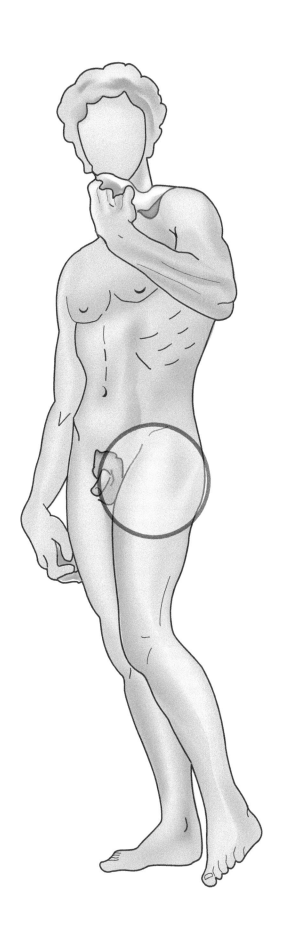

The hip: the joint at the root of the lower limb

The hip is the **proximal joint of the lower limb** located at its root and is responsible for its full orientation in space; hence its three axes and three degrees of freedom **(Fig. 1)**.

- A *transverse* axis XOX', lying in the coronal plane for movements of **flexion-extension**
- A *sagittal* axis YOY', located in an *anteroposterior* plane passing through the centre O of the joint and controlling movements of **abduction-adduction**
- A *vertical* axis OZ, which is collinear with the long axis OR of the lower limb when the hip is straight. It controls the movements of **lateral rotation** and **medial rotation** of the lower limb as a whole.

Hip movements occur in a single joint, the hip or coxofemoral joint. It is an enarthrosis, i.e. a tight-fitting *spheroidal* joint that differs from the shoulder joint, which is a loose-fitting enarthrosis with great mobility at the expense of stability. The hip joint has a more limited range of movements, partly offset by a contribution from the lumbar spine. Enhanced stability compensates for this shortcoming.

The hip joint is *subject to compressive forces* as it supports the body, whereas the shoulder joint is *subject to tensile forces*.

Although the hip, like the shoulder, is a triaxial joint with three degrees of freedom, its movements, particularly in abduction, do not have the range necessary to reproduce the Codman's paradox observed at the shoulder joint. Thus, this pseudo-paradox (see Volume 1) does not exist in the lower limb.

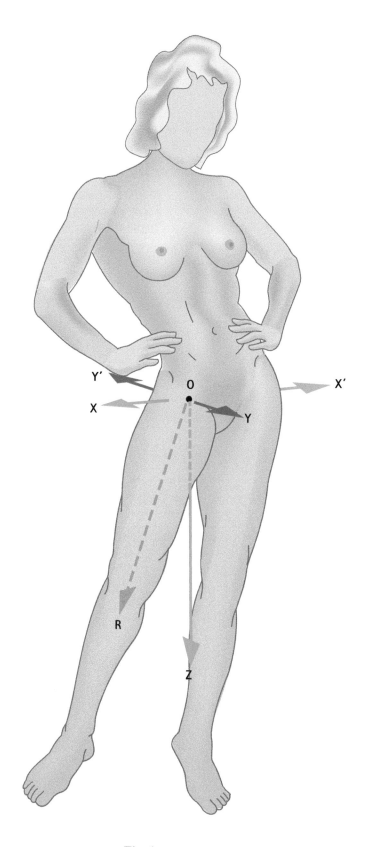

Fig. 1

5

Movements of flexion at the hip joint

Flexion at the hip joint is the movement that brings the anterior aspect of the thigh closer to the trunk so that the whole lower limb comes to lie anterior to the coronal plane passing through the joint. The **range of flexion** depends on multiple factors.

- On the whole, **active flexion** has a smaller range than passive flexion. The *position of the knee joint* also determines the range of hip flexion: with the *knee extended* **(Fig. 2)**, flexion reaches 90°; with the *knee flexed* **(Fig. 3)**, flexion can reach up to 120° or beyond.
- The range of **passive flexion** always exceeds 120° but is still dependent on the position of the knee. If the knee is *extended* **(Fig. 4)**, the range of flexion is clearly more limited than if the knee is *flexed* **(Fig. 5)**: **its amplitude is 145°**, and the thigh almost touches the thorax. It will be shown later (p. 146) how knee flexion allows a greater degree of flexion by relaxing the hamstrings.
- If both hips **are flexed passively at the same time** while the knees are already flexed **(Fig. 6)**, the anterior aspects of the thighs come into contact with the chest because hip flexion is compounded with posterior *tilting of the pelvis* due to flattening of the lumbar lordosis (arrow).

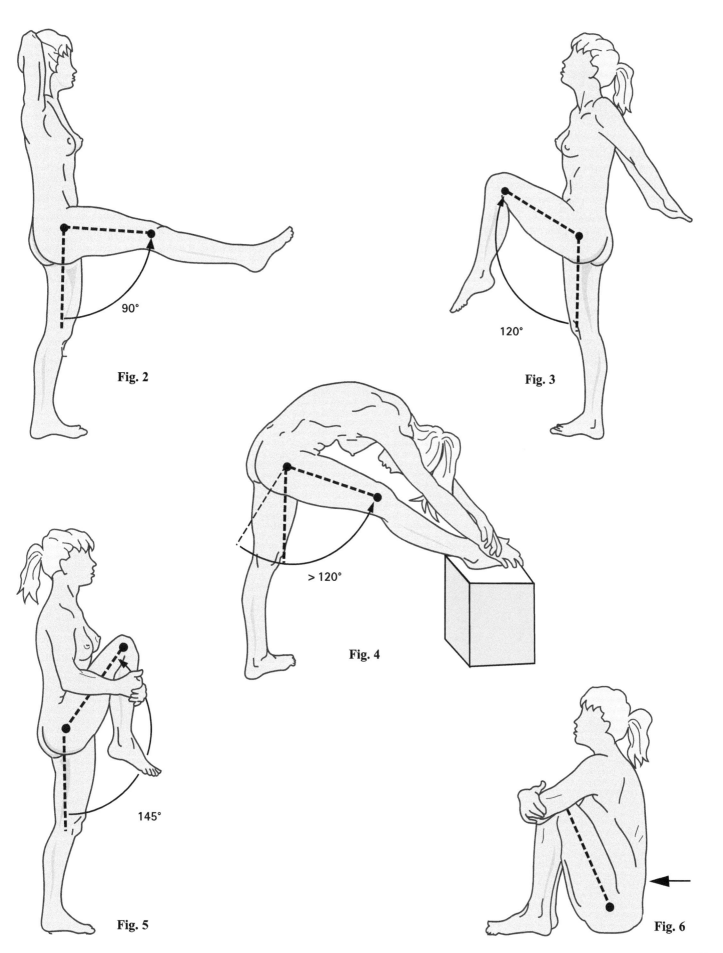

Fig. 2

90°

Fig. 3

120°

Fig. 4

> 120°

Fig. 5

145°

Fig. 6

Movements of extension at the hip joint

Extension takes the lower limb posterior to the coronal plane. The range of extension is notably less than that of flexion and is limited by the tension of the iliofemoral ligament (see p. 28). **Active extension** has a smaller range than passive extension. With the **knee extended (Fig. 7)**, hip extension has a greater range (20°) than with the **knee flexed**, when it is 10° **(Fig. 8)**. This follows from the fact that the hamstrings lose some of their efficiency as hip extensors because most of their contraction has been utilized to flex the knee (see p. 146).

Passive extension attains 20° **when the body makes a lunge (Fig. 9)** and 30° when the ipsilateral hand forcibly pulls the lower limb backwards **(Fig. 10)**.

Note that hip extension is appreciably increased by the anterior tilting of the pelvis that follows the concurrent *lumbar hyperlordosis*. This contribution of the lumbar spine can be measured **(Fig. 7 and 8)** as the angle between the vertical (Fine broken line) and the straight position of the thigh (medium broken line). The latter is easily determined because the angle between that position of the thigh and the line joining the centre of the hip joint to the anterior superior iliac spine is constant. This angle, however, varies with the individual as it depends on the static properties of the pelvis, i.e. the degree of anterior or posterior tilting.

The ranges given here apply to the normal untrained subject. They are considerably *increased by exercise and training*. Ballerinas, for example, can commonly do the *sideways splits* **(Fig. 11)**, even without resting on the ground, because of the flexibility of the iliofemoral ligament. It is worth noting, however, that they make up for the inadequate extension of the posterior thigh by a significant degree of forward pelvic tilting.

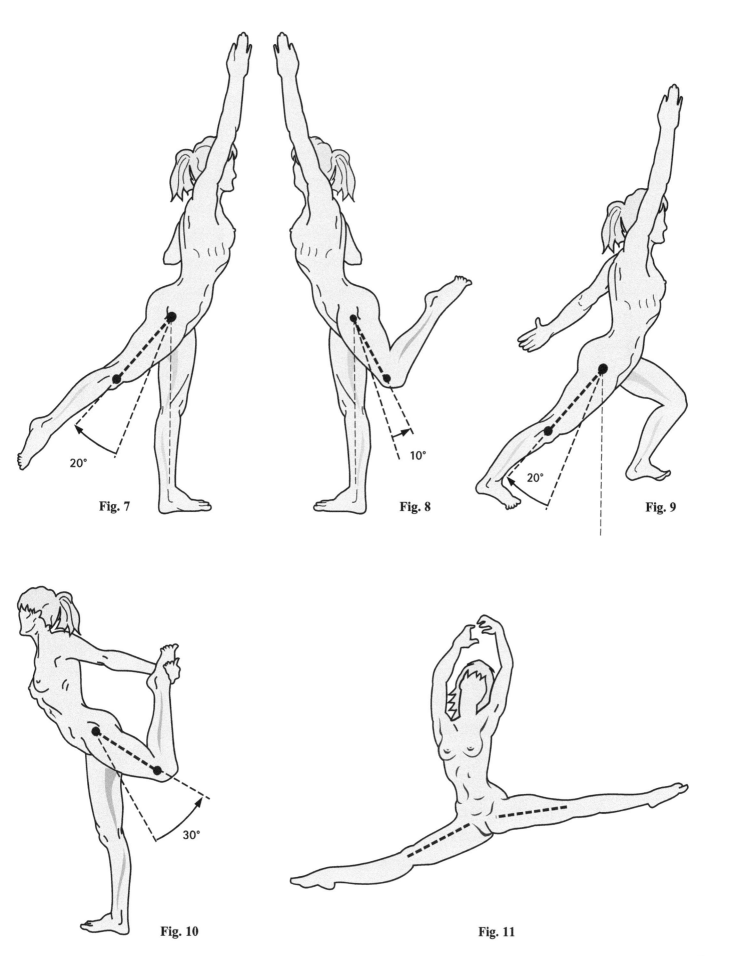

Fig. 7

Fig. 8

Fig. 9

Fig. 10

Fig. 11

Movements of abduction at the hip joint

Abduction displaces the lower limb *laterally and away from the plane of symmetry* of the body.

It is entirely possible theoretically to **abduct only one hip**, but in practice, abduction of one hip is automatically followed by a similar degree of abduction of the other hip. This becomes obvious after 30° abduction **(Fig. 12)**, when tilting of the pelvis is clearly observed as tilting of the line joining the surface markings of the two posterior iliac spines. If the long axes of the two lower limbs are produced, they can be seen to intersect on the axis of symmetry of the pelvis. This indicates that in this position, each hip has been abducted at 15°.

When abduction reaches an **absolute maximum (Fig. 13)** the angle between the two lower limbs is a right angle. Once more abduction can be seen to have occurred symmetrically at both hips, leading to the conclusion that each hip has a maximum of 45° abduction. Note that the pelvis is now tilted at an angle of 45° to the horizontal on the side of the supporting hip. The spinal column as a whole offsets this pelvic tilt by bending laterally towards the supporting limb. Here again the *spine is seen to participate* in hip movements.

Abduction is checked by the impact of the femoral neck on the acetabular margin (see p. 26), but well before this occurs, it has already been restrained by the adductor muscles and the ilio- and pubo-femoral ligaments (see p. 34).

Exercise and training can notably augment the maximal range of abduction: for example, ballerinas can achieve 120° **(Fig. 14)** to 130° **(Fig. 15)** active abduction without any support. Trained subjects can achieve 180° passive abduction by doing the splits sideways **(Fig. 16)**. In fact, this is no longer pure abduction, since, to slacken the iliofemoral ligaments, the pelvis is tilted anteriorly **(Fig. 17)**, while the lumbar spine is hyperextended (arrow); the hip is now in a position of abduction-flexion.

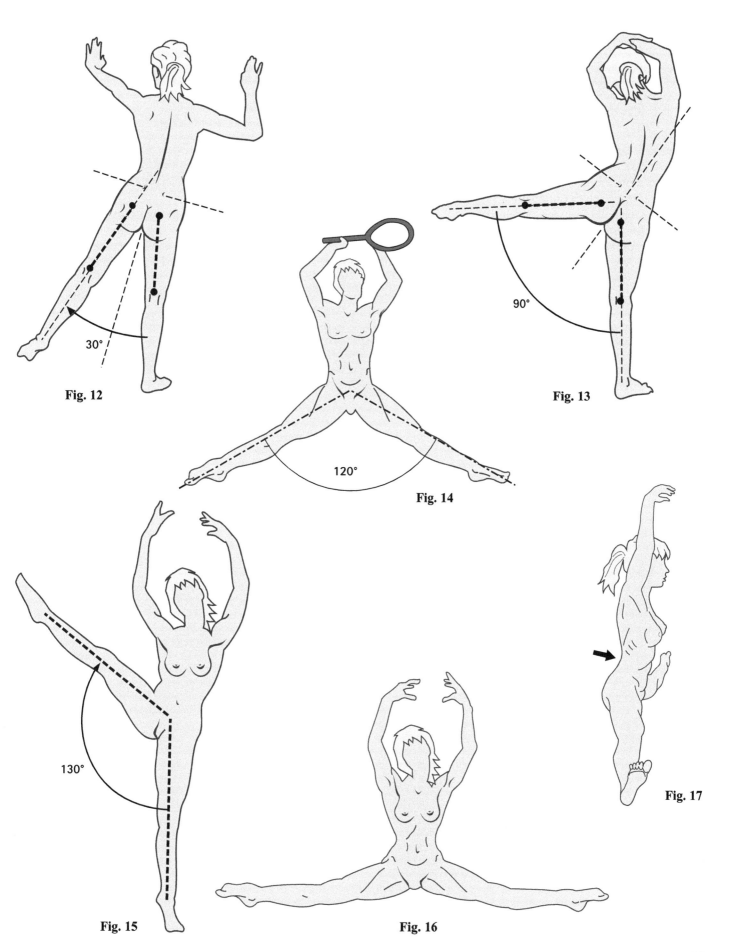

Fig. 12

Fig. 13

Fig. 14

Fig. 15

Fig. 16

Fig. 17

30°

90°

120°

130°

11

Movements of adduction at the hip joint

Adduction is the movement of the lower limb *medially towards the plane of symmetry of the body.* Since in the reference position both lower limbs are in contact there is no 'pure' adduction.

On the other hand, **relative adduction (Fig. 18)** occurs when the limb moves medially from any position of abduction.

There are also movements of **adduction combined with extension** of the hip **(Fig. 19)** and of **adduction combined with flexion** of the hip **(Fig. 20).**

Finally, there are also movements of **adduction at one hip combined with abduction at the other hip (Fig. 21)**; these are associated with tilting of the pelvis and hyperlordosis of the lumbar spine. Note that when the feet are set apart (as is necessary to maintain balance) the angle of adduction at one hip

is not equal to that of abduction at the other **(Fig. 22)**. The difference between these two angles is equal to the angle between the two axes of the lower limbs as they lie in the initial position of symmetry.

In all these combined movements involving adduction, the maximal range of adduction is 30°.

Of all these combined adduction movements, one is most common **(Fig. 23)**, as illustrated by the **cross-legged sitting position.** Adduction is then associated with flexion and external rotation. This is the position of maximal instability for the hip (see p. 38). It is often the posture adopted by front-seat passengers, thus exposing them to dashboard hip dislocation.

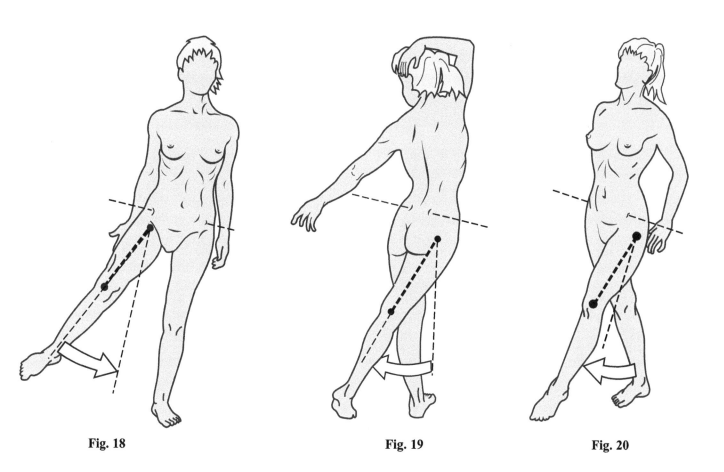

Fig. 18

Fig. 19

Fig. 20

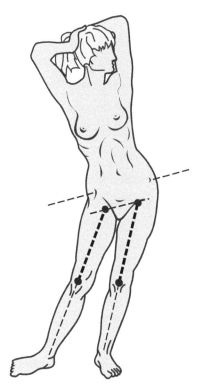

Fig. 21

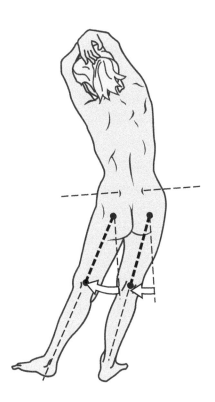

Fig. 22

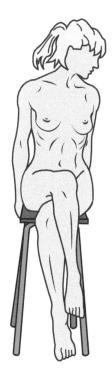

Fig. 23

Movements of axial rotation at the hip joint

These movements occur around the *mechanical axis of the lower limb* (see axis OR, **Fig. 1**). In the straight position this axis coincides with the vertical axis of the hip joint (see axis OZ, **Fig. 1**). Under these circumstances **lateral rotation** is the movement of the limb that brings the tips of the toes to face laterally, and **medial rotation** brings the tips of the toes to face medially. Since the knee is fully extended (see p. 136), the hip is the only joint responsible for this rotation.

Nevertheless, this is not the position used for the assessment of the range of rotational movements, which is better carried out with the subject lying prone or sitting on the edge of a table with the *knee flexed at 90°*.

When the subject is **lying prone**, the **reference position (Fig. 24)** is obtained when the leg is almost at right angles to the thigh and is vertical. From this position, when the leg swings *laterally*, *medial rotation* **(Fig. 25)** occurs with a total range of 30-40°. When the leg swings *medially*, *lateral rotation* **(Fig. 26)** occurs with a total range of 60°.

When the subject **sits on the edge of the table** with the hip and the knee flexed at 90°, the same criteria apply: when the leg swings *medially*, **lateral rotation** occurs **(Fig. 27)**; when the leg swings *laterally*, **medial rotation** occurs **(Fig. 28)**. In this position the total range of lateral rotation can be greater than in the lying-down position because hip flexion *relaxes the ilio- and pubo-femoral ligaments*, which are the main checks on lateral rotation (see p. 32).

In the **squatting position (Fig. 29)** lateral rotation is combined with abduction and flexion exceeding 90°. Yoga experts can achieve such a degree of lateral rotation that their two legs become parallel and horizontal ('the lotus position').

The range of rotation depends on the angle of anteversion of the femoral neck, which is quite marked in the child. As a result, the thigh is medially rotated, and the child displays an in-toeing gait, often coupled with a bilateral pes planovalgus. With growth, the angle of anteversion decreases to normal adult values, and these walking problems disappear. This wide angle of anteversion, however, can be maintained and even increased when children become accustomed (wrongly) to sitting on the ground with *their heels pressed against each other* and their hips *flexed*. This posture causes medial rotation of the femur and accentuates the angle of anteversion of both femoral necks because of the great plasticity of the young skeleton. This defect can be corrected by forcing the child to adopt the inverse sitting position, i.e. the squatting position or even better, the lotus position. Over time, this leads to remodelling of the femoral neck into a more retroverted position.

This **angle of anteversion of the femoral neck** was difficult to measure by routine radiology, but nowadays with the **CT scan** it can be measured easily and accurately. This method should be used to evaluate malrotations of the lower limb, which usually *start* at the hip.

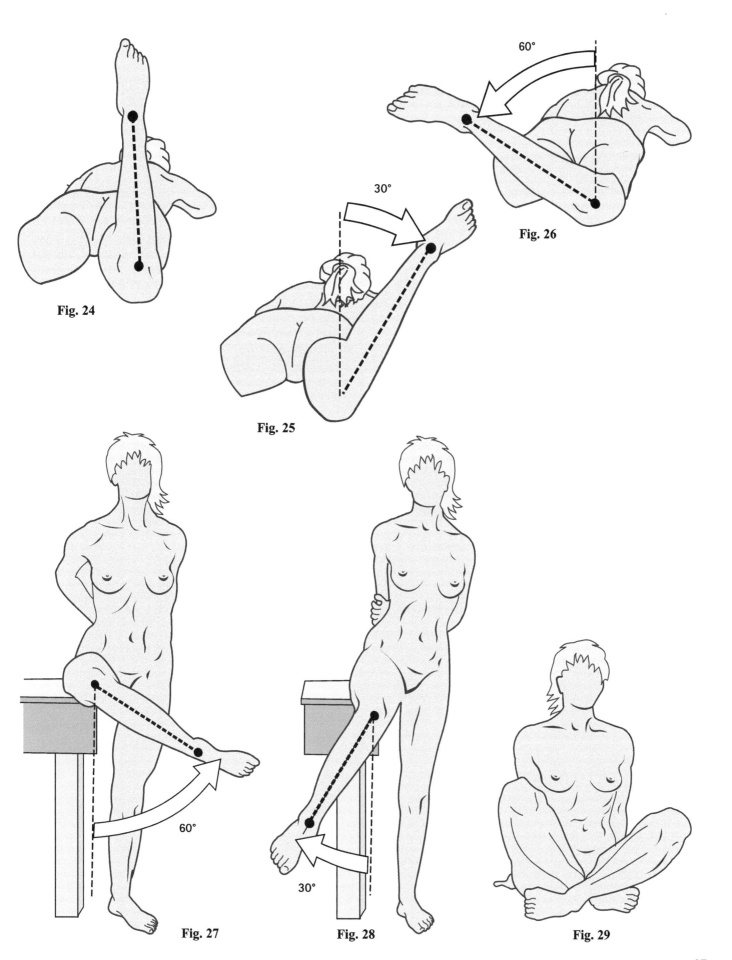

Fig. 24

Fig. 25

Fig. 26

Fig. 27

Fig. 28

Fig. 29

Movements of circumduction at the hip joint

As with all joints with three degrees of freedom, the movement of circumduction of the hip is defined as the *combination of elementary movements occurring simultaneously around the three axes*. When circumduction reaches its *maximal amplitude*, the axis of the lower limb traces in space a *cone* with its apex at the centre of the hip joint: this is the **cone of circumduction (Fig. 30)**.

This cone is far from symmetrical, as the maximal ranges of the various elementary movements in space are not equal. Thus the path traced by the extremity of the lower limb is not a circle but a *wavy curve* traversing the various sectors of space established by the *intersection of the three planes of reference:*

1. The sagittal plane (S), containing the movements of flexion-extension

2. The coronal plane (C), containing the movements of abduction-adduction

3. The horizontal plane (H).

The eight sectors of space are numbered I-VIII, and the cone traverses the following sectors successively: III, II, I, IV, V and VIII. Note how the curve skirts the supporting limb; if the latter were removed, the curve would be slightly shifted inwards. The arrow R, representing the distal, anterior and lateral prolongation of the lower limb in sector IV, is the **axis of the cone of circumduction** and corresponds to the *position of function and of immobilization of the hip.*

Strasser proposed that the **curve be inscribed on a sphere (Fig. 31)** with centre **O** lying at the centre of the hip joint, with radius **OF** equal to the length of the femur and with **LM** representing the equator. On this sphere can be determined the various range maxima with the use of a system of latitudes and longitudes (not drawn in the diagram).

He had also proposed a similar method for the shoulder, where it is more relevant because of the greater degree of axial rotation of the upper limb.

Starting from a chosen position, OL, of the femur, movements of abduction (arrow *Ab*) and of adduction (arrow (*Ad*) occur only along the horizontal meridian **HM**; movements of *medial rotation* (**MR**) and of *lateral rotation* (**LR**) take place around the axis OL. Movements of *flexion-extension* fall into two groups depending on whether they occur along a parallel **P**, i.e. *circumpolar* flexion **F1**, or along a large circle **C**, i.e. *circumcentral* flexion **F2**. Flexion **F2** can be resolved into **F1** and **F3** on the equator HM, an observation of little practical value.

More important, on the other hand, is that the pseudoparadox of Codman (see Volume 1) cannot occur at the hip because of the limited range of abduction.

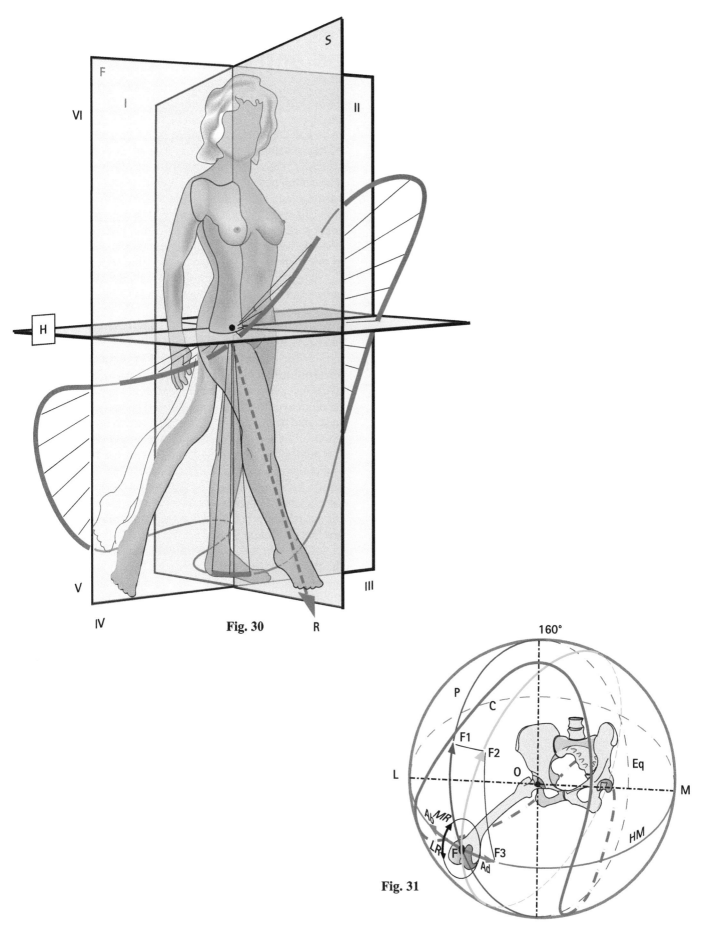

Fig. 30

R

Fig. 31

160°

17

Orientation of the femoral head and of the acetabulum

The hip joint is an **enarthrosis** (a **ball-and-socket** joint) with **spherical** articular surfaces.

The femoral head

The femoral head (**Fig. 32**, anterior view) is made up of two-thirds of a sphere of diameter 4-5 cm. Its geometrical centre is traversed by the three axes of the joint, horizontal axis **1**, vertical axis **2** and anteroposterior axis **3**.

The head is supported by the *femoral neck*, which joins the shaft. The axis of the neck (arrow A) is obliquely set and runs superiorly, medially and anteriorly. In the adult, the neck forms an angle D of 125° with the shaft (*angle of inclination*), and with the coronal plane an angle of 10-30° (*angle of anteversion*) open medially and anteriorly. Therefore (**Fig. 35**, postero-medial view) the vertico-coronal plane, passing through the centre of the femoral head and the axis of the femoral condyles, lies almost completely anterior to the femoral shaft and its upper extremity. This plane P contains the **mechanical axis MM'** of the lower limb, and this axis forms an angle of 5-7° with the axis **D** of the shaft (see p. 68).

The shape of the head and neck *varies considerably from person to person* and, according to anthropologists, this is the result of functional adaptation. Two extreme types are recognized (**Fig. 36**, inspired by Paul Bellugue):

*   The **rangy type**: the head exceeds two-thirds of a sphere; the neck-shaft angles are maximal (I = 125°; A = 25°); the femoral shaft is slender, and the pelvis is small and high-slung. This morphology favours a high degree of joint mobility and reflects *adaptation to speed in running* (a and c).
*   The **squat type**: the head barely exceeds one half of a sphere, the neck-shaft angles are narrower (I = 115°; A = 10°), the shaft is wider and the pelvis large and broad. The range of movements is reduced and the loss of speed is offset by a gain in strength. This is the *morphology of strength* (b and d).

The acetabulum

The acetabulum (**Fig. 33**, blue arrow; lateral view), located on the *lateral aspect of the hip bone* at the junction of its three constituent bones, *receives the femoral head*. It is hemispherical and is bounded by the acetabular margin (**Am**). Only the periphery of the acetabulum is coated by a lunate articular cartilage **Ca**, which is interrupted interiorly by the deep acetabular notch. The central part of the acetabulum lies deeper than the articular cartilage and is therefore not in contact with the femoral head. It is called the *acetabular fossa* (**Af**) and is separated from the inner surface of the hip bone by a thin layer of bone (**Fig. 34**; bone shown as transparent). The centre of the acetabulum **O** lies at the intersection of IP and ST (I = iliac tuberosity; P = pubis; S = anterosuperior iliac spine; T = ischial tuberosity). It will be shown later (p. 32) how the acetabular labrum (Al) is applied to the acetabular margin.

The acetabulum is not directed only *laterally* but also faces *inferiorly* and *anteriorly* (**Fig. 38**, arrow **A'** representing the axis of the acetabulum). In **Fig. 37** (**vertical section of the acetabulum**), it is quite clear that it faces inferiorly at an angle of 30-40° with the horizontal, so that the upper part of the acetabulum overhangs the femoral head laterally. This overhang is measured by the *angle of Wiberg, W*, which is normally 30°. The dome of the acetabulum is where the articular cartilage sustains the highest pressure from contact with the femoral head and where therefore the cartilage is thickest both in the acetabulum and on the femoral head. The **horizontal section (Fig. 38)** shows the acetabulum facing anteriorly at an angle of 30-40° between the acetabular axis **A'** and the coronal plane. Also included are the *acetabular fossa* **Af**, lying inside the *crescent-shaped articular cartilage* **Ca**; the acetabular labrum **Al**, applied to the transverse acetabular ligament (**TAL**) and the acetabular margin; and the *plane tangential* to the acetabular margin (**Pm**) and the parallel plane of the labrum (**Pl**), both running obliquely anteriorly and medially.

In clinical practice, these two sections of the joint can be duplicated as follows:

*   For the **vertico-frontal section** tomography gives a picture close to **Fig. 37**.
*   For the **two horizontal and vertico-frontal sections** a CT scan of the hip gives a picture close to **Fig. 38** and allows the angles of anteversion of the acetabulum and of the femoral neck to be measured. These measurements can be very useful in the *diagnosis* of *hip dysplasias*.

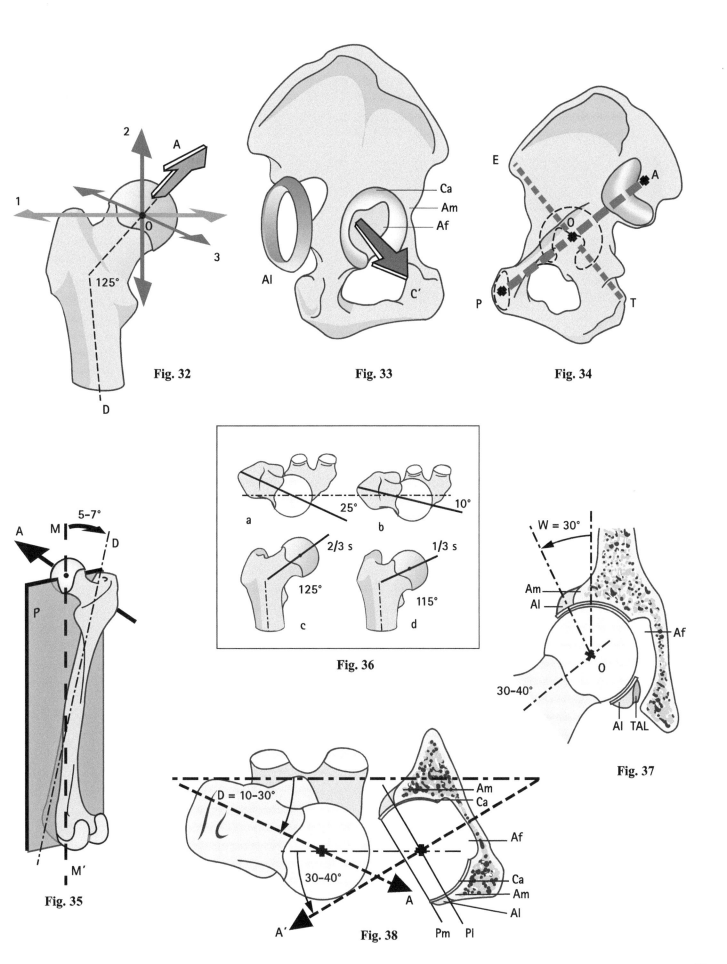

Fig. 32

Fig. 33

Fig. 34

Fig. 35

Fig. 36

Fig. 37

Fig. 38

19

Relationships of the articular surfaces

When the hip is in the **straight position**, which corresponds to the *erect posture* **(Fig. 40)**, the femoral head is not completely covered by the acetabulum, and its cartilage-coated antero-superior surface remains *exposed* **(Fig. 39**, white arrow). This results **(Fig. 45**: three-dimensional diagram of the reference axes of the right hip) from the fact that the *axis of the femoral neck* (A) running obliquely superiorly, anteriorly and medially is out of line with the *acetabular axis* (A'), which runs obliquely inferiorly, anteriorly and laterally. A **mechanical model of the hip (Fig. 41)** illustrates this arrangement as follows. On the one hand, a sphere is fixed to a shaft so bent as to mimic the angles of inclination and anteversion; the plane D represents the plane passing through the axis of the femoral shaft and the transverse axis of the femoral condyles. On the other hand, a hemisphere is suitably arranged relative to the *sagittal plane S*; a small plane C represents the *coronal plane* passing through the centre of the hemisphere.

In the **straight position**, the sphere is mostly exposed superiorly and anteriorly: the *dark greyish-blue crescent* represents the exposed part of the articular cartilage.

By appropriately turning the acetabular hemisphere relative to the femoral sphere **(Fig. 44)** complete coincidence of the articular surfaces can be achieved with disappearance of the exposed dark greyish-blue crescent. By using the reference planes S and C it is easy to realize that this coincidence is brought about by the combination of three elementary movements:
- flexion, approximately 90° (arrow 1)
- a small measure of abduction (arrow 2)
- a small measure of lateral rotation (arrow 3).

In this new position **(Fig. 46)**, the acetabular axis A' and that of the femoral neck A' are collinear.

On the skeleton **(Fig. 42)**, coincidence of the articular surfaces is achieved by the same movements of *flexion, abduction and lateral rotation* so that the femoral head is totally ensconced within the acetabular cavity. This hip position corresponds to the **quadruped position (Fig. 43)**, which is therefore the *true physiological position of the hip*. During evolution, the transition from quadruped to **biped locomotion** has led to the *loss of coincidence of the articular surfaces of the hip joint*. Inversely, this lack of coincidence can be considered as evidence in favour of man's origin from quadruped ancestors.

Following the transition to bipedalism, such a permanent lack of coincidence of the articular surfaces in the standing position can lead to osteoarthritis of the hip, especially when it is coupled with *abnormal orientation of the articular surfaces*, as observed in **hip dysplasias.**

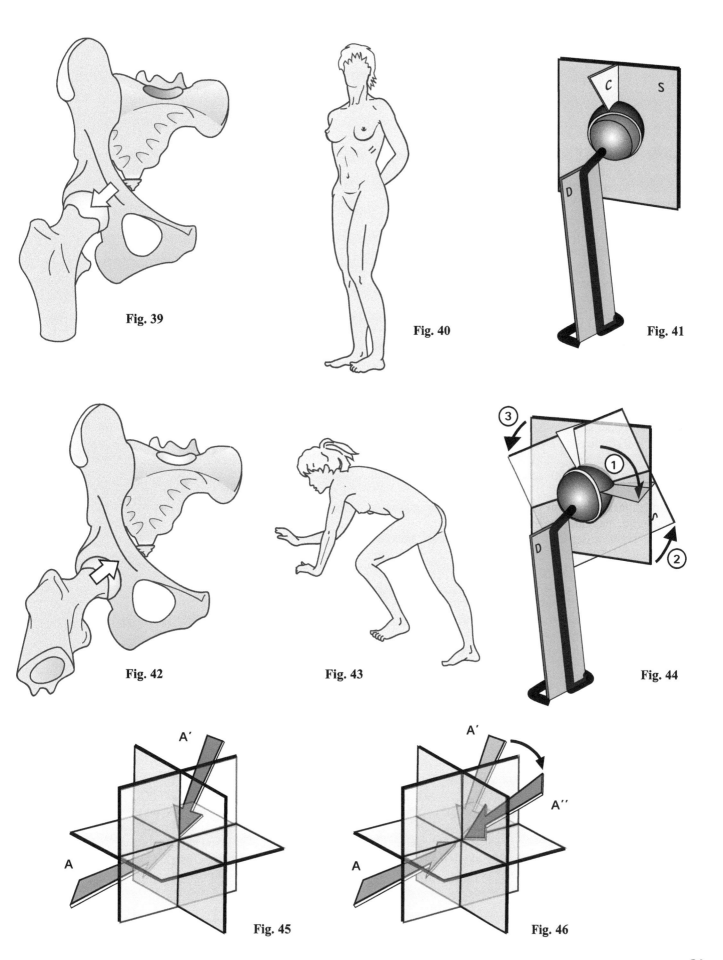

Fig. 39

Fig. 40

Fig. 41

Fig. 42

Fig. 43

Fig. 44

Fig. 45

Fig. 46

The architecture of the femur and of the pelvis

The head, neck and shaft of the femur constitute a **cantilever** in engineering terminology. In fact, the body weight, when applied to the femoral head, is transferred to the femoral shaft by a lever arm, *the femoral neck*. A similar set-up is seen in the **gibbet** (**Fig. 51**), where the weight acting vertically tends to shear off the horizontal beam at its junction with the shaft and thus close the angle between beam and shaft. To prevent this occurrence a *strut* is interposed obliquely.

The femoral neck represents the horizontal shaft of the gibbet and an *overall picture of the skeleton of the lower limb* (**Fig. 49**) shows that the mechanical axis of its three joints (heavy broken line) runs medial to the 'femoral gibbet'. Note also that the mechanical axis does not coincide with the vertical as shown by the line of alternating dashes and dots. The mechanical significance of this arrangement will emerge later (see p. 132).

To prevent the shearing off of the base of the femoral neck (**Fig. 52**), the upper end of the femur has a special structural pattern easily recognized in a **vertical section** of the desiccated bone (**Fig. 47**). The lamellae of spongy bone are arranged in **two trabecular systems** corresponding to the *mechanical lines of force*.

The **main trabecular system** consists of two sets of trabeculae fanning out into the femoral neck and head as follows:

- The **first set (1)** arises from the lateral cortex of the shaft and terminates on the inferior cortex of the head, the so-called *arcuate bundle of Gallois and Bosquette*.
- The **second set (2)**, arising from the medial cortex of the shaft and from the inferior cortex of the neck, fans out vertically upwards to terminate on the cortex of the head, the so-called *cephalic or supporting bundle*.

Culmann has shown that when a test-tube is loaded eccentrically and bent into the shape of a crook or a crane (**Fig. 50**) *two sets of lines of force* are generated:

- an *oblique set* on the convex aspect that corresponds to the *tensile forces* and is the counterpart of the arcuate bundle
- a *vertical set* on the concave aspect that corresponds to the compressive forces and is the counterpart of the supporting bundle (the strut of the gibbet).

The **accessory trabecular system** consists of two bundles fanning out into the greater trochanter:

- **the first bundle (3)** arising from the medial cortex of the shaft (the *trochanteric bundle*);
- **the second bundle (4)** consisting of vertical trabeculae running parallel to the lateral cortex of the shaft (the *subcortical bundle*).

- **Three points** are worth noting:

1. Inside the greater trochanter, the arcuate bundle (1) and the trochanteric bundle (3) form a *Gothic arch*, and their intersection creates a stronger *keystone* that runs down from the upper cortex of the neck. The inner pillar is less strong and weakens with age as a result of senile osteoporosis.

2. In the head and neck there is yet *another Gothic arch* formed by the intersection of the arcuate bundle (1) and the supporting bundle (2). At this intersection, the bone is denser and constitutes the nucleus of the femoral head. This trabecular system running from neck to head rests on an extremely strong support – the **thick cortex of the inferior aspect of the neck**, known as *Merkel's (M) inferior spur of the neck, Adams' arch* or the **calcar femorale (CF)**.

3. Between the trochanteric Gothic arch and the supporting bundle, there is a **zone of least resistance** exacerbated by *senile osteoporosis*; it is the site of *basal fractures of the femoral neck* (**Fig. 52**).

The structure of the **pelvic girdle** (**Fig. 47**) can also be studied in the same way, since it forms a completely closed ring that transmits vertical forces from the lumbar spine (double red arrow) towards the two hip joints.

Two *main trabecular systems* transmit the stresses from the *auricular surface* of the sacrum to the acetabulum on the one hand and to the ischium on the other (**Figs 47 and 48**).

The **sacro-acetabular trabeculae** fall into two sets:

1. The first set (**5**), arising from the upper part of the auricular surface, converges on to the posterior border of the greater sciatic notch to form the sciatic spur (**S**), whence it is reflected laterally before fanning out towards the inferior aspect of the acetabulum and then blending with the tensile lines of force in the femoral neck (1).

2. The second set (**6**) arising from the inferior part of the auricular surface, converges at the level of the pelvic inlet to form a **distinct bony ridge (BR)**, where it is reflected before fanning out on the upper aspect of the acetabulum and then blending with the compressive lines of force of the supporting bundle (2).

The **sacro-ischial trabeculae** (**7**) arise from the auricular surface together with the above-mentioned bundles and then run downwards to reach the ischium. They intersect the trabeculae arising from the acetabular margin (**8**). These ischial trabeculae support the weight of the body when sitting.

Finally, the trabeculae arising from the bony ridge and from the sciatic spur (**Fig. 47, S**) run together into the horizontal ramus of the pubis to complete the pelvic ring, which is further reinforced by subcortical trabeculae (4).

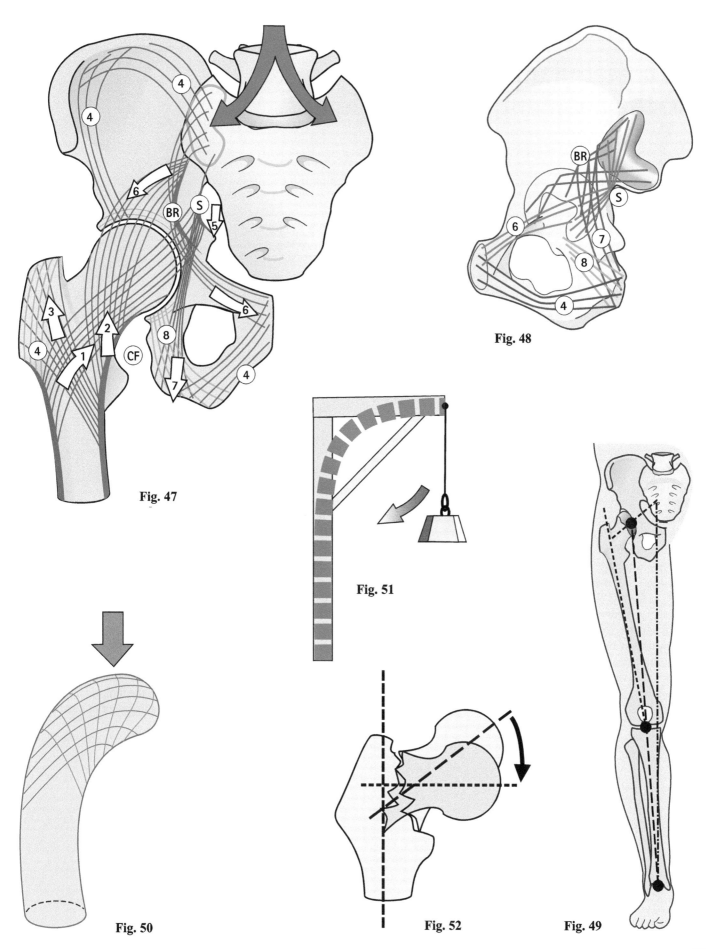

Fig. 47

Fig. 48

Fig. 51

Fig. 50

Fig. 52

Fig. 49

23

The acetabular labrum and the ligament of head of femur

The acetabular labrum (Al) is a fibrocartilaginous ring inserted into the **acetabular margin (Fig. 53)**; it deepens considerably the **acetabular cavity** (see p. 36) and fills out the irregularities of the acetabular margin. The anteroposterior part of the labrum has been removed revealing the *iliopubic notch* (IPN). The *acetabular notch* (An), the deepest of the three notches, is bridged by the labrum as it inserts into the **transverse acetabular ligament** (TAL), which is itself attached to the two sides of the notch. (In the diagram, the ligament and the labrum have been *separated*.) The straight head T1 of the rectus femoris tendon arises from the anterior inferior iliac spine, while its reflected head (T2) curves along the supra-acetabular grove, and its recurrent head (T3) runs towards the articular capsule to blend with it. The **vertico-frontal section of the hip (Fig. 54)** shows the labrum attached to the edge of the notch and to the transverse ligament (see also **Fig. 37**). In the upper part of **Fig. 54** can be seen, lying deep to the gluteus medius (Gme), the articular capsule (C), the superior band of the iliofemoral ligament (ILF) and the reflected tendon (T2) of the rectus femoris embedded within the capsule.

The **labrum** is in fact *triangular on cross-section* with three surfaces: a deep surface completely inserted into the acetabular margin and the transverse ligament; a medial surface facing the joint and coated with articular cartilage continuous with that of the acetabulum for articulation with the femoral head; a lateral surface receiving the insertion of the joint capsule (C) only at its base, so that the sharp edge of the labrum lies free within the joint cavity and forms a **perimarginal circular recess (Fig. 55, R, inspired by Rouvière)** in conjunction with the capsule.

The **ligament of the head of femur** (LHF) (Formerly called the **ligamentum teres**) is a flattened band 3-3.5 cm long **(Fig. 57)** running on the floor of the acetabular fossa **(Fig. 53)** to the femoral head **(Fig. 54)**. It is inserted into the upper part of the **fovea femoris capitis (Fig. 56)**, which lies just below and behind the centre of the articular cartilage, and it glides on the lower part of the fovea. The ligament consists of three bundles:

- *The posterior ischial bundle* (pi), which is the longest and runs through the acetabular notch under the transverse ligament **(Fig. 53)** to insert below and behind the posterior horn of the lunate articular cartilage
- *The anterior pubic bundle* (ap), inserted into the acetabular notch itself behind the anterior horn of the articular cartilage
- *The intermediate bundle* (ib), which is the thinnest and is inserted into the upper border of the transverse ligament **(Fig. 53**: the transverse ligament TAL and the labrum Al have been dismantled).

The ligament of head of femur lies embedded in fibro-adipose tissue **(Fig. 54)** at the back of the acetabular fossa (BAF), where it is covered by synovium **(Fig. 55)**. This synovial lining is attached on the one hand to the central border of the articular cartilage and the superior border of the transverse ligament and on the other to the femoral head around the foveal insertion of the ligament of head of femur. It has thus roughly the shape of a truncated cone; hence its name of '**tent of the ligament of head of femur**' (T).

The ligament of head of femur plays only a minor mechanical role, though it is extremely strong (Force needed for rupture = 45 kg), but it contributes to the **vascular supply of the femoral head**. **Fig. 58** (inferior view, inspired by Rouvière) shows the posterior branch of the obturator artery (**1**) sending an acetabular branch, i.e. the *artery of the ligament of head of femur* (**6**), which runs underneath the transverse ligament before entering the ligament of head of femur. The femoral head and neck also receive an arterial supply from the *capsular branches* (**5**) of the *anterior* (**3**) and *posterior* (**4**) circumflex arteries derived from the *deep femoral artery* (**2**). Thus, a neck fracture that interrupts the capsular arteries will *reduce the blood supply* to the femoral head, which is now supplied only by the artery of the ligament of head of femur.

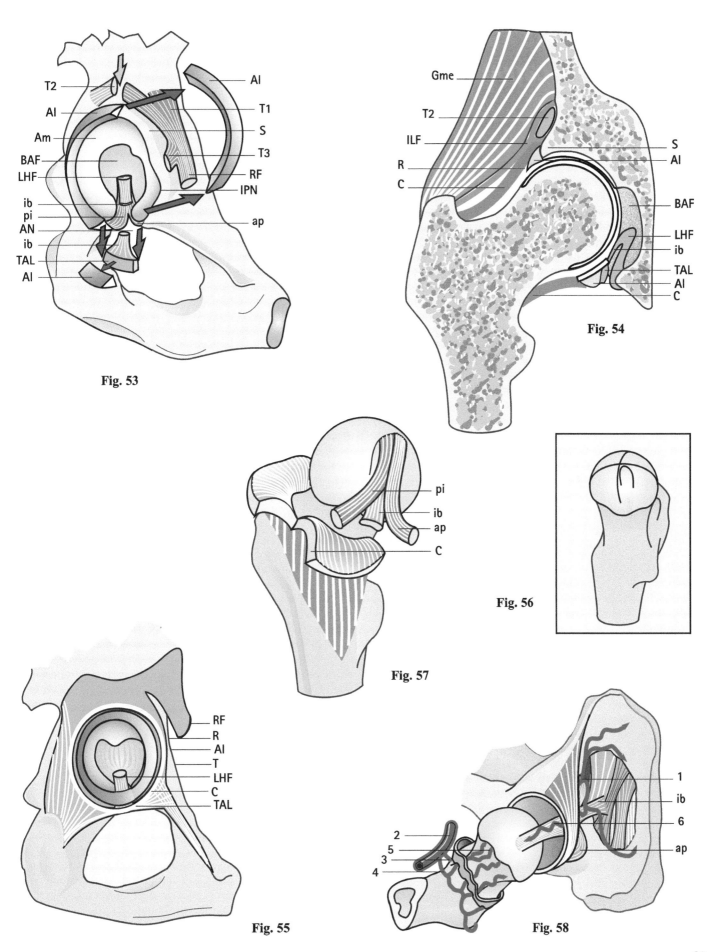

Fig. 53

T2
AI
Am
BAF
LHF
ib
pi
AN
ib
TAL
AI

AI
T1
S
T3
RF
IPN
ap

Fig. 54

Gme
T2
ILF
R
C

S
AI
BAF
LHF
ib
TAL
AI
C

Fig. 55

RF
R
AI
T
LHF
C
TAL

Fig. 56

Fig. 57

pi
ib
ap
C

Fig. 58

1
ib
6
ap
2
5
3
4

The articular capsule of the hip joint

The articular capsule is shaped like a **cylindrical sleeve (Fig. 59)** running from the hip bone to the upper end of the femur and made up of four types of fibres:

- **Longitudinal fibres (1)**, which help to unite the articular surfaces and run parallel to the axis of the cylinder
- **Oblique fibres (2)**, which also unite the articular surfaces and spiral around the cylinder
- **Arcuate fibres (3)**, which are attached to the hip bone and crisscross from one end of the acetabular margin to the other, forming an arc whose apex lies flush with the middle of the sleeve. These fibres buttonhole the femoral head and help to keep it within the acetabulum
- **Circular fibres (4)** with no bony attachments, which are particularly abundant in the middle of the sleeve, where they narrow it slightly. They stand out on the deep surface of the capsule and form the *zona orbicularis* (*Weber's ring*), which hugs the neck tightly.

Medially, the capsular ligament is inserted into the acetabular margin (**5**), the transverse ligament and the outer surface of the labrum (see p. 24). It is intimately related to the *tendon of the rectus femoris* (**Fig. 53**, RF) as described below.

The straight head of the rectus (T1), arising from the anterior inferior iliac spine, and the *reflected head* (T2), arising from the posterior part of the groove above the acetabulum, unite before running in a slit within the insertion of the capsule (**Fig. 54**), which is reinforced superiorly by the superior band of the ilio-femoral ligament (d) (see p. 28). Its *deep recurrent fibres* (e) strengthen the anterior aspect of the capsule.

Laterally, the capsule is inserted not into the edge of the cartilage coating the femoral head but into the *base of the neck* along a line running:

- anteriorly, along the *intertrochanteric line* (**6**)
- posteriorly (**Fig. 60**), not along the trochanteric crest (**7**) but at the junction of the lateral and middle thirds of the neck (**8**), just above the groove (**9**) of the obturator externus before its insertion into the trochanteric fossa (Tf) lying on the medial surface of the greater trochanter (Gt).
- The line of insertion of the capsule crosses obliquely both the inferior and superior surfaces of the neck. Inferiorly, it

runs above the fossa anterior to the lesser trochanter (**10**) and then 1.5 cm above and in front of the lesser trochanter (Lt). Its deepest fibres run upwards on the inferior surface of the neck to insert into the edge of the cartilage lining the femoral head. In so doing they raise synovial folds (**Frenula capsulae 11**), the most prominent being the *pectineofoveal fold of Amantini* (**12**).

These frenula are useful *during movements of abduction*. If during **adduction (Fig. 61)** the lower part of the capsule (1) slackens, while its upper part becomes taut (2), then during **abduction (Fig. 62)** the lower part of the capsule would be too short and would thus limit movement unless the frenula (3) *unpleated* and provided some extra length. Meanwhile, the upper part of the capsule (2) is thrown into folds, and the neck impinges on the acetabular margin *via the labrum* (4), *which is bent out of shape*. This explains why the labrum deepens the acetabulum *without limiting the movements at the joint*.

In extreme flexion the anterosuperior part of the neck hits the acetabular margin, and in some individuals the neck (**Fig. 59**) at this point bears an iliac impression (Ii) just below the edge of the cartilage.

After injection of a radio-opaque substance into the joint cavity **arthrographic images (Fig. 63)** can be obtained to highlight some features of the capsule and the labrum:

- The *zona orbicularis* (9) indents the capsule distinctly in the middle and divides the joint cavity into two chambers: a *lateral* (1) and a *medial* (2) chamber, which give rise to the *superior recesses* (3) above and the *inferior recesses* (4) below.
- The medial chamber also contains:
  - above, a spur-like recess with its apex pointing towards the acetabular margin, the so-called supramarginal recess (5) (compare with **Fig. 54**)
  - below, two rounded peninsulae separated by a deep gulf: these are respectively the two acetabular recesses (6) and the capsular impression of the *ligament of head of femur* (7).
- Finally, the *joint space* (8) can be seen between the femoral head and the acetabulum.

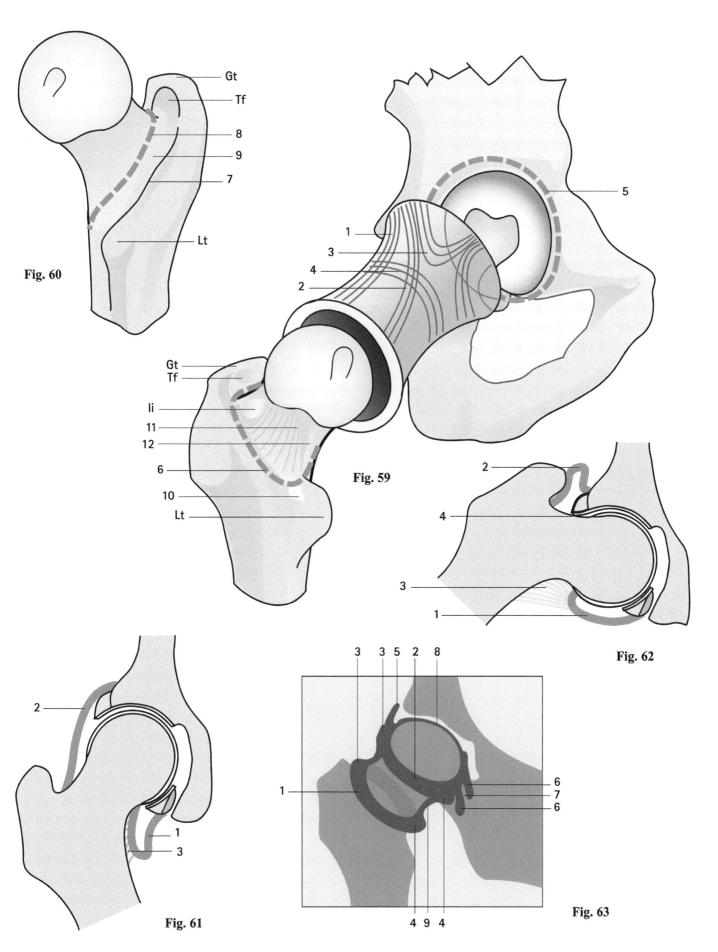

Fig. 60

Gt
Tf
8
9
7
Lt

Fig. 59

Gt
Tf
Ii
11
12
6
10
Lt

1
3
4
2

5

Fig. 62

2
4
3
1

Fig. 61

2
1
3

Fig. 63

3 3 5 2 8
1
6
7
6
4 9 4

The ligaments of the hip joint

(The numbers refer to the same structures in all the diagrams.) The capsule of the hip joint is strengthened by **powerful ligaments** anteriorly and posteriorly.

Fig. 64 shows the upper extremity of the femur with the insertions of the vastus lateralis (VL) and of the gluteus minimus (GM) and the **anterior aspect** of the hip joint covered by two ligaments:

- **the iliofemoral ligament** (1a and 1b), fan-shaped with its apex attached to the lower part of the anterior inferior iliac spine (also the origin of the rectus femoris, RF) and its base inserted into the whole length of the intertrochanteric line. Its central part (1c) is relatively thin and weak, while its two borders are strengthened by:
  - **The superior or iliotrochanteric band** (1a), which is the strongest of the ligaments of the joint with a thickness of 8-10 mm. It is attached laterally to the *upper part of the intertrochanteric line* and to the *pretrochanteric tubercle*. It is strengthened superiorly by another ligament, called *the ilio-tendino-trochanteric ligament* (1d), which, according to Rouvière, is formed by the fusion of the *deep recurrent fibres of the rectus femoris* (e) and a *fibrous band arising from the acetabular margin* (f). The deep surface of the gluteus minimus (GM) sends off an aponeurotic expansion (g) to blend with the external aspect of the superior band.
  - **The inferior band** (1b), with the same site of origin as the former, but with an insertion laterally into *the lower part of the intertrochanteric line.*
- The **pubofemoral ligament** (2) is attached medially to the *anterior aspect of the iliopubic eminence*, and the *anterior lip of the pubic arch*, where its fibres blend with the origin of the pectineus muscle, and it is inserted into the *anterior surface of the fossa* anterior to the lesser trochanter.

Taken as a whole (Fig. 65), these two ligaments, lying in front of the hip joint, resemble a letter N lying on its side (Welcker) or better a letter Z with its *upper limb* (1a), i.e. the iliotrochanteric band, nearly horizontal, its *middle limb* (1b), i.e. the inferior band, running nearly vertically and its *inferior limb* (2), i.e. the pubofemoral ligament, coursing almost horizontally to complete the letter Z. Between the pubofemoral ligament and the iliofemoral ligament (×) the capsule is thinner and is related to the bursa between the capsule and iliopsoas tendon (IP). Occasionally the capsule is perforated at this level and the joint cavity communicates with the bursa.

Posteriorly (Fig. 66) there is only one ligament, **the ischiofemoral ligament (3)**, arising from the posterior surface of the acetabular margin and the labrum. Its fibres, running inferiorly and laterally, cross the posterior surface of the neck (h) **(Fig. 67)** to gain insertion into the inner surface of the greater trochanter *in front of the trochanteric fossa*, where is also inserted the tendon of the obturator externus after traversing the groove that borders the capsular insertion. **Fig. 67** also shows some of its fibres (i) blending directly with the *zona orbicularis* (j).

During the change from the quadruped to the biped erect posture the pelvis moved into a position of extension relative to the femur (see p. 20), and all the ligaments **became coiled around the femoral neck in the same direction (Fig. 68**: right hip seen from the outside) and now run clockwise from the hip bone to the femur. Thus **extension winds the ligaments around the neck**, tightening them, and **flexion unwinds** and relaxes them.

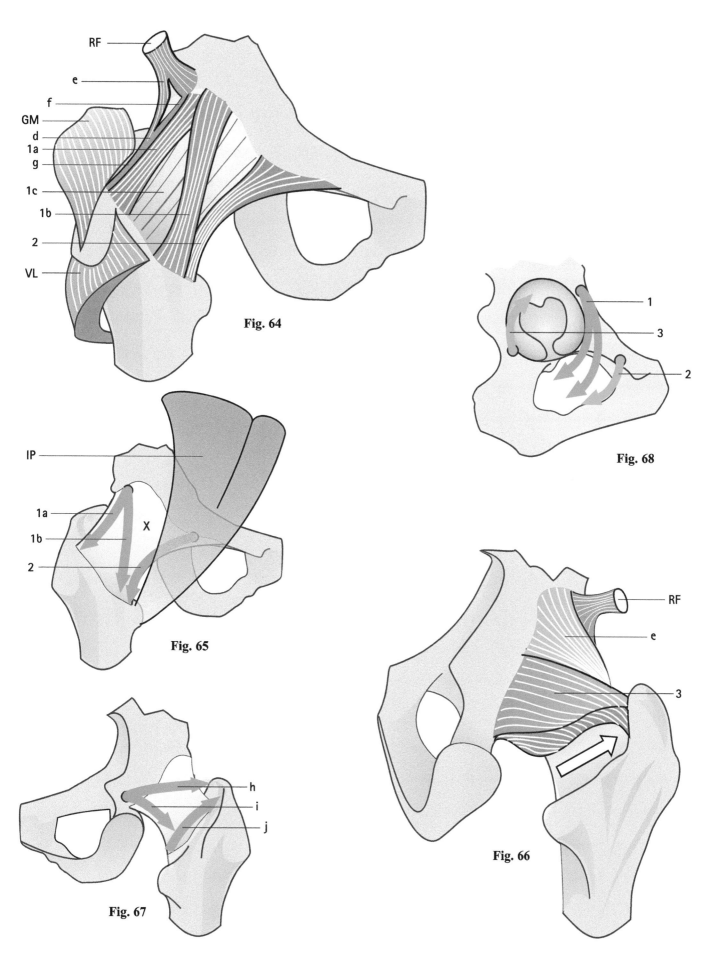

RF

e

f

GM

d

1a

g

1c

1b

2

VL

Fig. 64

IP

1a

1b

X

2

Fig. 65

1

3

2

Fig. 68

RF

e

3

Fig. 66

h

i

j

Fig. 67

Role of the ligaments in flexion-extension

Fig. 69 (hip in the straight position) is a diagrammatic representation of the *moderately tensed* ligaments, i.e. the two bundles of the iliofemoral ligament (ILF), and the pubofemoral ligament (PF). (Note that the posteriorly located ischiofemoral ligament is not included.) In **Fig. 70** the blue margin represents the acetabulum, and the circle in the centre represents the femoral head and neck. The ligaments, drawn as springs, run between the margin and the circle: they are the iliofemoral ligament (ILF) in front and the ischiofemoral ligament (IsF) at the back. (For simplification, the pubofemoral ligament is not included in this diagram.)

During hip extension (**Fig. 71**: the iliac bone rotates backwards while the femur stays put) *all the ligaments become taut* (**Fig. 72**) as they wind round the femoral neck. Of all these ligaments, the inferior band (ILF) of the iliofemoral ligament is stretched the most as it runs nearly vertically (**Fig. 71**) and is thus responsible for checking the *posterior tilt of the pelvis.*

During hip flexion (**Fig. 73**: the iliac bone tilts forward while the femur stays put) the opposite holds true and all the anterior ligaments are relaxed (**Fig. 74**) including the ischiofemoral, the pubofemoral and the iliofemoral. This relaxation of the ligaments is one of the factors responsible for the *instability* of the hip in this position.

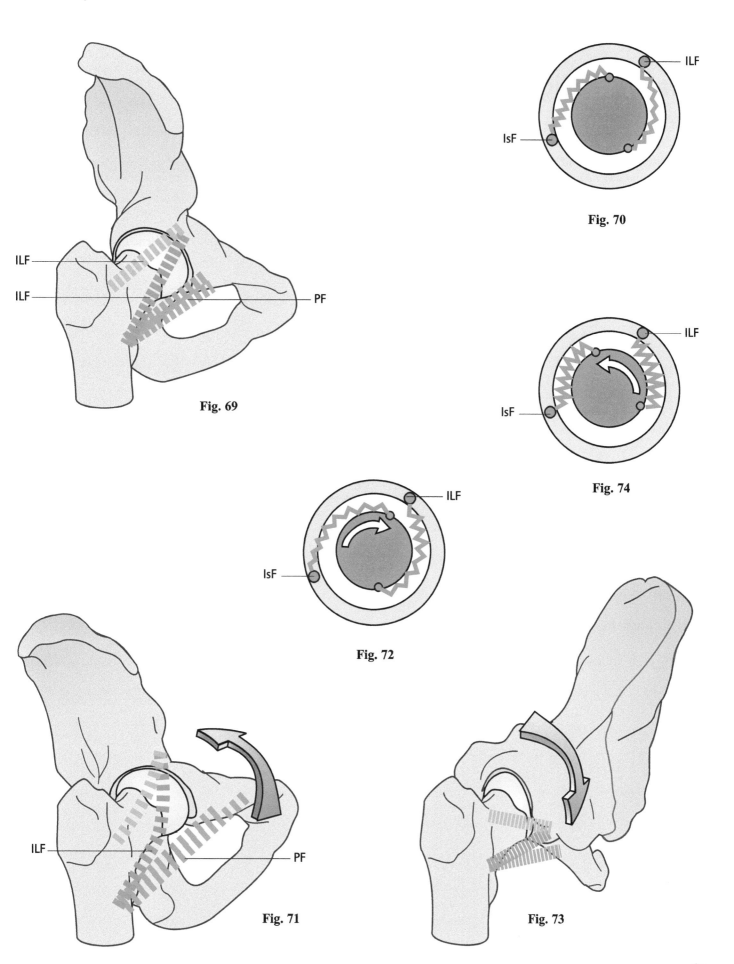

ILF

ILF

PF

Fig. 69

IsF

ILF

Fig. 70

ILF

Fig. 72

IsF

ILF

Fig. 74

ILF

PF

Fig. 71

Fig. 73

Role of the ligaments in lateral-medial rotation

During lateral rotation of the hip (Fig. 75) the intertrochanteric line moves away from the acetabular margin with the result that all the anterior ligaments of the hip are tightened, especially the bands running horizontally, i.e. the superior band of the *iliofemoral ligament* (ILF) as well as the pubofemoral (PF). **A horizontal section of the joint seen from above (Fig. 76) and a posterosuperior view of the joint (Fig. 77)** clearly show tightening of the anterior ligaments and slackening of the ischiofemoral ligament (IsF).

During medial rotation (Fig. 78) the opposite occurs: all the anterior ligaments running horizontally are slackened, especially the superior band of the iliofemoral ligament (ILF) and the pubofemoral ligament (PF), while the ischiofemoral ligament (IsF) becomes taut **(Fig. 79 and 80)**. The vertical inferior band of the iliofemoral ligament is tightened considerably during extension, as shown in **Fig. 71** (p. 31).

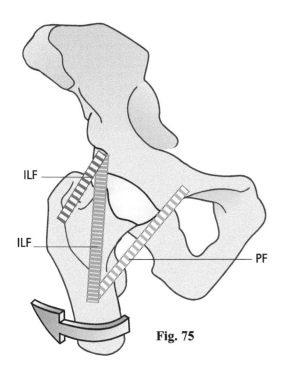

ILF

ILF

PF

Fig. 75

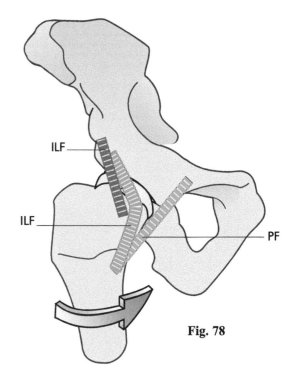

ILF

ILF

PF

Fig. 78

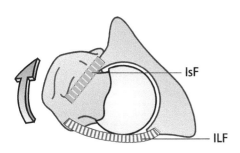

IsF

ILF

Fig. 76

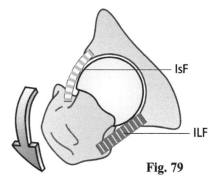

IsF

ILF

Fig. 79

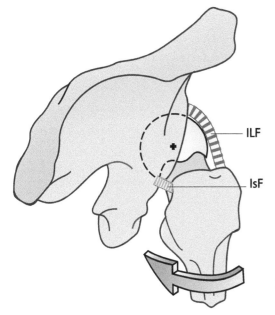

ILF

IsF

Fig. 77

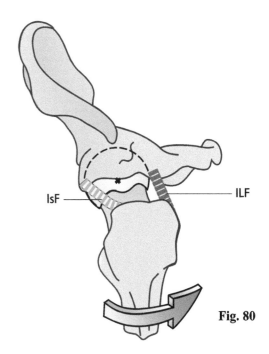

IsF

ILF

Fig. 80

Role of the ligaments in adduction-abduction

Fig. 81 shows that in the **straight position** the anterior ligaments, i.e. the *superior* (sb) *and inferior* (ib) *bands* of the iliofemoral ligament are moderately tensed, as is the pubofemoral ligament (PF).

During adduction (Fig. 82) the superior band (sb) is tightened considerably, and the inferior band (ib) only slightly, while the pubofemoral ligament (PF) relaxes.

During abduction (Fig. 83) the opposite obtains: the *pubofemoral ligament* PF is tightened considerably, while the *superior* and, to a lesser extent, the *inferior bands* are relaxed.

The **ischiofemoral ligament** (IsF), seen **only from the back**, is stretched during adduction **(Fig. 84)** and tenses up during abduction **(Fig. 85)**.

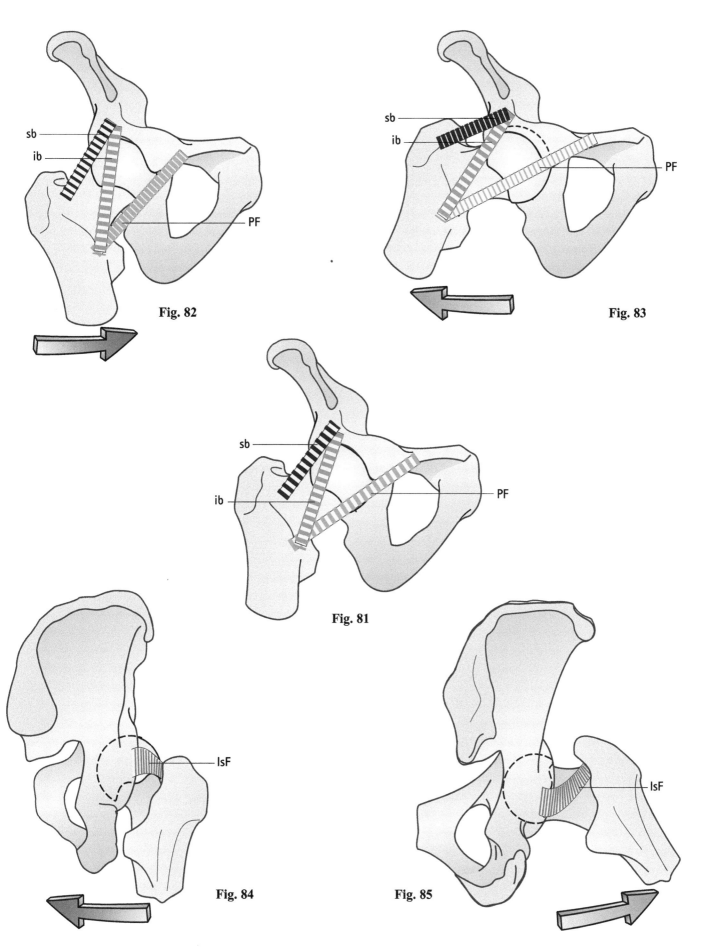

Fig. 82

Fig. 83

Fig. 81

Fig. 84

Fig. 85

The functional anatomy of the ligament of head of femur

This *anatomical vestige* (formerly known as ligamentum teres) plays a minor role in restricting hip movements, but it carries the artery of the head of femur, which is critical in supplying blood to the femoral head.

In the **straight position (Fig. 86**, vertico-coronal section) it is moderately tensed, and its femoral insertion lies in its *intermediate position* (**1**) in the *depths of the acetabular fossa* (**Fig. 87**: diagram of the acetabular fossa showing the *various positions of the fovea capitis femoris*), i.e. slightly below and behind the centre of the fossa (×).

During hip flexion (Fig. 88) the ligament of head of femur is twisted round itself, and the fovea (**Fig. 87**) comes to lie above and in front of the centre of the acetabular fossa (**2**). Hence the ligament *plays no part in limiting flexion.*

During medial rotation (Fig. 89: coronal section, viewed from above) the fovea is displaced posteriorly, and the femoral insertion of the ligament comes into contact with *the posterior part of the articular cartilage* (**3**). The ligament stays moderately taut.

During lateral rotation (Fig. 90) the fovea moves anteriorly, while the ligament comes into contact with the *anterior part of the articular cartilage* (**4**) and is only moderately stretched. Note how the posterior surface of the femoral neck comes to hit the acetabular margin via the acetabular labrum, which becomes *flattened and everted.*

During abduction (Fig. 91) the fovea moves inferiorly towards the acetabular notch (**5**), and the ligament is *folded back on itself.* The labrum is flattened between the superior border of the neck and the acetabular margin.

Finally, **during adduction (Fig. 92)** the fovea moves *superiorly* (**6**) to touch the roof of the acetabular fossa. This is the only position where the ligament is really under tension. The inferior border of the neck pushes back slightly the labrum and the transverse acetabular ligament.

It appears therefore that all the *possible positions of the fovea* are encompassed within the acetabular fossa, including its posterior (**7**) and anterior (**8**) bulges, which correspond to the foveal positions during adduction-extension-medial rotation (**7**) and adduction-flexion-medial rotation (**8**). Between these two bulges the articular cartilage, shaped like a shallow recess, *corresponds to the position where adduction is minimal* because of the impact of one lower limb on the other in the coronal plane. Thus, the inner profile of the articular cartilage is not due to chance but reflects the *locus of the extreme positions* taken by the foveal insertion of the ligament of head of femur.

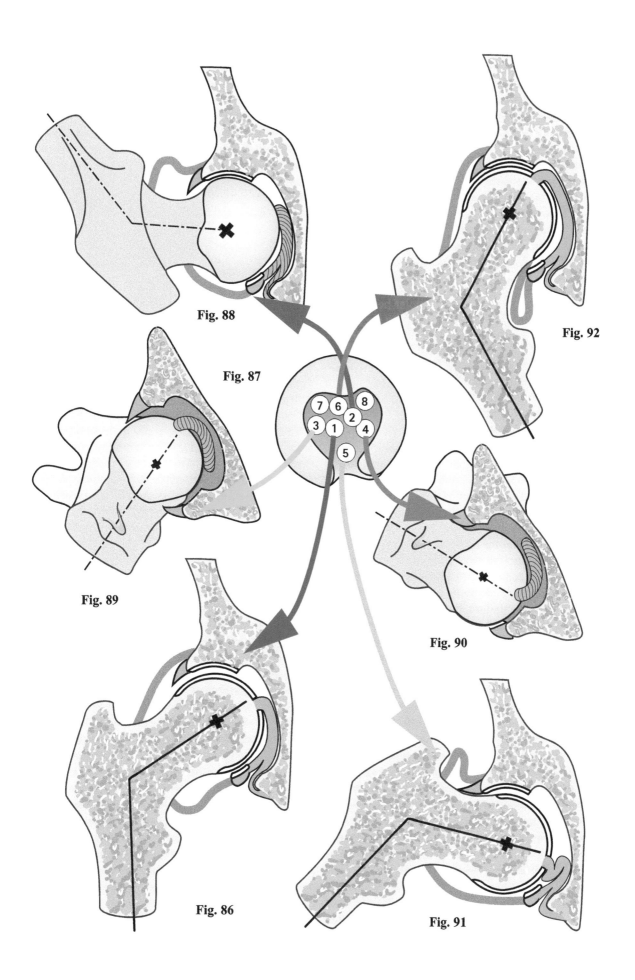

Fig. 88

Fig. 87

Fig. 92

Fig. 89

Fig. 90

Fig. 86

Fig. 91

Coaptation of the articular surfaces of the hip joint

In contrast with the shoulder, which tends to be dislocated by the force of gravity, the hip joint is assisted by **gravity**, at least in the straight position **(Fig. 93)**. To the extent that the acetabular roof adequately covers the femoral head, the latter is pressed against the former by a force (ascending white arrow) opposite to the body weight (descending white arrow).

It is known that the acetabulum is no more than a hemisphere, and so cannot form part of what is known in mechanics as a **retaining interlocking system.** The femoral head cannot be mechanically retained within the bony acetabular hemisphere, as can easily be observed on a dry skeleton. The acetabular labrum, however, widens and deepens the acetabulum so that *its cavity exceeds a hemisphere* (black arrows), setting the stage for a fibrous **interlocking and retaining system.** The labrum retains the femoral head with the help of the zona orbicularis of the fibrous capsule, which buttonholes the femoral neck tightly (shown in section as small blue arrows).

Atmospheric pressure plays an important part in securing the articular coaptation of the hip joint, as *proved by the experiments of the Weber brothers.* They noted that, if all the connections (including the capsule) between hip bone and femur were severed, the femoral head did not fall out of the acetabulum spontaneously and in fact could only be pulled out with the help of a strong force **(Fig. 94)**. If, on the other hand, **(Fig. 95)** *a small hole was drilled into the depths of the acetabulum*, the femoral head and the lower limb fell away under their own weight. The *reverse experiment*, consisting of plugging the hole after the head had been replaced in the acetabulum, showed that the head stayed inside the acetabulum as it had done originally. This experiment is comparable to the *classic experiment of Magdebourg*, showing that it is impossible to separate the two hemispheres after creation of a vacuum inside **(Fig. 96)**, whereas it is easy to do so once air has been allowed back in through a tap **(Fig. 97)**. This experiment is a perfect demonstration of the role of atmospheric pressure.

The **periarticular ligaments and muscles** are vital in maintaining the coaptation of the articular surfaces. Note **(Fig. 98,** horizontal section) that their functions are reciprocally balanced. Thus anteriorly the muscles are very few (blue arrow) and the ligaments (black arrows) are strong, while posteriorly the muscles (red arrow) predominate. This coordinated activity keeps the femoral head (green arrow) closely applied to the acetabulum. It is noteworthy that the action of the ligaments varies **according to the position of the hip. In extension (Fig. 99)** the ligaments are tensed and are efficient in securing coaptation. **In flexion (Fig. 100)** the ligaments are slack (see p. 31), and the femoral head is not as strongly applied against the acetabulum. This mechanism can be easily understood using the mechanical model **(Fig. 101)**, where parallel strings run between two wooden circles (a). When one circle is rotated relative to the other (b) they are brought closer together.

The position of flexion is therefore a **position of instability** for the joint because of the slackness of the ligaments. When a measure of adduction is added to the flexion, as in the sitting position with legs crossed **(Fig. 102)**, a relatively mild force applied along the femoral axis (arrow) is enough to cause posterior dislocation of the hip joint *with or without fracture of the posterior margin of the acetabulum*, e.g. dashboard hip dislocation in a car accident.

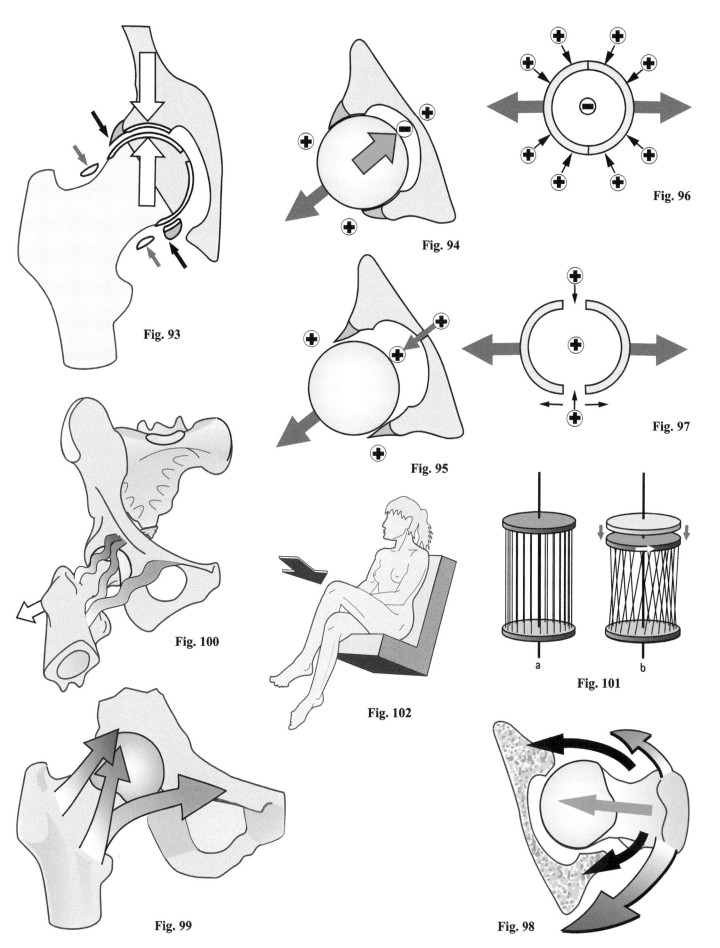

Fig. 93

Fig. 94

Fig. 96

Fig. 95

Fig. 97

Fig. 100

Fig. 102

Fig. 101

a

b

Fig. 99

Fig. 98

Muscular and bony factors maintaining the stability of the hip joint

The periarticular muscles are **essential for hip joint stability** on condition, however, that they *run transversely*. Thus the muscles **(Fig. 103)** running roughly parallel to the femoral neck *keep the femoral head in contact with the acetabulum*, such as the pelvitrochanteric muscles (only the piriformis (1) and the obturator externus (2) shown here), and the glutei, especially the minimus and the medius, which generate a powerful component (3) of force (blue arrow) ensuring coaptation. For this reason these muscles are called the *muscular fasteners of the hip joint*.

Conversely, the *longitudinal muscles*, like the *adductors* (4), tend to dislocate the femoral head above the acetabulum (left side, **Fig. 103**), especially if the acetabular roof is everted, a congenital malformation that can easily be detected in anteroposterior radiographs of the pelvis **(Fig. 104)**. Normally, the *angle of Hilgenreiner*, between the horizontal Hilgenreiner line joining the y-shaped triradiate cartilages (the y line) and the tangent to the acetabular roof, is 25° in the neonate and 15° at the end of the first year; when this angle exceeds 30°, there is congenital malformation of the acetabulum. Dislocation is recognized by *upward displacement of the ossification centre of the femoral head above the Hilgenreiner line and by inversion of the centre-edge (CE) angle of Wiberg* (see **Fig. 37**, p. 27). In cases of acetabular malformation, the dislocating action of the adductors 4' is enhanced when the hip is already *adducted* **(Fig. 103)** and is *diminished during hip abduction* **(Fig. 105)** until *they eventually produce coaptation in full abduction*.

The orientation of the femoral neck in both the coronal and horizontal planes is of considerable importance in securing joint stability. It has been shown (p. 18) that in the **coronal plane** the axis of the neck forms an *angle of inclination* of **120-125°** with the axis of the shaft (a, **Fig. 106**: diagram of the hip from the front).

In congenital hip dislocation, this angle of inclination can reach up to 140°, producing a coxa valga, so that during adduction **c** the axis of the neck has already a *head start* of 20° on its normal counterpart. Therefore a 30° adduction in an abnormal hip P corresponds to a 50° adduction in a normal hip, and this degree of adduction only *reinforces the dislocating action of the adductors*. Hence coxa valga promotes pathological dislocation of the hip. Conversely, this abnormal hip will be *stabilized in abduction*; hence abduction at 90° is the first of the various positions of immobilization used in the surgical *treatment of congenital hip dislocation* **(Fig. 107**: positions of immobilization used in the prevention of hip dislocation in the neonate).

In the horizontal plane (Fig. 108: diagram of the hip from above) the mean value of the angle of anteversion is 20° (**a**) because bipedalism has led to the divergence of the femoral neck and acetabulum (p. 20), so that the anterior part of the femoral head lies outside the acetabulum. If the neck is more anteverted with an increase of the angle of anteversion to 40° for example (**b**), this condition is called *anteversion of the neck*, and the even more exposed head is more prone to anterior dislocation. In fact, for a lateral rotation of 25° (**c**), the axis of the normal neck still passes through the acetabulum (N), whereas the axis of the anteverted neck (P), with a head start of 20°, will pass through the acetabular margin, setting the stage for *anterior hip dislocation*. Thus *neck anteversion favours pathological hip dislocation*. Conversely, neck retroversion is a stabilizing factor like medial rotation (d), which explains why the third position of surgical reduction of congenital hip dislocation combines the straight position and *medial rotation* **(Fig. 107)**.

These architectural and muscular factors are extremely important in maintaining the **stability of prostheses**. Hence, during total hip replacement the surgeon must secure the following:

- *the proper orientation of the neck* without excessive anteversion, especially when the anterior approach is used, and vice versa
- *the correct orientation of the acetabular prosthesis*, which, like the natural acetabulum, must face inferiorly at an angle not exceeding 45-50° with the horizontal and slightly anteriorly at an angle of 15°
- *the restoration of the 'physiological length' of the femoral neck* by ensuring the normality of the lever arm of the gluteal muscles, which are essential for the stability of a prosthesis.

Emphasis must also be placed on the *choice of the surgical approach* to ensure minimal disruption of the balanced activity of the periarticular muscles.

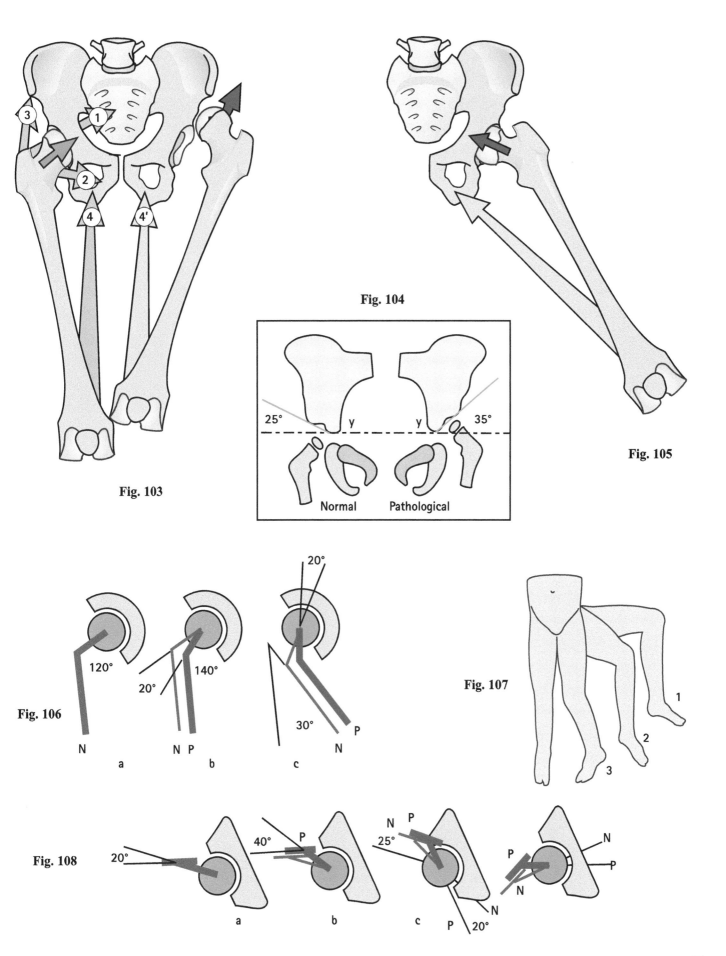

Fig. 103

Fig. 104

Fig. 105

Fig. 106

Fig. 107

Fig. 108

41

The flexor muscles of the hip joint

The **hip flexors** lie *anterior to the coronal plane* passing through the centre of the joint **(Fig. 109)** and also anterior to the axis of flexion-extension XX' lying in the same coronal plane.

The numerous hip flexors include the following (**Fig. 110**: pelvis shown as transparent):

- The **ilio-psoas** (1) and the **iliacus** (2) share a common tendon of insertion into the *lesser trochanter* after bending sharply at the level of the iliopubic eminence. The iliopsoas is the most powerful of the flexors and has the longest range with the highest fibres of the psoas arising from T12. Its action as an adductor is challenged by many authors, although its tendon runs medial to the anteroposterior axis since the apex of the lesser trochanter *falls on the mechanical axis of the lower limb* (see **Fig. 49**, p. 23). In support of its adductor action, however, is the observation that on the skeleton the lesser trochanter is nearest to the iliopubic eminence during flexion-adduction-lateral rotation. The iliopsoas also produces *lateral rotation*.
- The **sartorius** (3) is mainly a *hip flexor* and secondarily produces *abduction-lateral rotation* (**Fig. 111**: the leg kicking the ball); it acts also on the *knee*, producing flexion-medial rotation (see p. 149, **Fig. 253**). It is quite powerful, with a muscle pull equivalent to 2 kg, and nine-tenths of its power is expended in producing flexion.
- The **rectus femoris** (4) is a powerful flexor (equivalent to 5 kg), but its action on the hip *depends on the degree of knee* flexion, with its efficiency *being directly proportional to the degree of knee flexion* (see p. 145). It is especially active in movements combining knee extension and hip flexion, as when the swinging limb moves forwards during walking **(Fig. 112)**.
- The **tensor fasciae latae** (5) is a strong *flexor* in addition to being a stabilizer of the pelvis (see p. 50) and an adductor of the hip.

Some muscles are only *accessory hip flexors*, but their contribution to flexion is not negligible. These include the following:

- **the pectineus** (6): above all an adductor
- **the adductor longus** (7): primarily an adductor but also partially flexor (see p. 54)
- the most anterior fibres of the **glutei minimus and medius** (9).

All these hip flexors can produce *adduction-abduction* and *lateral-medial rotation* as accessory movements, and they can be divided into two groups according to their actions.

The **first group** comprises the **anterior fibres of the glutei minimus and medius** (9) and the **tensor fasciae latae** (5), which produce *flexion-abduction-medial rotation* (**Fig. 113**: right thigh) and are involved alone or predominantly in the production of the soccer player's movement shown in **Fig. 113**.

The **second group** comprises the **iliopsoas** (1 and 2), the **pectineus** (6) and the **adductor longus** (7), which produce *flexion-adduction-lateral rotation*; this complex movement is illustrated in **Fig. 114**.

During **pure flexion**, as in *walking* (**Fig. 112**), these two groups must act as a *balanced set of synergists and antagonists*. In **flexion-adduction-medial rotation (Fig. 115)**, the adductors and the tensor fasciae latae need to play a dominant role assisted by the medial rotators, i.e. the glutei minimus and medius.

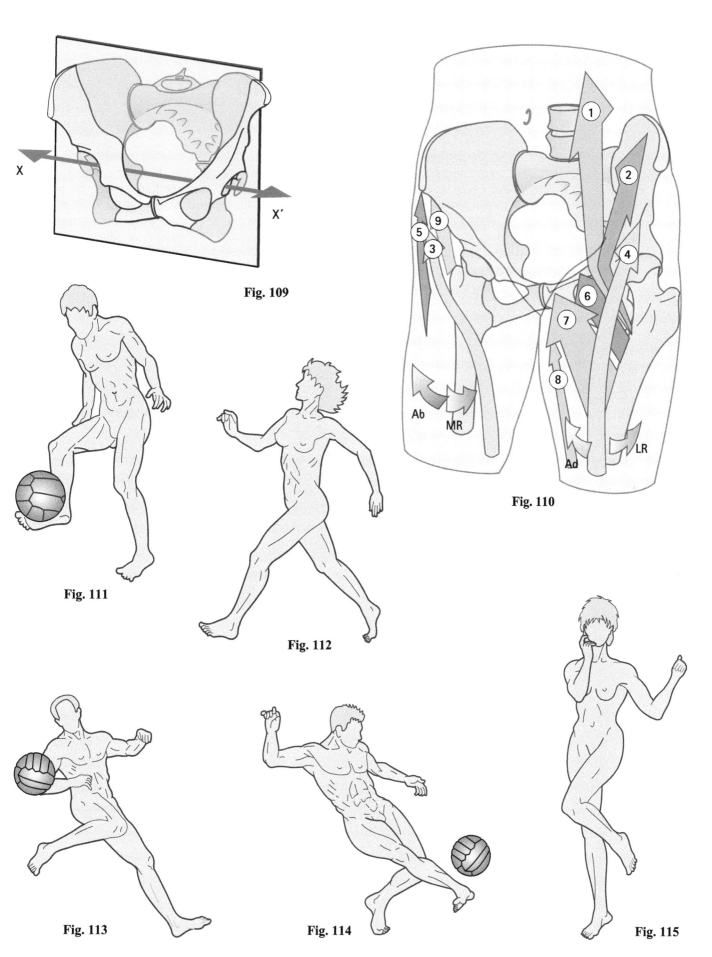

Fig. 109

Fig. 110

Fig. 111

Fig. 112

Fig. 113

Fig. 114

Fig. 115

The extensor muscles of the hip joint

The **hip extensors** lie posterior to the coronal plane passing through the centre of the joint **(Fig. 116)** and containing the *transverse axis* XX' of flexion-extension. There are **two groups** of extensor muscles: one inserted into the upper extremity of the femur and the other in the vicinity of the knee **(Fig. 117)**.

Of the **first group**, located at the root of the lower limb, the most important is the **gluteus maximus (1 and 1')**, which is the most powerful muscle in the body with a force equivalent to 34 kg for an excursion of 15 cm. It is also the *largest and the thickest* (66 cm² in cross-section) and therefore the strongest (Force equivalent to 238 kg). It is assisted by the most posterior fibres of the **glutei minimus and medius** (3). These muscles are also *lateral rotators* (see p. 58).

The **second group** consists essentially of the **hamstring muscles**, i.e. the **biceps femoris** (4), the **semitendinosus** (5) and the **semimembranosus** (6) with a force equivalent to 22 kg (only two-thirds of that of the gluteus maximus). As *biarticular muscles*, their efficiency at the hip *depends on the position of the knee*, and locking of the knee in extension enhances their extensor action on the hip, suggesting an *antagonism-synergism* relationship between the hamstrings and the quadriceps femoris, especially *the rectus femoris*. Also included in this group are some of the *adductors* (see p. 54), particularly the *adductor magnus* (7), which is an *accessory hip extensor*.

The hip extensors have secondary actions depending on their position relative to the anteroposterior axis YY' of abduction-adduction.

- Those running **above the YY' axis** produce *abduction along with extension*, as in the dancing movement illustrated in **Fig. 118**. They include the **most posterior fibres of the glutei minimus (3) and medius (4)** and **the highest fibres of the gluteus maximus (1')**.

- Those running **below the axis YY'** produce *adduction* and *extension* simultaneously, as in the movement illustrated in **Fig. 119**. They include the **hamstrings**, the **adductors** lying behind the coronal plane and the bulk of the **gluteus maximus** (1). To produce **pure extension (Fig. 120)**, i.e. without associated abduction or adduction, these two muscle groups must be thrown into balanced contraction as synergists-antagonists.

The hip extensors play a vital role in **stabilizing the pelvis anteroposteriorly.**

- When the pelvis is tilted posteriorly **(Fig. 121)**, i.e. in the direction of extension, it is stabilized only by the tightening of the iliofemoral ligament (ILF), which limits extension **(Fig. 71**, p. 31).

- There is a position **(Fig. 122)** where the centre of gravity C lies *exactly above the centre of the hip joint*, as a result, neither the flexors nor the extensors are active, but the equilibrium of the pelvis is *unstable*.

- When the pelvis is tilted anteriorly **(Fig. 123)** the centre of gravity C comes to lie *in front of the transverse axis of the hip joints*, and the hamstrings (H) are the first to contract in order to straighten the pelvis.

- When the markedly tilted pelvis needs to be straightened **(Fig. 124)**, the *gluteus maximus* (G) contracts powerfully along with the *hamstrings* (H), which are more efficient the greater the degree of knee extension, as in standing with trunk bent forwards and hands touching the feet.

During **normal walking**, extension is produced by the hamstrings without help from the *gluteus maximus*, but during running, jumping or walking up a slope the gluteus maximus plays an essential role, which explains why it is such a powerful muscle.

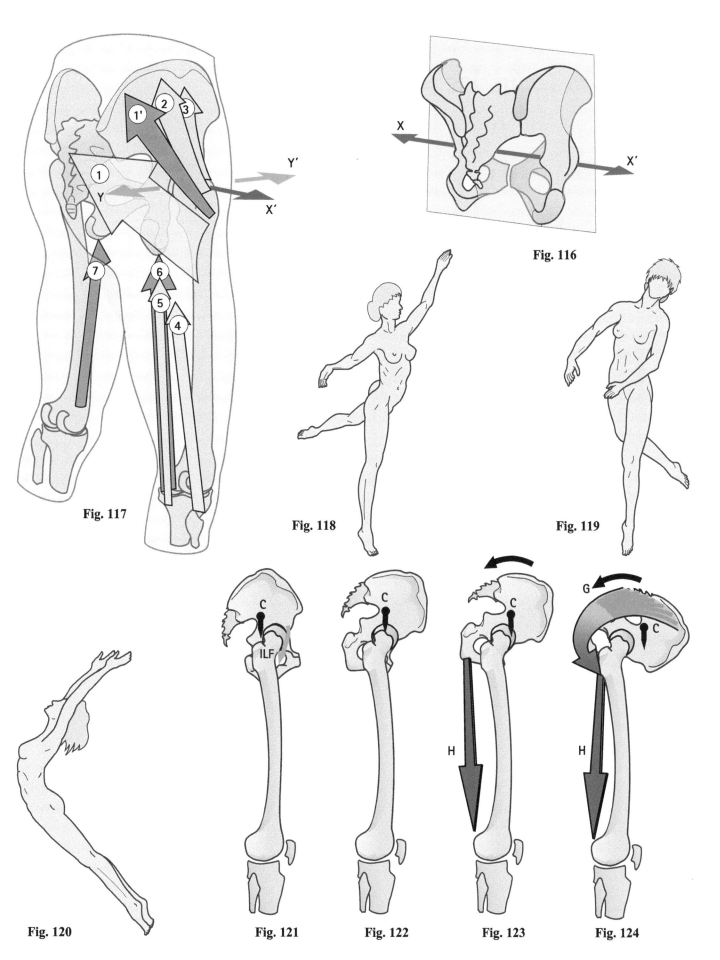

Fig. 117

Fig. 116

Fig. 118

Fig. 119

Fig. 120

Fig. 121

Fig. 122

Fig. 123

Fig. 124

The abductor muscles of the hip joint

The **hip abductors** generally lie *lateral to the sagittal plane* passing through the centre of the joint **(Fig. 125)** and run laterally and superiorly to the anteroposterior axis YY' of abduction-adduction contained in that plane.

The *main abductor muscle* is the **gluteus medius** (1), which has a cross-section area of 40 cm², an excursion of 11 cm and a force equivalent to 16 kg. It is highly efficient because it is almost perpendicular to its lever arm OT **(Fig. 126)**. It is also essential, along with the gluteus minimus, for the transverse stabilization of the pelvis (see p. 50).

The **gluteus minimus** (2) is essentially an abductor **(Fig. 127)** with a cross-sectional area of 15 cm², an excursion of 9 cm and a force equivalent to 4.9 kg, i.e. three times less than that of the gluteus medius.

The **tensor fasciae latae** (3) is a powerful abductor of the hip in the straight position. It has a force equivalent to half that of the gluteus medius (7.6 kg), but its lever arm is much longer than that of the medius. It also *stabilizes the pelvis.*

The **gluteus maximus** (4) only abducts with its *highest fibres*, and so the bulk of the muscle produces adduction. Its superficial fibres, which contribute to the 'deltoid of the hip' **(Fig. 131)**, also abduct the hip.

The **piriformis** (5) is undeniably an abductor despite the fact that its importance cannot be demonstrated experimentally because of its deep location (6).

According to their secondary roles in producing flexion-extension and abduction-adduction, these abductors can be classified into two groups:

- The **first group** includes all the muscles *anterior to the coronal plane* passing through the centre of the joint, i.e, tensor fasciae latae and nearly all the anterior fibres of the glutei medius and minimus. These muscles, contracting alone or in conjunction with weaker partners, produce *abduction-flexion-medial rotation* **(Fig. 128)**.

- The **second group** comprises those *posterior fibres of the glutei minimus and medius* lying behind the coronal plane, as well as the *abductor fibres of the gluteus maximus*. These muscles, contracting alone or in conjunction with weaker partners, produce *abduction-extension-lateral rotation* **(Fig. 129)**.

To obtain **pure abduction (Fig. 130)**, i.e. without interference from other movements, these two muscle groups must be *activated as a balanced couple of synergists-antagonists.*

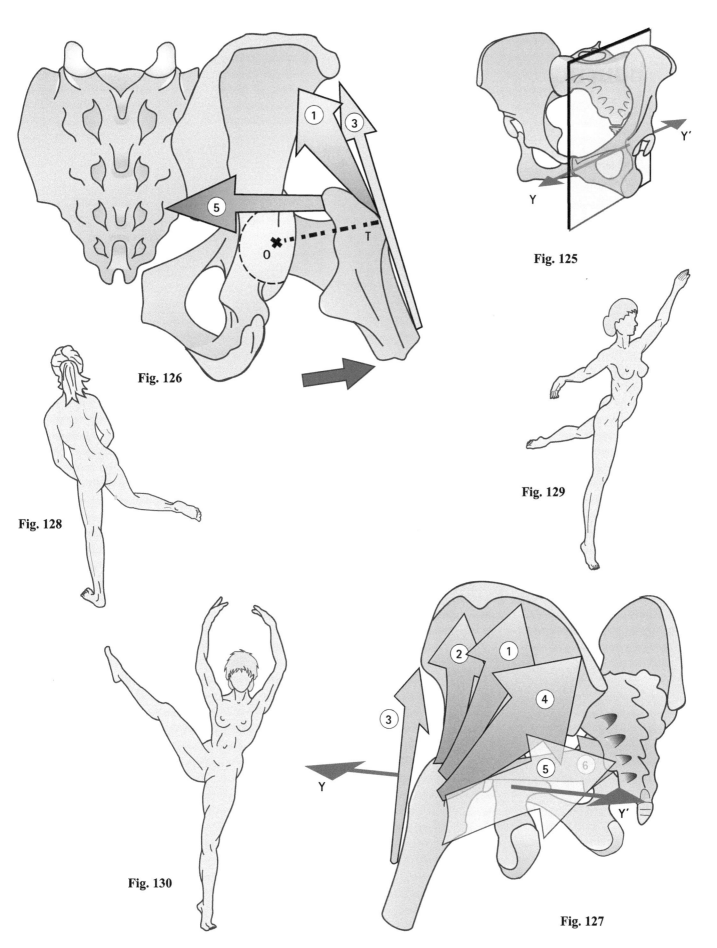

Fig. 125

Fig. 126

Fig. 128

Fig. 129

Fig. 130

Fig. 127

47

Hip abduction

The 'deltoid of the hip' (Farabeuf) forms a wide muscular fan (Fig. 131) on the lateral aspect of the hip joint. It owes its name to its *triangular shape*, with apex pointing inferiorly, and to its anatomical and functional resemblance to the deltoid muscle of the shoulder joint. It is made up, however, not of a continuous sheet of muscle but of two *muscle bellies*, which form the anterior and posterior borders of the triangle: *anteriorly*, the **tensor fasciae latae** (1) arising from the *anterior superior iliac spine* (2) and running obliquely inferiorly and posteriorly; *posteriorly*, the **superficial fibres of the gluteus maximus** (3) arising from the posterior third of the iliac crest and the dorsum of the sacrum and coccyx and running inferiorly and anteriorly. These two muscles are inserted respectively into the **anterior and posterior borders of the iliotibial tract (4)**, a longitudinal condensation of the **fascia lata**, which is the superficial layer of the deep fascia of the thigh. After receiving the insertion of the tensor fasciae latae and gluteus maximus, the iliotibial tract becomes the tendon of insertion of the 'deltoid' (5), which is attached to (6) *Gerdy's tubercle on the lateral surface of the lateral tibial condyle*. Between these two muscles the deep fascia of the thigh (7) covers the gluteus medius. These two muscles can contract separately, but, when they contract in a balanced fashion, their tendon is pulled along its long axis and the 'deltoid' then produces *pure abduction*.

The efficiency of the glutei minimus and medius depends on the **length of the femoral neck (Fig. 132)**. If the head were '*placed*' directly on to the shaft, the total range of abduction would be increased considerably, but the lever arm OT' of the gluteus medius would be three times shorter and its efficiency three times less. This observation therefore *explains logically* why the femoral head is cantilevered on the shaft by the femoral neck (see pp. 19, 21 and 23): this mechanical arrangement is weaker and decreases the range of abduction, but it *increases the efficiency of the gluteus medius*, which is essential for the transverse stabilization of the pelvis.

The action of the **gluteus medius** on the lever arm of the femoral neck varies with the degree of abduction. When the hip is in the straight position **(Fig. 133)** the muscular pull F is not perpendicular to the lever arm OT and so can be resolved into two vectors:

- vector f'' acting towards the centre of the joint, i.e. *centripetally*, and promoting **articular coaptation (Fig. 133)**
- vector f' acting at right angles, i.e. *tangentially* and providing the *effective force* of the muscle at the start of abduction.

Subsequently, as abduction proceeds **(Fig. 134)**, the vector f'' tends to decrease as the vector f' increases. Therefore the gluteus medius becomes *progressively less efficient in securing coaptation and more efficient as an abductor*. It attains maximal efficiency at approximately 35° abduction, when the direction of its force is *perpendicular to the lever arm OT2* and f' coincides with F *when the full force of the muscle is devoted to abduction*. The muscle is now shorter by a length T1T2, i.e. about one-third of its total length, but it still has the remaining two-thirds of its excursion available for contraction.

The **action of the tensor fasciae latae (Fig. 135)** can be studied in the same way. Its force F acting on the iliac spine C1 can be resolved into a centripetal vector $f1''$ and a pelvis-tilting tangential vector $f1'$. As abduction proceeds **(Fig. 136)**, $f2'$ increases but never equals the total force F of the muscle. On the other hand, the diagram clearly shows that the muscle is shortened (C1'C2) only by a tiny fraction of its total length from the iliac spine to Gerdy's tubercle. This explains why the belly of the muscle is so short compared with the length of its tendon, since it is well known that the maximal excursion of a muscle does not exceed one half of the length of its contractile fibres.

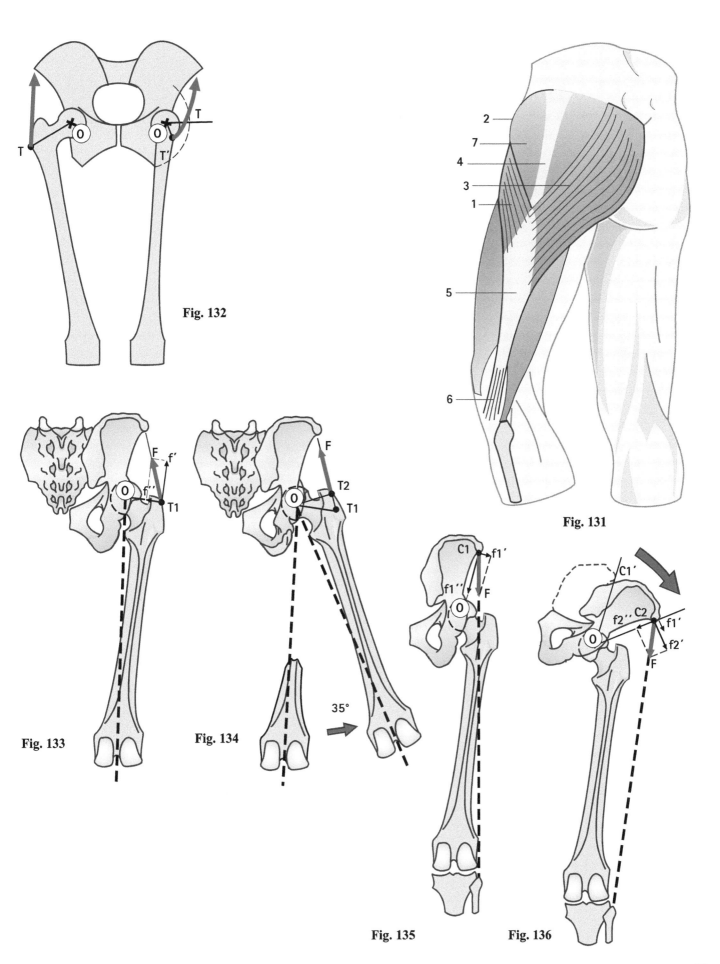

Fig. 132

Fig. 131

Fig. 133

Fig. 134

35°

Fig. 135

Fig. 136

49

The transverse stability of the pelvis

When the **pelvis is in double-limb support**, its transverse stability is secured by the simultaneous and bilateral contraction of the adductors (red arrows) and abductors (green arrows). When these antagonistic actions are properly balanced **(Fig. 137)**, the pelvis is *stabilized symmetrically*, as in the military position of standing to attention. If the abductors predominate on one side and the adductors on the other side, **(Fig. 138)**, the pelvis is *tilted laterally* towards the side of adductor predominance. Unless muscular balance can be restored at this point, the subject will fall to that side.

When the **pelvis is in single-limb support (Fig. 139)**, transverse stability is ensured solely by the action of the abductors on the supporting side, since the body weight W, acting through the centre of gravity, will tend to tilt the pelvis at the supporting hip. Thus the pelvis can be likened to a *type I lever* **(Fig. 141)**, where the fulcrum is the supporting hip O, the resistance is the body weight W acting through the *centre of gravity* G and the force is the pull of the gluteus medius (GMe) acting from the lateral aspect L of the iliac fossa towards the greater trochanter T. To keep the pelvis horizontal when supported by one limb, the force of the gluteus medius must be adequate to cancel that of the body weight, taking into account that the lever arms OE and OG are unequal in length. In thus balancing the pelvis, the

gluteus medius and gluteus minimus (Gme) are strongly assisted **(Fig. 139)** by the *tensor fasciae latae* (TFL).

If there is insufficiency of any of these muscles **(Fig. 140)**, the effect of gravity is not properly counterbalanced, and the pelvis tilts to the opposite side, forming an **angle a** directly proportional to the severity of the muscular insufficiency. The tensor fasciae latae stabilizes not only the pelvis but *also the knee* and behaves **(Fig. 154**, p. 113) like a true *active lateral collateral ligament*, so that its paralysis in the long run will cause the knee joint space to *gap laterally* **(angle b)**.

Stabilization of the pelvis by the glutei medius and minimus and the tensor fasciae latae is essential for **normal walking (Fig. 142)**. While the pelvis is in single-limb support, the *inter-iliac line* stays horizontal and more or less parallel to the line joining the shoulders. If these muscles are paralysed on the side supporting the pelvis **(Fig. 143)**, the pelvis tilts towards the opposite side with a similar tilting of the line joining the shoulders. This typical stance during single-limb support, i.e. tilting of the pelvis on the opposite side and *bending of the upper trunk towards the supporting side*, corresponds to the **Duchenne-Trendelenburg's** sign, which indicates *paralysis or insufficiency of the glutei minimus and medius*.

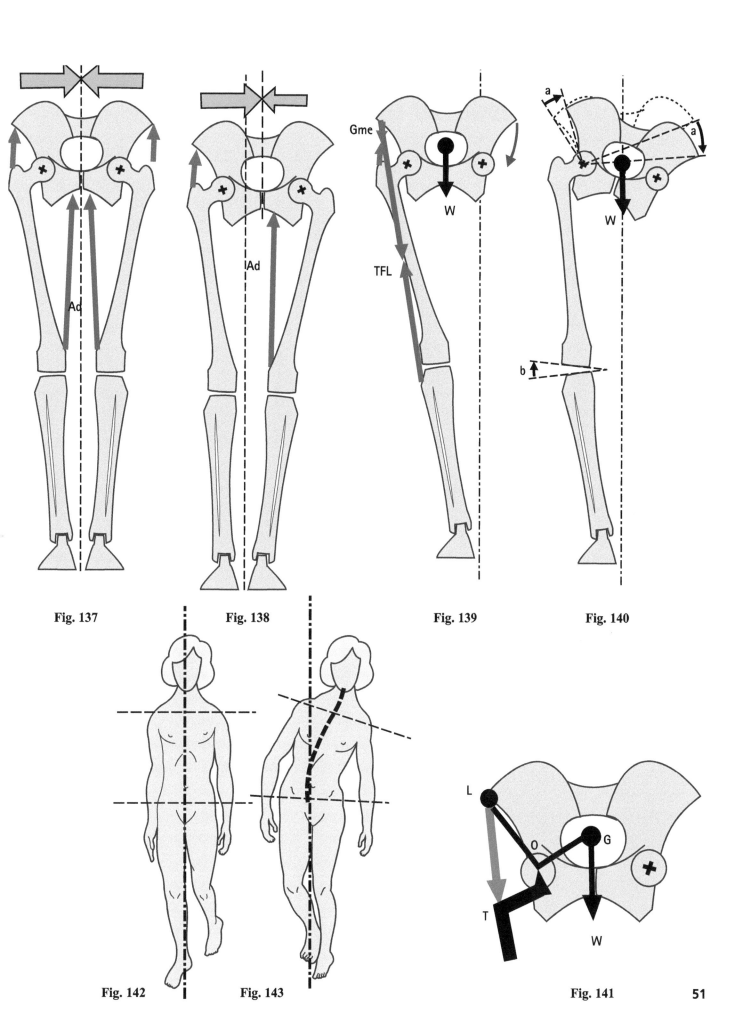

Fig. 137

Fig. 138

Fig. 139

Fig. 140

Fig. 142

Fig. 143

Fig. 141

51

The adductor muscles of the hip joint

The hip adductors lie generally medial to the sagittal plane passing through the centre of the joint **(Fig. 144)**. In any case, they *run inferior and medial* to the anteroposterior axis yy' of abduction-adduction located in the same sagittal plane.

The adductors are particularly *numerous and powerful*. **Fig. 145** (posterior view) shows them forming a large fan spanning the whole length of the femur. The **adductor magnus** (1) is the *most powerful* (Force equivalent to 13 kg). Its peculiar arrangement **(Fig. 146)** is due to the fact that its most medial fibres, arising from the ramus of the pubis and the ramus of the ischium, are inserted the most proximally into the femur, whereas its most lateral fibres from the ischial tuberosity are inserted the most distally into the linea aspera. As a result, its *superior* (2) *and intermediate (1) fibres form a sort of gutter concave posterolaterally*, which can be seen in the diagram because the superior fibres are considered transparent and the hip has been disarticulated with lateral rotation of the femur. In this gutter (insert representing a section taken at the level of the arrow) runs a third set of fibres (the *inferior* fibres), constituting a distinct fusiform muscle belly, also known as the **adductor minimus** or the **third adductor** (3).

This fibre arrangement *reduces the relative lengthening of the muscle during abduction* and *allows a greater range of abduction* to occur while retaining the efficiency of the muscle. This idea is illustrated in **Fig. 147**, which shows the following:

- Side A: the real direction of the fibres
- Side B: the real direction of the fibres and their 'simplified' direction in the absence of any abduction-induced torsion

(broken lines), i.e. with the most medial fibres having the most distal insertion and the most lateral fibres having the most proximal insertion (the exact opposite of their arrangement in life)

- These two arrangements are shown in adduction (Ad) and in abduction (Ab). The lengthening of the fibres from adduction to abduction is obvious and is indicated by the difference between the lengths of the arcs of the circles described during movement: **u** for the fibres arising from the pubis, **v** for the fibres arising from the ischium and **z** for the fibres inserting into the greater trochanter.

Fig. 145 also illustrates the other muscles that contribute to adduction:

- The **gracilis** (4) forms the internal border of the muscular fan
- The **semimembranosus** (5), the **semitendinosus** (6) and the **long head of the biceps femoris** (7) are primarily hip extensors and knee flexors but also have an important adductor component
- The **gluteus maximus** (8): the bulk of its fibres (i.e. the fibres lying below axis YY'), produce adduction
- The **quadratus femoris** (9) and the **pectineus** (10) produce adduction and lateral rotation
- The **obturator internus** (11), assisted by the gemelli (not shown) and the **obturator externus** (12), are secondary adductors.

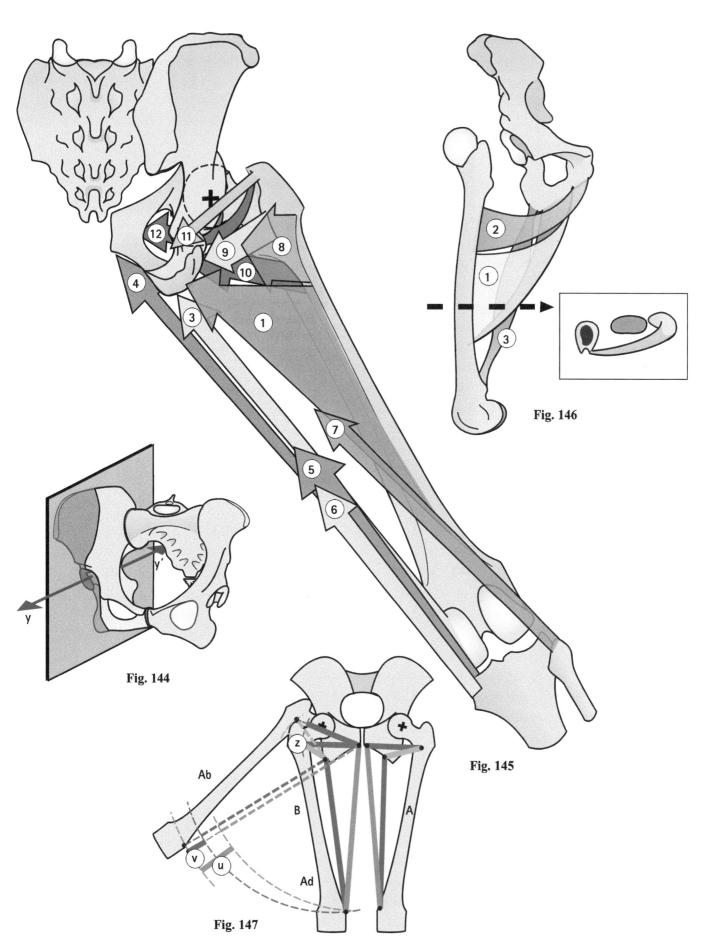

Fig. 146

Fig. 144

Fig. 145

Fig. 147

The adductor muscles of the hip joint (*continued*)

Fig. 148 (anterior view) shows diagrammatically the following adductors:

- the **adductor longus** (13), whose muscular power (equivalent to 5 kg) falls short of half of that of the adductor magnus
- the **adductor brevis** (14), whose two bundles are covered inferiorly by the adductor longus and superiorly by the pectineus (10)
- the **gracilis** (4), which forms the medial border of the adductor compartment.

In addition to their main adductor function these muscles also produce some degree of *flexion-extension and axial rotation*.

Their **role in flexion-extension (Fig. 149**, medial view) depends on their site of origin. If the muscles arise from the ischium and pubis *posterior* to the coronal plane passing through the centre of the joint (line of alternating dots and dashes), they are hip extensors; in particular, the lower fibres of the adductor magnus, the adductor minimus, and, of course, the hamstrings. When the muscles arise from the hip bone *anterior* to the coronal plane, they are simultaneous adductors and flexors, e.g. the pectineus, the adductor brevis, the adductor longus, the superior bundle of the adductor magnus and the gracilis. Note, however, that their role in flexion-extension also depends on the initial position of the hip.

The adductors, as already shown, are essential for the stabilization of the pelvis in double-limb support, and they play an essential role in **certain postures** or in certain movements in sports like skiing **(Fig. 150)** or horse-riding **(Fig. 151)**.

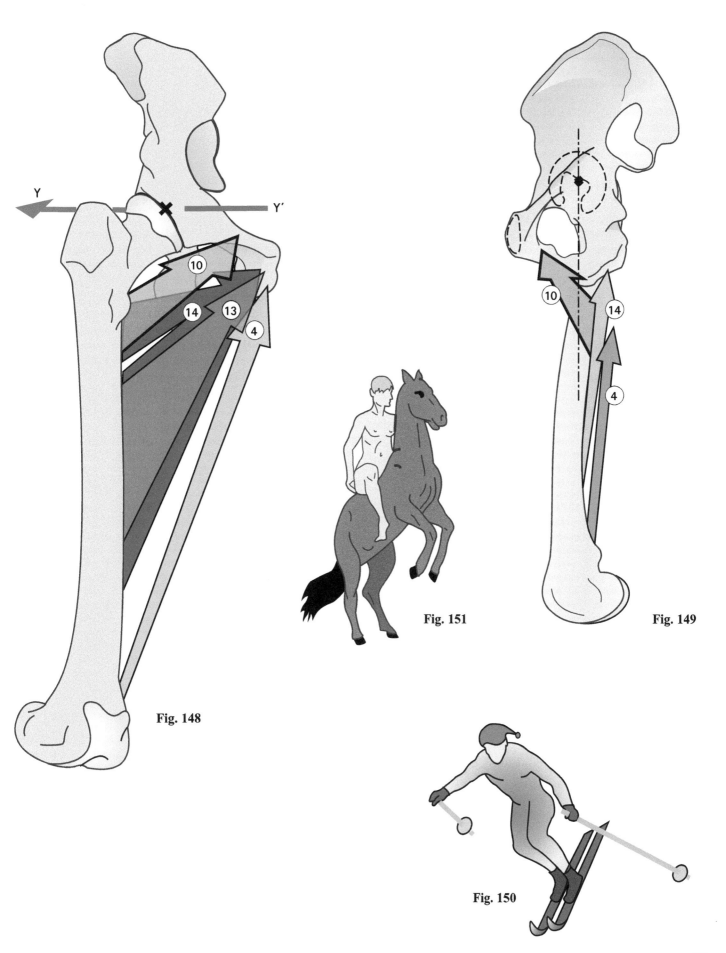

Y — X ····· Y'

⑩
⑭ ⑬
④

Fig. 148

⑩
⑭
④

Fig. 151

Fig. 149

Fig. 150

The lateral rotator muscles of the hip joint

The lateral rotators are *numerous* and *powerful* and cross *the vertical axis of the hip posteriorly*, as is well shown in the **horizontal section of the pelvis (Fig. 152**, superior view, right side), passing slightly above the centre of the joint. This diagram shows all the lateral rotators as follows:

- **The pelvitrochanteric muscles** with lateral rotation as their primary function
  - **The piriformis** (1) arises from the anterior surface of the sacrum, runs posteriorly and laterally and emerges through the greater sciatic notch **(Fig. 153**, right postero-superior view) to insert into the superior border of the greater trochanter.
  - The **obturator internus** (2) runs more or less parallel to the piriformis, but it is reflected at a right angle on the posterior border of the ischium above the ischial spine **(Fig. 153)**. The first (2') part of its course at its origin from the margin of the obturator foramen is *intrapelvic*. In the second part of its course, it is flanked by the tiny superior and inferior gemelli, which arise from the ischial spine and the ischial tuberosity and skirt its superior and inferior borders respectively. The obturator internus and the gemelli insert by common tendon into the medial surface of the greater trochanter. They have similar actions.
  - **The obturator externus** (3) arises from the *external surface of the margins of the obturator foramen*, and its tendon winds posteriorly below the hip joint and runs upwards behind the femoral neck to its insertion in the floor of the trochanteric fossa. On the whole, the muscle spirals round the femoral neck and can only be seen in its entirety when the pelvis is considerably tilted on the femur **(Fig. 154**: posterior-infero-lateral view of the pelvis with the hip flexed). This explains its two main actions: it is above all a lateral rotator when the hip is flexed (see also p. 58), and it is a weak hip flexor because of its winding course around the femoral neck.

- Some **adductor muscles** are also lateral rotators:
  - The **quadratus femoris** (4), arising from the ischial tuberosity and inserted into the posterior intertrochanteric line **(Fig. 153)**, can also extend or flex the hip **(Fig. 152)**, depending on the position of the hip.
  - The **pectineus** (6), arising from the horizontal ramus of the pubis and inserted into the intermediate line of the trifurcate linea aspera **(Fig. 154)**, produces adduction, flexion and lateral rotation.
  - The most posterior fibres of the **adductor magnus (Fig. 155**, 3) also produce lateral rotation, like the hamstrings.
  - The **glutei:** the whole of the **gluteus maximus**, including both its superficial (7) and its deep fibres (7'); the posterior fibres of the **gluteus minimus** and especially of the **gluteus medius** (8) **(Figs 152 and 153)**.

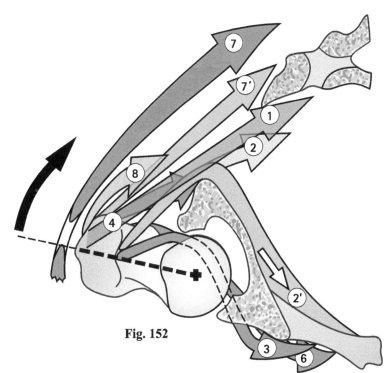

Fig. 152

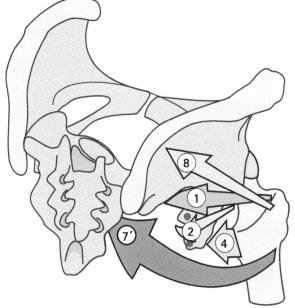

Fig. 153

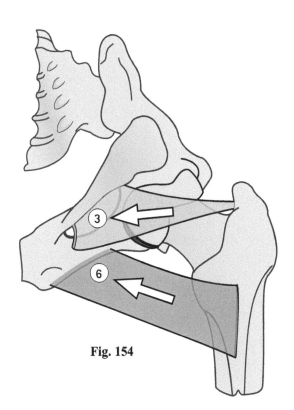

Fig. 154

Rotator muscles of the hip joint

The **horizontal section (Fig. 155)**, passing just below the femoral head, shows the lateral rotational component of force of the hamstrings and adductors. The horizontal projections of the long head of the biceps femoris (1), the semitendinosus, the semimembranosus (2), the adductor magnus (3) and even of the adductor longus and **adductor brevis** (4) all run posterior to the vertical axis; hence these muscles are lateral rotators (LR) when the lower limb turns on its long axis **(Fig. 23)**, i.e with knee extended and hip and foot acting as pivots. Note that during medial rotation (MR) some of the adductors run anterior to the *vertical axis* and so become *medial rotators*.

The medial rotators are *less numerous* than the external rotators, and their pull is about one-third of that of the lateral rotators (equivalent to 54 kg for the medial rotators and 146 kg for the lateral rotators). These muscles run *anterior to the vertical axis of the hip joint*. The **horizontal section (Fig. 156)** shows the three medial rotators of the hip:

• the **gluteus medius** (5): only its anterior fibres rotate the hip
• the **gluteus minimus** (6): virtually all its fibres rotate the hip
• the **tensor fasciae latae** (7): runs above the anterior superior iliac spine (ASIS).

After a moderate degree of medial rotation, i.e. 30-40° **(Fig. 157)**, the obturator externus (8) and the pectineus (9) run exactly inferior to the centre of the joint; hence they are no longer lateral rotators, while the glutei minimus and medius (6) are still medial rotators.

Conversely **after full medial rotation (Fig. 158)** the **obturator externus** (8) and the **pectineus** (9) become medial rotators because they now run anterior to the vertical axis, while the **tensor fasciae latae** (7) and the **glutei minimus** and **medius** (5) become lateral rotators. This is the case only when medial rotation is maximal. It is an example of the inversion of muscular action according to the position of the joint, and it is the result of a change in the direction of the muscle fibres as well illustrated in **Fig. 159 (antero-supero-lateral view in perspective)**. With the hip in forced medial rotation, the **obturator externus** (8) and the **pectineus** (9) run anterior to the vertical axis (double arrow), while the glutei minimus and medius (5) take an oblique course superiorly and posteriorly.

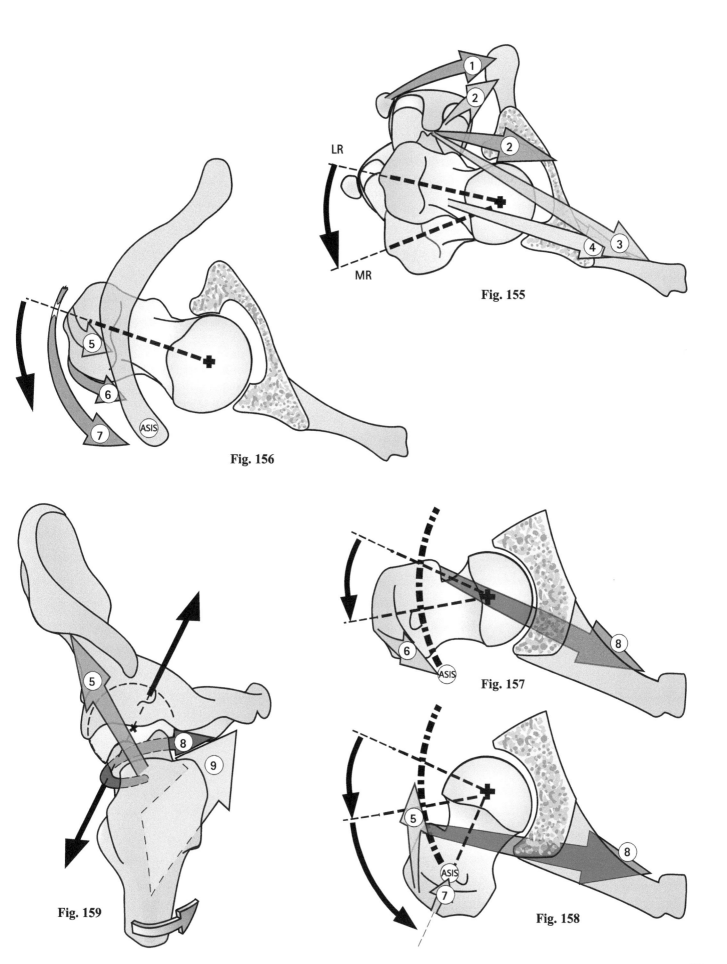

Fig. 155

Fig. 156

Fig. 157

Fig. 158

Fig. 159

Inversion of muscular actions

The actions of the motor muscles of a joint with three degrees of freedom vary according to the position of the joint, as their secondary actions are altered and even reversed. The most typical example is **the inversion of the flexor component of the adductor muscles (Fig. 160)**. Starting from the straight position (0°) *all the adductors are flexors*, except the posterior fibres of the adductor magnus (AM), which remains an extensor right up to –20° extension, but the flexor component persists only if the limb stays below the site of origin of each muscle. Thus the adductor longus (AL) is *still a flexor* at +50° extension, but it becomes an extensor after +70° flexion. Likewise, the adductor brevis is only a flexor up to +50° and then becomes an extensor, while for the gracilis the limit for flexor action is +40°.

The diagram clearly shows that only the true flexors can produce flexion right up to their limits of action: at +120° flexion the excursion of the **tensor fasciae latae** (TFL) is completed, since it is now shorter by a distance of aa' equivalent to half of its length; and the iliopsoas (IP) loses most of its efficiency since its tendon *tends to move away from the iliopubic eminence*. This diagram explains why the lesser trochanter (LT) is located *very far posteriorly*, the excursion of the iliopsoas tendon is thereby *increased* by a length equal to the thickness of the femoral shaft.

The **quadratus femoris** also shows very clearly the inversion of its flexor component **(Fig. 161**: the transparent hip bone makes the femur and the course of the quadratus visible). In *extension* **E** the quadratus is a flexor (blue arrow) and becomes an extensor (red arrow) in *flexion* **F** with the position of transition corresponding to the straight position of the hip.

Muscle efficiency itself depends largely on joint position. When the **hip is already flexed (Fig. 162)**, the hip extensors are stretched. With **120° flexion (F)** the **gluteus maximus** is passively elongated *by a distance of gg'*, which equals 100% for some of its fibres and the hamstrings by a distance of **hh'**, which is about 50% of their length in the straight position of the hip, provided the knee stays extended. This observation explains the **starting position of runners (Fig. 163)**: maximal hip flexion followed by knee extension (this second phase is not illustrated here) that tenses the hip extensors appropriately for the strong impulse needed at the start. It is this tension of the hamstrings that checks hip flexion when the knee is extended.

Fig. 162 shows also that from the straight position to –20° extension the change in length of the hamstrings hh" is small, supporting the idea that *the hamstrings work at their best advantage when the hip is half-flexed*.

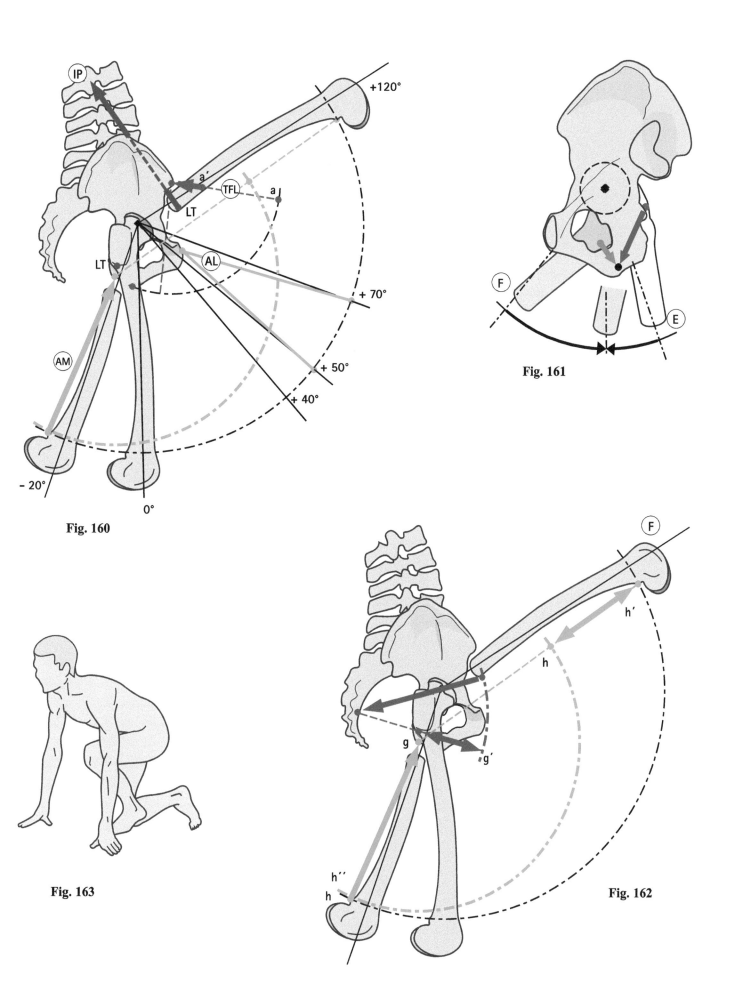

Fig. 160

+120°

IP

TFL

a'

a

LT

LT

AL

AM

+ 70°

+ 50°

+ 40°

– 20°

0°

Fig. 161

F

E

Fig. 163

Fig. 162

F

h'

h

g

g'

h''

h

Inversion of muscular actions *(continued)*

When **the hip is markedly flexed (Fig. 164)**, the **piriformis** also shows inversion of its actions (**Fig. 165**, posterolateral view). With the hip in the straight position it is a combined lateral rotator-flexor-abductor (red arrow), but with the hip markedly flexed (blue arrow) it becomes a medial rotator-extensor-abductor: the point of inversion corresponds to 60° flexion, where it is only an abductor.

In **marked flexion (Fig. 166**: posterolateral view of the flexed hip) the **piriformis** (1) is still an abductor, while the obturator internus (2) and the *entire gluteus maximus* (3) also become abductors; these muscles allow the knees to be spread apart (blue arrow) and the hip to be rotated laterally (green arrow) when the hips are flexed at 90°. The gluteus minimus (4) is very clearly a medial rotator (red arrow) and becomes an adductor (**Fig. 167**) like the tensor fasciae latae (5). These muscles produce an overall movement of combined flexion-adduction-medial rotation (**Fig. 168**).

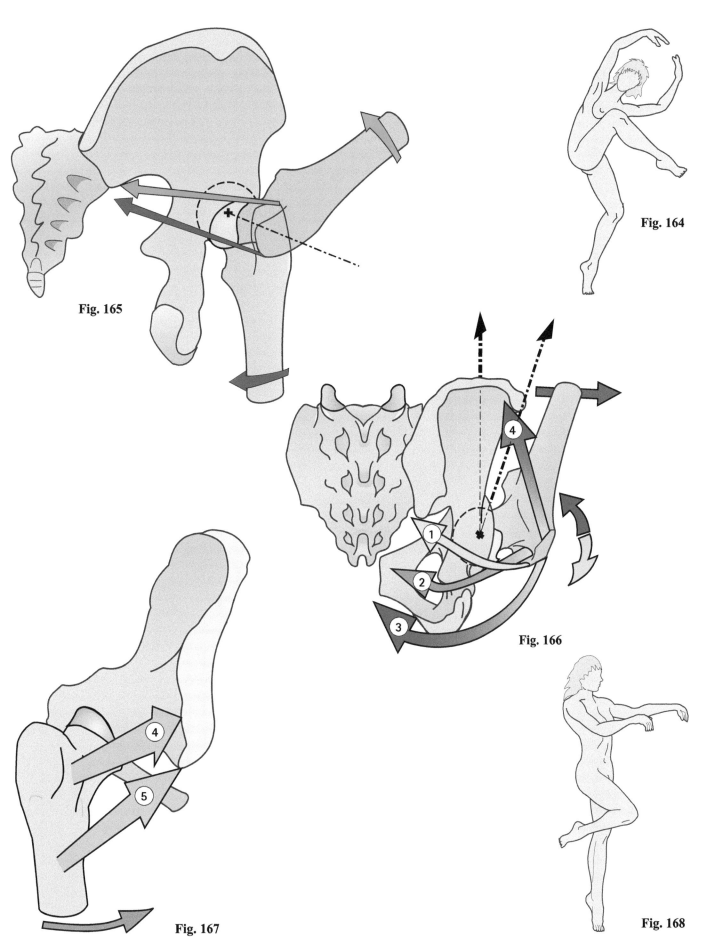

Fig. 164

Fig. 165

Fig. 166

Fig. 167

Fig. 168

Successive recruitment of the abductor muscles

Depending on the degree of hip flexion, the pelvis, on single-limb support, is stabilized by different abductor muscles.

With the hip in **full extension (Fig. 169, red arrow)**, i.e. in the straight position, the centre of gravity of the body 'falls' behind the line joining the two hips, with the result that the pelvis is tilted posteriorly. This tilt is prevented by the tension of the iliofemoral ligament (see also p. 31) and by the contraction of the tensor fasciae latae (1), which is also a hip flexor; *hence the tensor corrects simultaneously posterior and lateral tilting of the pelvis.* As an abductor the tensor acts synergistically with the *superficial fibres of the gluteus maximus* (2) as part of the '*deltoid of the hip*'.

When the pelvis is **only slightly tilted posteriorly (Fig. 170)**, the centre of gravity still falls behind the line joining the hips, and the *gluteus minimus* (3) is recruited. Note that this muscle is also an abductor-flexor like the tensor fasciae latae.

When the pelvis is **in equilibrium anteroposteriorly (Fig. 171)**, the centre of gravity falls on the line joining the hips, and the pelvis is stabilized laterally by the gluteus medius (4).

As soon as the pelvis is **tilted anteriorly**, the **gluteus maximus** is called into action, followed in succession **(Fig. 172)** by the **deep fibres of the gluteus maximus** (5), the **piriformis (6)** and **(Fig. 173)** the **obturator internus** (7). During this entire process, including extreme hip flexion **(Fig. 174)**, the **gluteus maximus** (2) operates as an *antagonist-synergist* with the tensor fasciae latae (1), as an abductor and also as a moderator of hip flexion. The obturator externus (7) is also called into action.

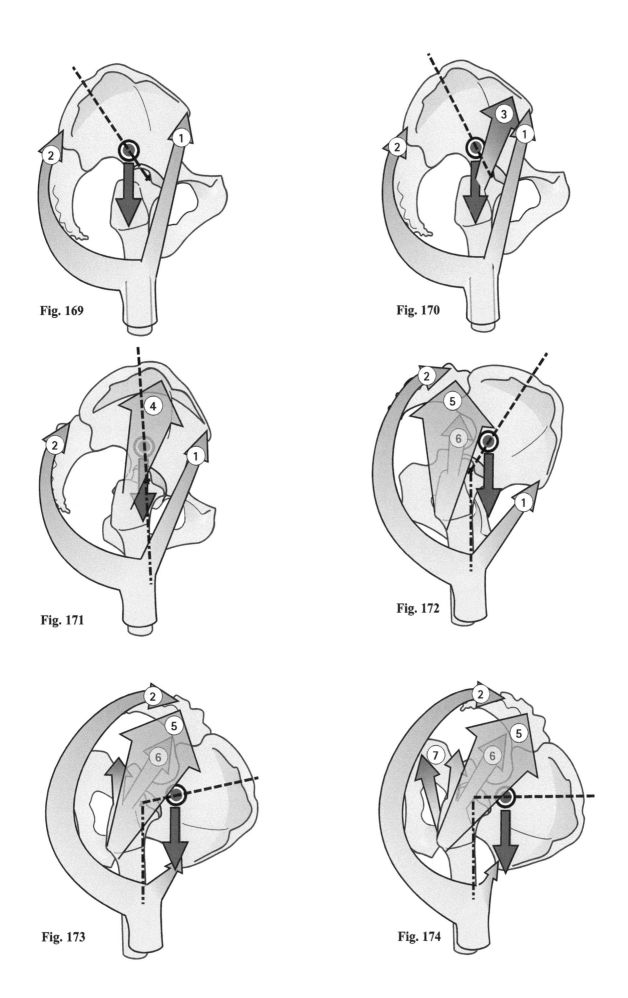

Fig. 169

Fig. 170

Fig. 171

Fig. 172

Fig. 173

Fig. 174

Chapter 2

THE KNEE

The knee is the **intermediate joint** of the lower limb. It is mainly a joint with *one degree of freedom* for flexion-extension, thus allowing the extremity of the limb to be *moved towards or away from* its root, which is the same as *controlling the distance between the body and the ground.* The knee works essentially by **axial compression** under the action of gravity.

The knee has an *accessory or second degree of freedom,* i.e. rotation around the axis of the leg only when *the knee is flexed.* The knee faces the *mechanical challenge* of reconciling *two contradictory requirements*:

* to have *great stability in full extension* when the knee is severely stressed as a result of the weight of the body and the length of the lever arms involved

* to display *great mobility in flexion,* as needed for running and for the *optimal orientation of the foot* relative to the irregularities of the ground.

The knee solves these problems by using highly ingenious mechanical devices, but the *small degree of interlocking of the articular surfaces* - essential for mobility - renders it liable to *sprains and dislocations.*

During **flexion**, the knee is unstable, and the *ligaments and menisci* are most susceptible to injury, but it is in **extension** that the knee is most vulnerable to *fractures of the articular surfaces and ligamentous tears.*

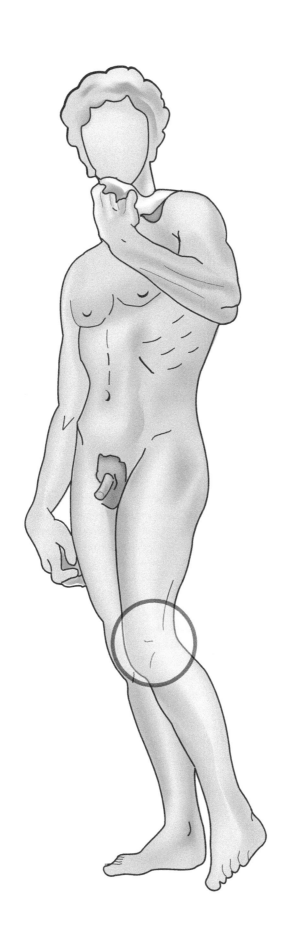

The axes of the knee joint

The **first degree of freedom** is related to the *transverse axis XX'* (**Fig. 1**: anteromedial view and **Fig. 2**: anterolateral view of the semi-flexed knee), around which occur movements of flexion-extension in a sagittal plane. This axis XX', lying in a coronal plane, passes horizontally through the femoral condyles. Because the long neck of the femur displaces the shaft laterally (**Fig. 3**: overview of the skeleton of the lower limb) the long axis of the shaft does not coincide with that of the leg but forms an obtuse angle of 170-175° open laterally. This is the **physiological valgus** of the knee.

Conversely, the centres of the three joints, i.e. the hip (H), the knee (K) and the ankle (A) lie on the same straight line HKA, which is the mechanical axis of the lower limb. In the leg it coincides with that of the leg, but in the thigh it forms an angle of about 6° with the femoral axis.

On the other hand, because the hips are wider apart than the ankles, the mechanical axis of each lower limb is slightly oblique interiorly and medially at an angle of 3° with the vertical. This angle is greater the wider the pelvis, as in women. This observation also explains why the *physiological valgus of the knee is more marked in women than in men*.

The flexion-extension axis XX' is *horizontal* and so does not coincide with Kb, the bisector of the angle of valgus. The angle between XX' and the femur is 81°, and that between XX' and the axis of the leg is 93°. As a result, during full flexion the axis of the leg does not come to rest immediately *posterior* to the femoral axis but rather *slightly posterior and medial to it*, so that the heel moves medially towards the plane of symmetry of the body. Thus *extreme flexion brings the heel into contact with the buttock at the level of the ischial tuberosity*.

The **second degree of freedom** is related to rotation around the long axis YY' of the leg (**Figs 1 and 2**), which is clearly defined with the knee flexed. The structure of the knee makes **axial rotation impossible when the knee is fully extended:** the axis of the leg then coincides with the mechanical axis of the lower limb and *axial rotation takes place not at the knee but at the hip joint, which comes to the rescue of the knee.*

In Figures 1 and 2 an axis ZZ' is shown running anteroposteriorly at right angles to the other two axes. This axis does not really represent a third degree of freedom but, because of a measure of play in the joint due to relaxation of the collateral ligaments, it allows the occurrence of small **valgus and varus movements** of 1-2 cm observed at the ankle; but, when the knee is fully extended, these movements disappear completely as the collateral ligaments become taut. If they still persist, they must be viewed as abnormal, i.e. an indication of collateral ligament injury.

In fact, these movements occur normally as soon as the knee is bent. To determine whether they are abnormal they must be compared with those of the other knee, provided the latter is unscathed.

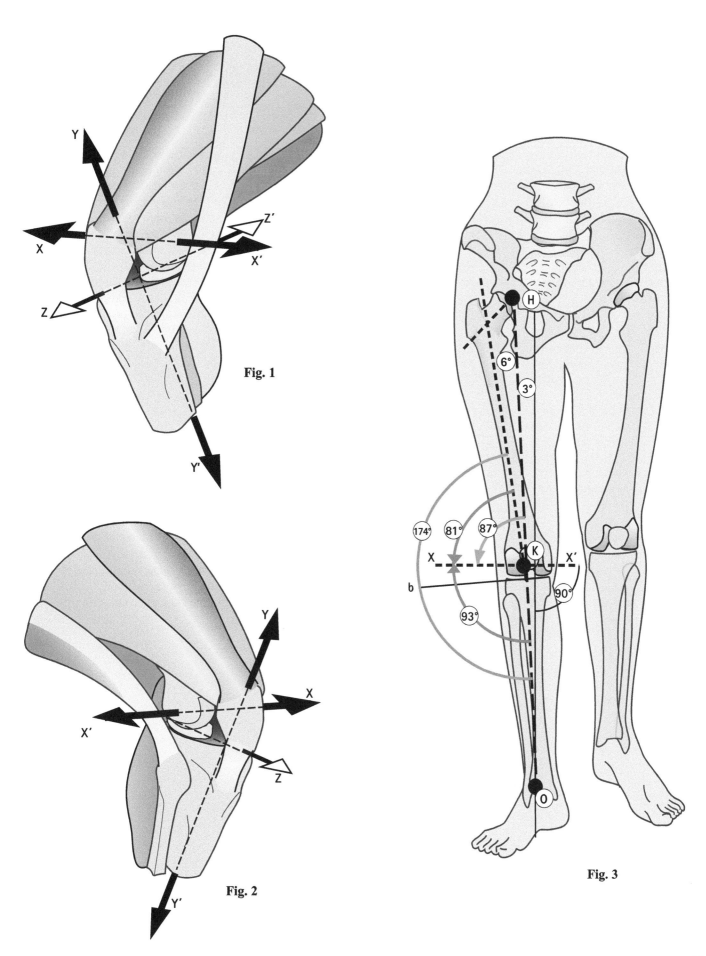

Fig. 1

Fig. 2

Fig. 3

Medial and lateral deviations of the knee

In addition to its sex-related physiological variations, the angle of valgus can exhibit individual pathological variations (**Fig. 4**: frontal view of the skeleton of the lower limbs).

Inversion of the angle of valgus produces the **genu varum** (**Fig. 4**: **Var** in left knee), i.e. *bandy legs* (**Fig. 6**). The centre of the knee joint, corresponding to the tibial intercondylar eminence and the femoral intercondylar fossa, is displaced laterally. Genu varum can be quantitated in two ways:

- by measuring the *angle between the long axes of the femoral and tibial shafts*, it is present if the angle (e.g. 180-185°) exceeds the normal value (170°) and inverts the normally obtuse angle
- by measuring the **lateral displacement (Fig. 5**, Id) of the centre of the joint relative to the mechanical axis of the lower limb, (e.g. 10-15 or 20 mm): lateral displacement (Id) is recorded as 15 mm.

Conversely, closure of the angle of valgus gives rise to the **genu valgum (Fig. 4)**, i.e. *knock knees* (**Fig. 8**). There are also two ways of quantitating genu valgum:

- by measuring the *angle between the long axes of the femoral and tibial shafts:* it is present if the angle is less (e.g. 165°) than the normal value of 170°
- by measuring the **medial displacement (Fig. 7**, md) of the centre of the joint with respect to the mechanical axis of the lower limb (e.g. 10-15 or 20 mm): the medial displacement (md) is recorded as 15 mm.

Measurement of these **lateral and medial displacements** is more precise than that of the angle of valgus, but it requires high-quality **comprehensive radiographs of the lower limb**, known as *goniometric* radiographs (**Fig. 4**). In the diagram, the subject is exceptionally unlucky in having a *right genu valgum* and a *left genu varum*. In most cases, the deformity is similar on both sides but not necessarily symmetrical in severity, with one knee being more affected than the other. There are, however, only rare cases of deviation of both knees in the same direction, as in the diagram. This combined deformity is very uncomfortable, since it leads to loss of stability of the genu valgum. It can also arise when a corrective osteotomy procedure has overcorrected a genu varum into a genu valgum. A second osteotomy is then required without delay to restore the normal balance.

Varus or valgus (Var, Val) deviations of the knee are not harmless as they *cause osteoarthritis with time*. In effect, the mechanical loads are not evenly spread over the lateral and medial two compartments of the knee joint, leading to premature erosion of their respective articular surfaces and culminating in **medial femorotibial osteoarthritis in the presence of genu varum** or **lateral femorotibial osteoarthritis in the presence of genu valgum.** Appropriate treatment requires a tibial (or femoral) valgization osteotomy for genu varum and a tibial (or femoral) varization for genu valgum. It is precisely to prevent these complications that more attention is now devoted to the **surveillance of medial or lateral deviations of the knee in young children.** It is a fact that bilateral genu varum is very common in children and disappears progressively with growth. Nevertheless, this favourable outcome needs to be followed with comprehensive radiographs of the lower limbs. If a significant deviation were to persist at the end of childhood, the need might arise for medial or lateral tibiofemoral epiphysiodesis for genu valgum and genu varum, respectively. These operations work by inhibiting the growth of the more 'convex' side of the knee in favour of that of the more 'concave' side.

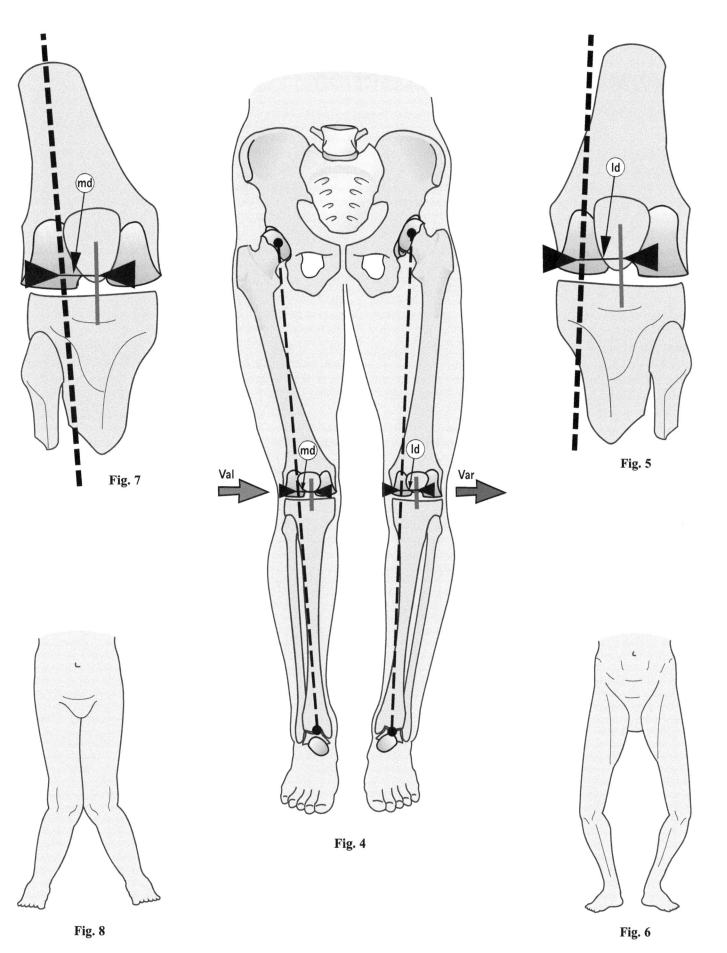

Fig. 7

Fig. 5

Val

Var

Fig. 4

Fig. 8

Fig. 6

Movements of flexion-extension

Flexion-extension is the main movement of the knee. Its range is measured from the reference position defined by the following criterion: the *collinearity of the long axis of the leg with that of the thigh* (**Fig. 9**, left leg). As seen from the side the femoral axis is directly continuous with that of the leg. In this position the lower limb is at its longest.

Extension is defined as the movement of the posterior surface of the leg away from the posterior surface of the thigh. There is strictly no absolute extension, since in the reference position the lower limb is already maximally extended. It is, however, possible to produce passive extension of 5-10° from the reference position (**Fig. 11**), wrongly called 'hyperextension'. It can be abnormally exaggerated in some people, leading to the *genu recurvatum*.

Active extension goes beyond the reference point rarely and then only slightly (**Fig. 9**), and its occurrence depends essentially on the position of the hip. In fact, the efficiency of the rectus femoris as a knee extensor increases as the hip is extended (see p. 144), indicating that pre-existing hip extension (**Fig. 10**: right leg lying posterior) sets the stage for knee extension.

Relative extension is the movement that brings the knee into full extension from any position of flexion (**Fig. 10**: left leg lying anterior). It takes place normally during walking, when the *swing* limb moves forwards to resume contact with the ground.

Flexion is the movement of the posterior surface of the leg towards the posterior surface of the thigh. Flexion can be *absolute*, starting from the reference position, and *relative*, starting from any position of flexion.

The range of knee flexion varies according to the position of the hip and the modalities of the movement itself.

Active flexion reaches 140° if the hip is already flexed (**Fig. 12**), and only 120° if the hip is extended (**Fig. 13**). This difference in amplitude is due to the fact that the hamstrings lose some of their efficiency with hip extension (see p. 146). It is nevertheless possible to exceed 120° with the hip extended because of the *brisk ballistic contraction of the hamstrings*. When the hamstrings contract abruptly and powerfully, they propel the leg into a flexion that culminates in passive flexion.

Passive flexion of the knee has a range of 160° (**Fig. 14**) and allows the heel to touch the buttock. This movement underlies an important clinical test for freedom of movement during knee flexion. The range of passive flexion can be measured as the distance between the heel and the buttock. Normally it is limited only by the elastic impact of the calf and thigh muscles. Pathologically, passive flexion is checked by shortening of the extensor muscles, especially the quadriceps, or fibrotic contraction of the joint capsule (see p. 102). It is always possible to quantitate a flexion deficit by either computing the difference between the flexion achieved and the maximal flexion expected (160°) or by measuring the distance between the knee and the buttock. In contrast an *extension deficit* is reckoned as a negative angle. For example, an extension deficit of –60° is the same as that measured between the position of maximal passive extension and the straight position. Thus Figure 13 can be taken to mean that the left leg is flexed at 120°, or, if it cannot be extended farther, that it shows an extension deficit of –120°.

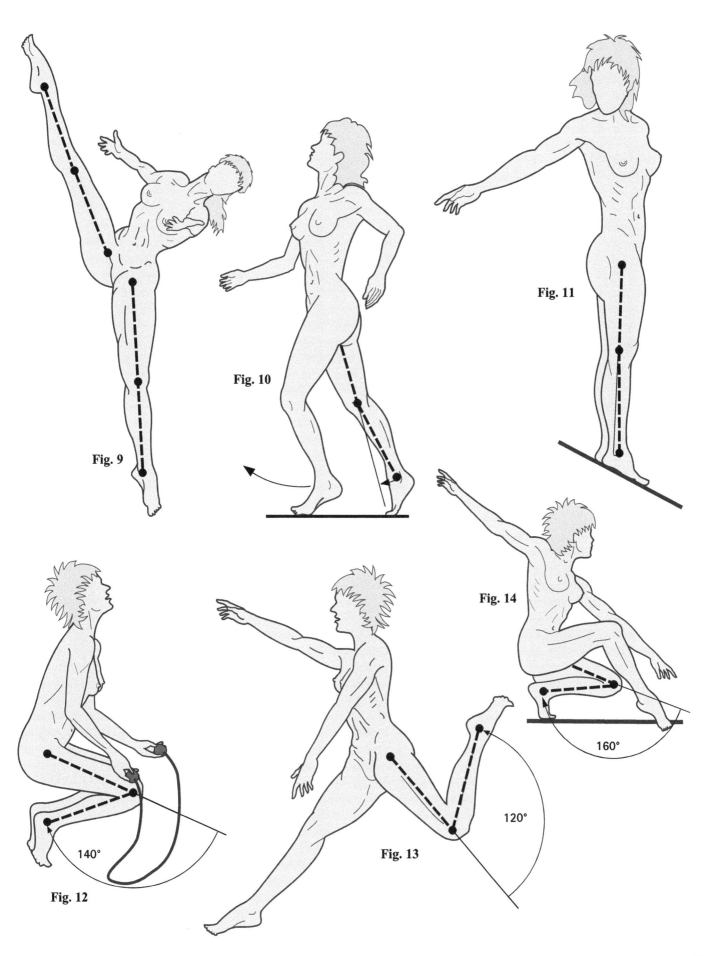

Fig. 9

Fig. 10

Fig. 11

Fig. 12

140°

Fig. 13

120°

Fig. 14

160°

73

Axial rotation of the knee

The movement of **rotation of the knee around its long axis** can only be performed with the *knee flexed*, since with knee extension and the interlocking of the joint the tibia becomes one with the femur.

To measure **active axial rotation** the knee must first be flexed at right angles while the subject is sitting *on a table with legs hanging down over the edge* **(Fig. 15)**, since knee flexion prevents hip rotation. In the *reference position* the toes face slightly laterally (see p. 78).

Medial rotation (Fig. 16) brings the toes to face medially and contributes significantly to adduction of the foot (see pp. 158 and 180).

Lateral rotation (Fig. 17) brings the toes to face laterally and also contributes to abduction of the foot.

According to Fick, the range of lateral rotation is 40° and that of medial rotation 30°, and the range varies with the degree of knee flexion, since, according to the same author, it is 32° for lateral rotation when the knee is flexed at 30° and 40° when the knee is flexed at 90°.

Passive axial rotation is measured with the subject lying prone *with the knee flexed at 90°*. The examiner grasps the foot with both hands and rotates it until the toes face laterally **(Fig. 18)** and medially **(Fig. 19)**. As expected, this passive rotation has a greater range than active rotation.

Finally, there is also a type of **axial rotation called 'automatic'** because it is inevitably and involuntarily *linked to movements of flexion-extension*. It occurs above all at the end of extension or at the start of flexion. When the knee is *extended* the foot is *laterally (EXternally) rotated* **(Fig. 20)**; hence the mnemonic EXtension = EXternal rotation. Conversely, when the knee is flexed the leg is *medially rotated* **(Fig. 21)**. The same movement occurs when, with the lower limbs tucked under the body, the toes automatically move to face medially, as in the *fetal position*.

The mechanism of this automatic axial rotation will be discussed later.

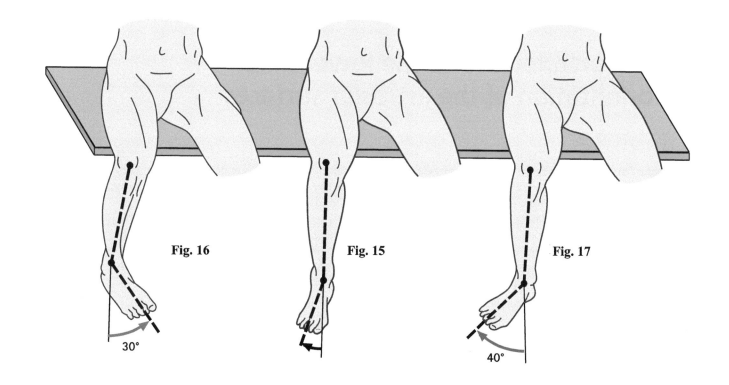

Fig. 16   Fig. 15   Fig. 17

30°   40°

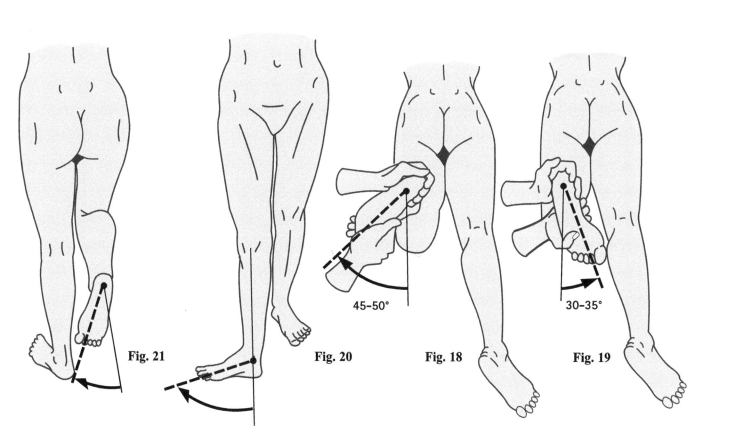

Fig. 21   Fig. 20   Fig. 18   Fig. 19

45–50°   30–35°

General architecture of the lower limb and orientation of the articular surfaces

The orientation of the femoral condyles and of the tibial articular surfaces promotes knee flexion. Two bony extremities, moving relative to each other **(Fig. 22)**, become moulded in accordance with their movements **(Fig. 23)** as demonstrated by *Fick's experiment*. Nevertheless, flexion will fall short of 90° **(Fig. 24)** unless a small fragment **(Fig. 25)** is removed from the upper bone so as to delay the impact of the lower bone. This zone of weakness thus created in the femur is offset by anterior displacement of the shaft so that the condyles become bent posteriorly **(Fig. 26)**. Reciprocally, the tibia is thinned posteriorly and reinforced anteriorly, *causing the tibial plateau to bend posteriorly.* Thus, during extreme flexion **(Fig. 27**: the femorotibial skeleton in flexion) the muscles can be lodged between tibia and femur.

The overall curvatures of the bones of the lower limb reflect the stresses applied and obey *Euler's laws governing the behaviour of columns eccentrically loaded* (quoted by Steindler).

If a column is jointed at both ends **(Fig. 29a**: free column loaded at the extremities), it is bent along its entire length, as is the case with the posteriorly concave femoral shaft **(Fig. 29b**: profile of the femur).

If a column is fixed below and mobile above **(Fig. 30a)**, two bends with opposite curvatures will result in the higher bend taking up two-thirds of the column; these bends correspond to the curvatures of the femur in the coronal plane **(Fig. 30b**: femur from the front).

If a column is fixed at both ends **(Fig. 31a)**, the bend occupies its two middle fourths and corresponds to the bend of the tibia in the coronal plane **(Fig. 31b)**.

In the sagittal plane, the tibia displays the following three features **(Fig. 32b)**:

- **retrotorsion** (t): a posterior bend
- **retroversion** (v): the tibial plateau shows a 5-6° slope posteriorly (this needs to be taken into account during total knee arthroplasties)
- **retroflexion** (f): a bend concave posteriorly corresponding to that seen in a column mobile at both ends **(Fig. 32a)**, like the femur.

The **opposite concavities of the femur and of the tibia** increase the available space to accommodate a *larger volume of muscle* **(Fig. 28**: femorotibial skeleton in flexion). This *arrangement resembles that seen at the elbow* (see Volume 1), where the curving of the articular ends of the bones provides a greater space for the muscles during flexion.

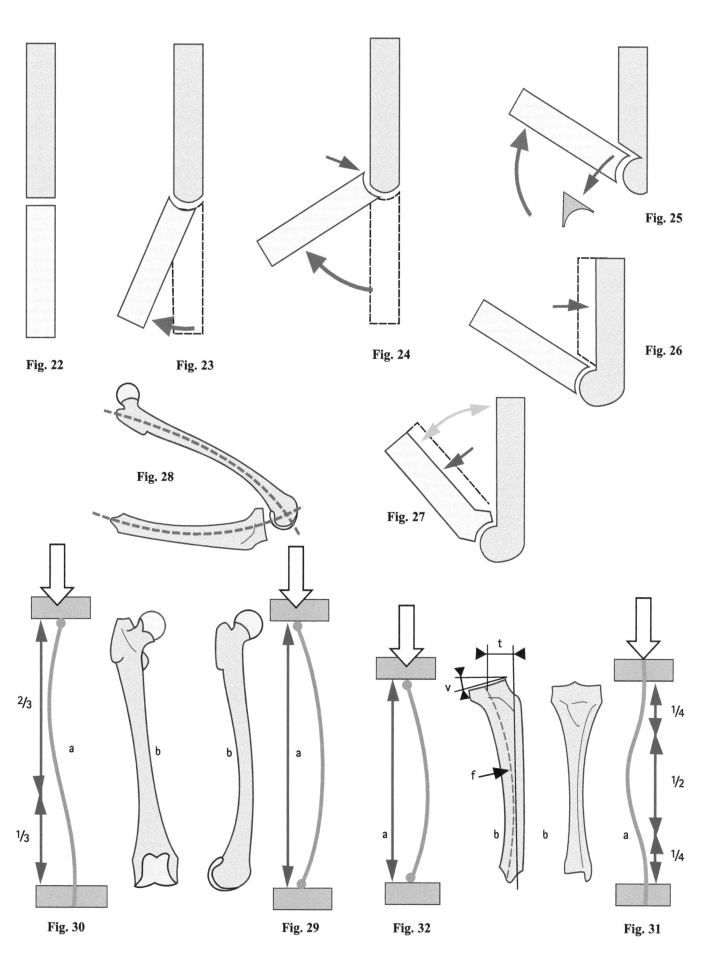

Fig. 22

Fig. 23

Fig. 24

Fig. 25

Fig. 26

Fig. 27

Fig. 28

Fig. 30

Fig. 29

Fig. 32

Fig. 31

General architecture of the lower limb and orientation of the articular surfaces *(continued)*

The axial torsions of the skeletal elements of the lower limb are explained in the diagrams on the next page using a sort of 'anatomical algebra'.

The successive segments of the lower limb are shown diagrammatically as seen from above.

Torsion of the femur is shown diagrammatically using its two extremities **(Fig. 33)**:

- In the normal position (a), the cervicocephalic extremity containing the head and neck A (in blue) and the lower extremity containing the condyles B (in red)
- Without torsion (b), the axis of the neck is parallel to that of the condyles, but in reality the axis of the neck forms an angle of 30° with the coronal plane (c)
- Therefore, if the condylar axis is to stay in the coronal plane (d), the femoral shaft must be twisted –30° by internal rotation corresponding to the anteversion angle of the neck.

Torsion at the level of the knee

The knee brings into contact **(Fig. 34a)** the femoral condyles (B, in red) and the tibial plateaus (C, in green). It looks as if both axes should be parallel and lie in the coronal plane (b), but in reality the automatic axial rotation (c) causes the tibia to rotate externally 5° below the femur during full knee extension.

Torsion at the level of the tibia

The tibia is represented diagrammatically **(Fig. 35a)** by the tibial plateau (C, in green) and by the tibiofibular mortise containing the talar pulley (D, in brown). The axes of these two articular surfaces are not parallel (b), but because of the torsion of the tibia, they form an angle of +25° due to a lateral rotation.

The result of these torsions

These torsions, staggered **(Fig. 36)** along the whole length of the lower limb (a), cancel out (–30° + 25° + 5° = 0°), so that the axis of the ankle has roughly the same orientation as that of the femoral neck, i.e. *laterally rotated +30°*. As a result, the axis of the foot is also bent laterally +30° in the erect posture with heels together and the pelvis (in red) symmetrically supported (b).

During walking, the forward movement of the swing limb *brings the ipsilateral hip forwards* (c); if the pelvis turns by 30° the *axis of the foot then points directly forwards* in the direction of walking. This optimizes the conditions for the loading phase to proceed.

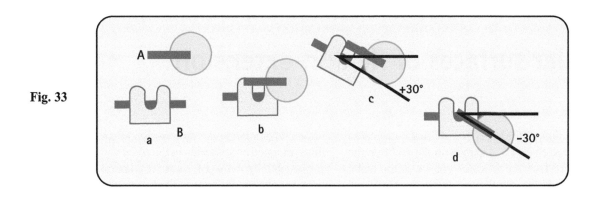

Fig. 33

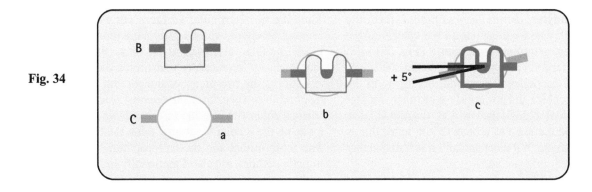

Fig. 34

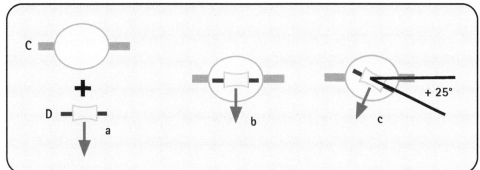

Fig. 35

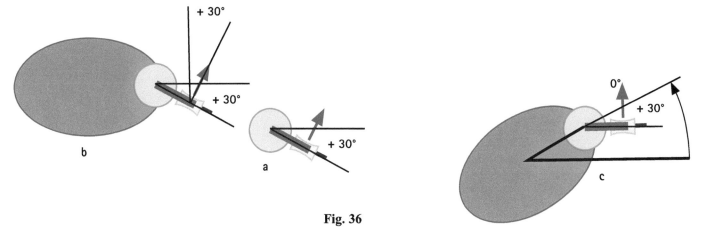

Fig. 36

The articular surfaces of flexion-extension

The main degree of freedom of the knee, that of flexion-extension occurring around a transverse axis, depends on the fact that the knee is a **hinge joint**. In fact, the articular surface of the distal end of the femur is shaped like a pulley or, more exactly, like a segment of a pulley **(Fig. 37)**, somewhat reminiscent structurally of the twin undercarriage of an aeroplane **(Fig. 38)**.

The **two femoral condyles**, *convex in both planes*, form the two cheeks of the pulley and correspond to the wheels of the undercarriage; they are continuous anteriorly **(Fig. 39)** with the two cheeks of the femoral pulley-shaped patellar surface or trochlea. The neck of the pulley corresponds anteriorly to the central groove of the trochlea and posteriorly to the intercondylar fossa, whose mechanical significance will be discussed later. Some authors describe the knee as a bicondyloid joint; this is true anatomically speaking, but mechanically it is indisputably a special type of hinge joint (see later).

The **tibial superior articular surfaces**, reciprocally modelled on those of the femur, consist of two curved and concave parallel gutters separated by the blunt intercondylar eminence running anteroposteriorly **(Fig. 40**: superomedial view in perspective). The *lateral articular surface* (LAS) and the *medial articular surface* (MAS) lie in two gutters on the surface (S) of the tibial plateau and are separated by the blunt intercondylar eminence with its *two intercondylar tubercles*. Anteriorly, the prolongation in space of this eminence corresponds to the *blunt vertical ridge on the deep surface of the patella* (P), whose two lateral borders correspond to the prolongation in space of the two concave tibial surfaces. This aggregate of surfaces has a transverse axis (I), which coincides with the intercondylar axis (II) when the joint is locked.

Thus the tibial articular surfaces correspond to those of the femoral condyles, while the tibial intercondylar tubercles lodge inside the femoral intercondylar fossa; this aggregate of articular surfaces functionally constitutes the **tibiofemoral joint**. Anteriorly, the two facets of the patellar articular surface correspond to *the cheeks of the femoral trochlea*, and the patellar vertical ridge fits into the *intercondylar fossa*. These surfaces make up the second functional joint, the **femoropatellar joint**. The femorotibial and the femoropatellar joints, though functionally distinct, are also functionally linked and are *contained within a single anatomical joint*, i.e. the knee joint.

To a first approximation, the knee joint, when *viewed only from the angle of flexion-extension*, can be represented by a pulley-shaped surface gliding on a twin set of curved and concave gutters **(Fig. 41)**. In real life, however, the situation is more complex, as will become obvious later.

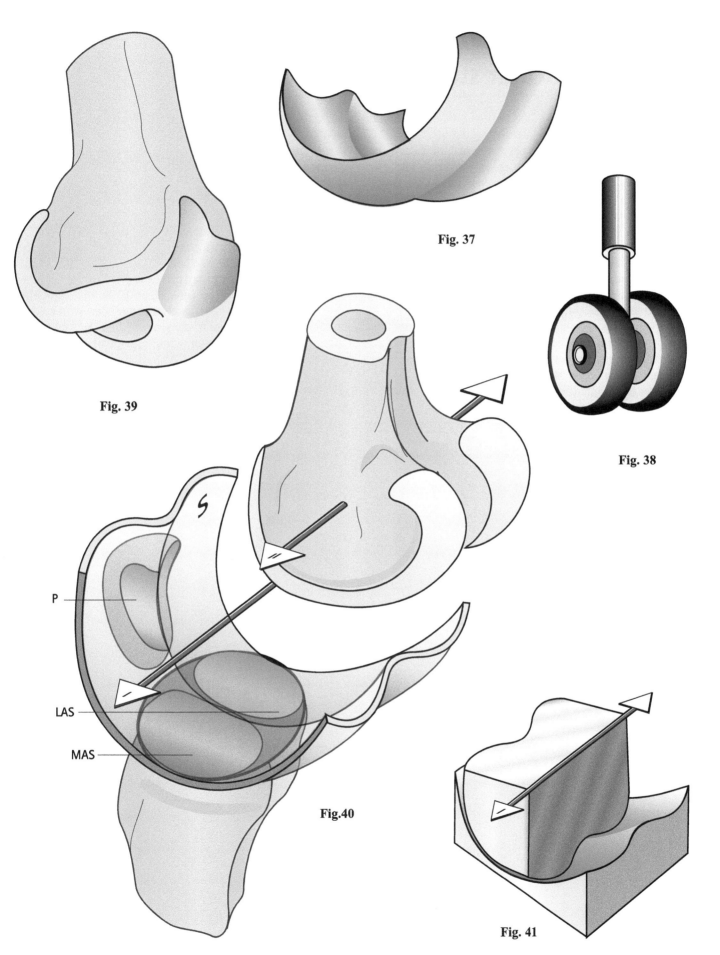

Fig. 37

Fig. 38

Fig. 39

P

LAS

MAS

S

Fig.40

Fig. 41

81

The tibial articular surfaces in relation to axial rotation

As described on the preceding page, the articular surfaces allow only one movement, i.e. flexion-extension. In fact, the blunt tibial intercondylar eminence, by lodging snugly inside the full length of the femoral patellar groove, precludes any axial rotation of the lower tibial surface on the upper femoral surface.

Hence, **for axial rotation to take place**, the tibial surface **(Fig. 42)** must be altered in such a way that its blunt central ridge is shortened and acts as a pivot. This is achieved by planing **(Fig. 43)** the two extremities of this ridge and leaving behind its middle part to act as a *pivot*, which, by lodging snugly inside the femoral patellar groove, allows the tibia to rotate around it. This pivot corresponds to the **intercondylar eminence with its two tubercles**, which border laterally the medial tibial articular surface and medially the lateral tibial articular surface. The vertical axis (R), around which occur the movements of axial rotation, passes through this central pivot, or more correctly through the medial intercondylar tubercle. Some authors give the label of central pivot to the two cruciate ligaments, which they consider to be the axis of longitudinal rotation of the knee. This terminology does not seem to be appropriate, since *conceptually*

a pivot suggests a **solid fulcrum**, which is more in-keeping with the **medial intercondylar tubercle** as the *true mechanical pivot of the knee*. As for the cruciate ligaments, the term *central link* seems more suitable.

This alteration of the articular surfaces is more easily understood with the help of a **mechanical model.**

Let us start with two structures **(Fig. 44)**, the one above containing a groove and the one below a tenon of the same size on the inside as the groove. They can *slide on each other* (arrows) but cannot turn relative to each other. If the two ends of the tenon are removed, leaving intact its central part with no diameters exceeding the width of the groove **(Fig. 45)**, we have now obtained a *cylindrical tenon* acting as a **pivot** able to fit into the groove.

Now **(Fig. 46)** these two structures can perform *two types of movement* relative to each other:

- a **sliding movement** of the central pivot along the groove (upper arrows), corresponding to flexion-extension
- a **rotational movement** of the pivot inside the groove (lower arrows), regardless of its location, corresponding to axial rotation of the leg.

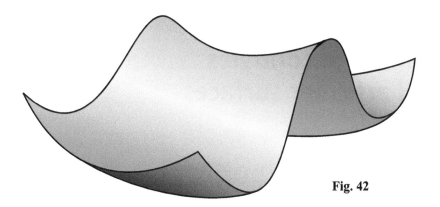

Fig. 42

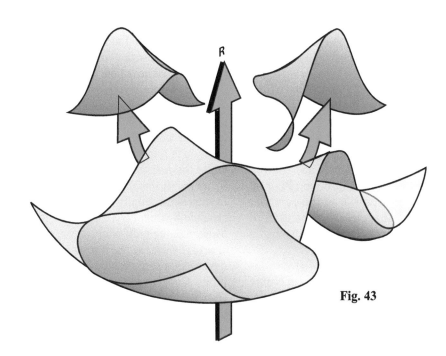

Fig. 43

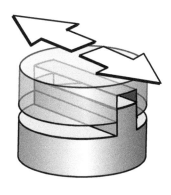

Fig. 44

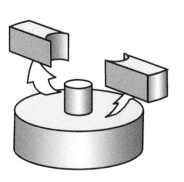

Fig. 45

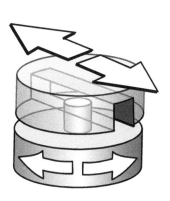

Fig. 46

Profiles of the femoral condyles and of the tibial articular surfaces

The **inferior surfaces (Fig. 47)** of the femoral condyles form two biconvex prominences longer anteroposteriorly than transversely. The condyles are not strictly identical: their long anteroposterior axes are not parallel but *divergent posteriorly.* Moreover, the medial condyle (M) juts out far more and is *narrower* than the lateral condyle (L). Between the trochlea and the condylar articular surfaces run the *medial and lateral oblique grooves* (og), the medial one being the more prominent.

The axes of the trochlear groove (**tg**) and of the intercondylar fossa (**f**) are collinear. The lateral cheek of the trochlea is more prominent than its medial cheek.

Figure 48 (**coronal section**) shows that the convexity of the condyles in the transverse plane matches the concavity of the tibial articular surfaces.

To study the *curvature of the femoral condyles and of the tibial articular surfaces in the sagittal plane*, it is convenient to study vertical sagittal sections taken at levels **aa'** and **bb'** (**Fig. 48**). These sections taken from a fresh bone (**Figs 50 and 52**, 51 and 53) provide an exact profile of the condylar and of the tibial articular surfaces. It is clear that the radii of curvature of the femoral condyles are not uniform but vary in a *spiral* fashion.

In geometry, the **spiral of Archimedes (Fig. 49)** is constructed from a point called the centre C, so that every time the radius R sweeps over an angle R' its length is correspondingly increased.

The spirals of the femoral condyles are quite different, though their radii of curvature increase regularly posteroanteriorly, i.e. from 17 to 38 mm for the medial condyle (**Fig. 50**) and 12-60 mm for the lateral condyle (**Fig. 51**), but each spiral does not have only one centre, but a series of centres, which lie on another spiral mm' for the medial condyle and nn' for the lateral condyle. Thus the curvature of each condyle represents a **spiral of a spiral**, as shown by Fick, who gave it the name of *evolute curve.*

On the other hand, starting from a point **t** on the condylar profile, the radius of curvature begins to decrease anteroposteriorly from 38 mm to 15 mm for the medial condyle (**Fig. 50**) and from 60 mm to 16 mm for the lateral condyle (**Fig. 51**).

The **anteroposterior profiles of the tibial articular surfaces (Figs 52 and 53)** differ from one another:
- The medial articular surface (**Fig. 52**) is **concave** superiorly, with its centre of curvature located above it and its radius of curvature equal to 80 mm.
- The lateral articular surface (**Fig. 53**) is **convex** superiorly with its centre of curvature O' located below it and its radius of curvature equal to 70 mm.

Whereas the medial articular surface is biconcave, the lateral articular surface is concave transversely and convex sagittally (as observed on a fresh bone). As a result, the medial femoral condyle is relatively stable on its corresponding tibial surface, while the *lateral condyle is unstable on the 'hump' presented by its corresponding tibial surface*, so that its stability during motion is essentially dependent on the intactness of the anterior cruciate ligament (ACL, **Fig. 84** p. 95).

Moreover, the radii of curvature of the condylar and of the tibial articular surfaces are not equal, leading to non-congruence of the articular surfaces: the knee is the prototype of non-congruent joints. Congruence is restored by the **menisci** (see p. 97).

Here again the centres of curvature lie on a spiral m'm" for the medial condyle and n'n" for the lateral condyle. On the whole, the lines joining these centres form two back-to-back spirals with very sharp apices (m' and n'), which correspond to the transition point between the two segments of the condylar profile:
- posterior to point t, the segment belonging to the *femorotibial joint*
- anterior to point t, the segment of the condyle and of the trochlea belonging to the *femoropatellar joint.*

The transition point t is thus the *most extreme point of the condyle* able to contact the tibial surface.

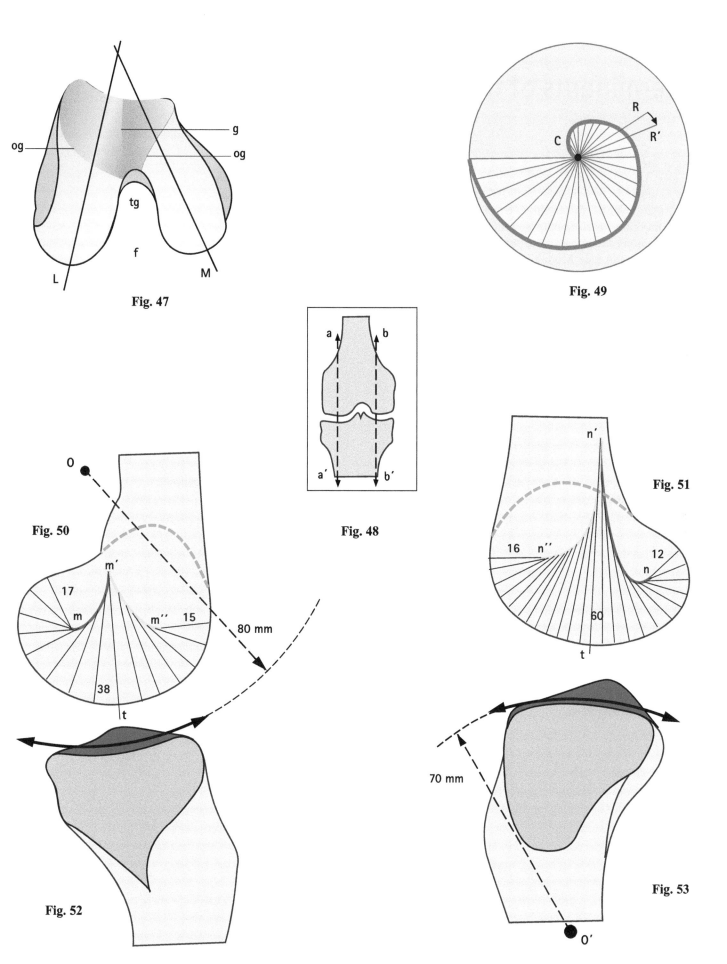

Fig. 47

og

g

og

tg

f

L

M

Fig. 49

C

R

R′

Fig. 48

a

b

a′

b′

Fig. 50

O

m′

17

m

m″

15

38

t

80 mm

Fig. 51

n′

16

n″

12

n

60

t

Fig. 52

Fig. 53

70 mm

O′

Determinants of the condylotrochlear profile

Using a **mechanical model (Fig. 54)**, I demonstrated (A.I. Kapandji, 1966) that the outlines of the femoral trochlea and condyles are geometrical surfaces determined, on the one hand, by the relationship between the cruciate ligaments and their femoral and tibial attachments, and on the other, by the relationships among the ligamentum patellae, the patella and the patellar retinacula (see Model 2 at the end of this volume). **When this model is set in motion (Fig. 55)** the *profiles of the femoral condyles and trochlea* are outlined by the **envelope** of the successive positions of the tibial articular surfaces and of the patella **(Fig. 56)**.

The posterior tibial part of the condylotrochlear profile (Fig. 57) is determined by the successive positions (1-5) of the tibial articular surfaces, 'slavishly' bound to the femur by the anterior (red) and the posterior (blue) cruciate ligaments; each ligament sweeps an arc of a circle with a centre located at its femoral insertion and radius equal to its length. Thus in extreme flexion, the femorotibial joint space gaps anteriorly owing to relaxation of the anterior cruciate ligament and stretching of the posterior ligament at the end of flexion.

The anterior patellar part of the condylotrochlear profile (Fig. 58), is determined by the successive positions (1-5 and all the intermediate positions) of the patella, which is bound to the femur by the retinacula and to the tibia by the ligamentum patellae.

Between the anterior patellar and the posterior tibial parts of the condylotrochlear profile there is a **transition point** t **(Figs 50 and 51**, p. 85) indicating the boundary between the femorotibial and femoropatellar joints.

By altering the geometrical relationships of the cruciate ligaments, it is possible to trace a family of curves for the condyles and the trochlea, and this underlies the unique 'personality' of every knee. Geometrically speaking, no two knees are alike; hence the *difficulty of producing a perfect prosthesis for a particular knee*. Prostheses can only be *more or less faithful approximations.*

The same problems arise when the cruciate ligaments are subjected to plastic operations or to **prosthetic replacements.** For example **(Fig. 59)**, if the tibial insertion of the anterior cruciate is shifted anteriorly, the circle described by its femoral insertion will also be shifted anteriorly **(Fig. 60)**, giving rise to a new condylar profile within the original profile. This will lead to some mechanical play in the joint with undue erosion of the articular cartilages.

A. Menschik of Vienna has since 1978 reproduced these findings by using a purely geometrical analysis.

This theoretical basis for the geometrical determination of the condylar trochlear profile is obviously based on the **isometry hypothesis**, i.e. the *invariance of the lengths of the cruciate ligaments*, which has not been confirmed (see below) by actual observations. Nonetheless, it explains many findings and can serve as a guide for the development of new operations on the cruciate ligaments.

More recently, Frain et al., using a mathematical model based on an anatomical study of 20 knees, have confirmed the concept of the *curve-envelope* and the *multiplicity of centres of curvature of instantaneous movements*, while emphasizing the constant functional relationships between the cruciate and collateral ligaments. The computer tracing of the velocity vectors at each point of contact between femur and tibia reproduces exactly the envelope of the condylar profile.

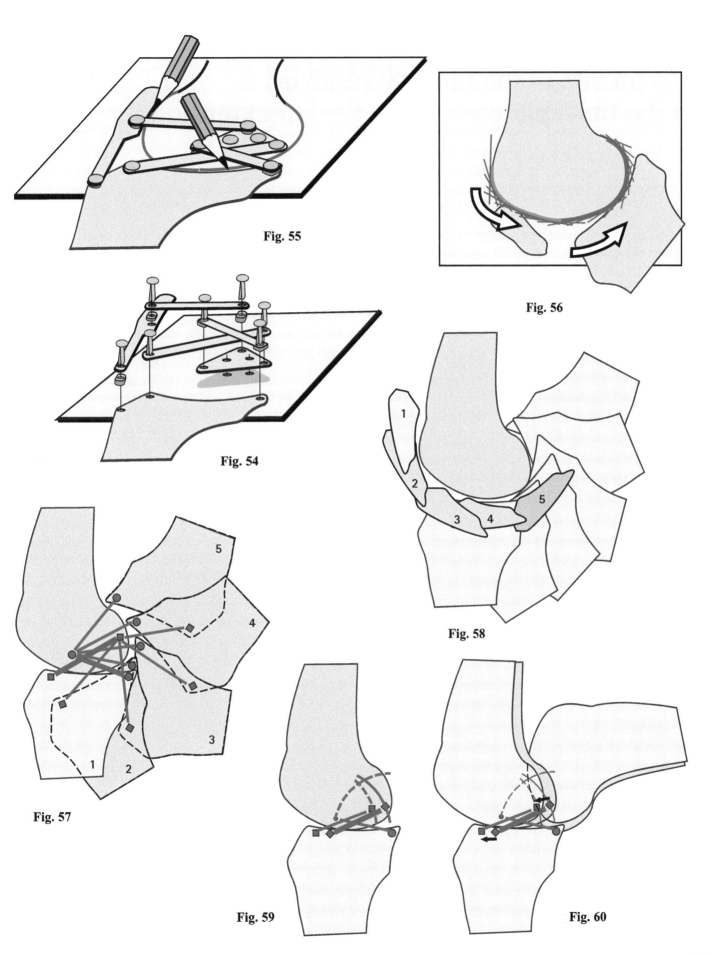

Fig. 55

Fig. 56

Fig. 54

Fig. 58

Fig. 57

Fig. 59

Fig. 60

87

Movements of the femoral condyles on the tibial plateau during flexion-extension

The rounded shape of the condyles could suggest wrongly that they roll over the tibial plateau. In fact, *when a wheel rolls on the ground without sliding* **(Fig. 61)**, each point on the ground corresponds to a single point on the wheel, so that the distance covered on the ground (OO") is exactly equal to the portion of the circumference that has rolled over the ground, i.e. the distance between the point marked by the triangle and that marked by the diamond. If the **condyle only rolled (Fig. 62)** after a certain degree of flexion (position II), it would topple over behind the tibial plateau, which is equivalent to dislocation of the joint, or else the tibial plateau would need to be longer posteriorly. The possibility of a pure rolling movement of the condyle is thus precluded by the fact that the full length of its circumference is *twice* that of the tibial surface.

If we assume that the **wheel slides without rolling (Fig. 63)**, then a single point on the ground corresponds to a whole segment of its circumference. This is what happens when the wheel of a car spins as it starts to move on ice. If **such a pure sliding movement of the condyle on the tibial plateau** were to occur **(Fig. 64)**, a single point on the tibial plateau would correspond to all the points on the condylar surface, but this occurrence would check flexion prematurely because of the impact of the condyle on the posterior margin of the tibial plateau (arrow).

It is also possible to imagine that the wheel **rolls and slides simultaneously (Fig. 65)**: it spins but still advances. Therefore, the distance covered on the ground (OO') corresponds to a greater length on the surface of the wheel (between the blue diamond and the blue triangle), which can be measured by unrolling the wheel on the ground (between blue diamond and white triangle).

In 1836 the **Weber brothers demonstrated experimentally (Fig. 66)** that this last mechanism actually operates in life. For various positions between extreme extension and extreme flexion they marked on the cartilage the corresponding points of contact between the femoral condyle and the tibial articular surface. They were able to observe, on the one hand, that the point of contact on the tibia moved backwards with flexion (black triangle for extension; black diamond for flexion), and

on the other hand that the distance between the corresponding points of contact marked on the femoral condyle was twice as great as the distance between the corresponding points of contact marked on the tibial surface. **This experiment proves indisputably that the femoral condyle rolls and slides simultaneously over the tibial plateau.** This is after all, the only way that posterior dislocation of the condyle can be avoided while permitting a greater range of flexion, i.e. 160° (compare flexion in **Figs 64 and 66**). Note that these experiments can be repeated using Model 3, printed at the end of this volume.

Later experiments (Strasser 1917) showed that the rolling to sliding ratio varied during the entire movement of flexion-extension. Starting from extreme extension the condyle begins to roll without sliding, and then sliding becomes progressively greater, so that at the end of flexion the condyle slides without rolling. Finally, the length over which pure rolling takes place varies with the condyle:

- for the medial condyle **(Fig. 67)** rolling occurs only during the first 10-15° degrees of flexion
- for the lateral condyle **(Fig. 68)** rolling continues up to 20° flexion.

Therefore, the lateral condyle rolls far more than the medial condyle, partly explaining why the distance covered by the lateral condyle over the tibial plateau is greater than that covered by the medial condyle. This important observation will be discussed later to *explain automatic rotation* (see p. 150).

It is also interesting to note that these 15-20° of initial rolling correspond to the *usual range of flexion-extension during ordinary walking.*

Frain et al. have shown that to every point along the path traced by the curved condylar profile there corresponds, on the one hand, the centre of the *osculatory circle* representing the centre of curvature of the condyle at this point and, on the other hand, the centre of the path of motion representing the point around which the femur rotates with respect to the tibia. It is only when these two circles coincide that a pure rolling movement occurs; otherwise the sliding to rolling ratio varies directly with the distance between these two centres.

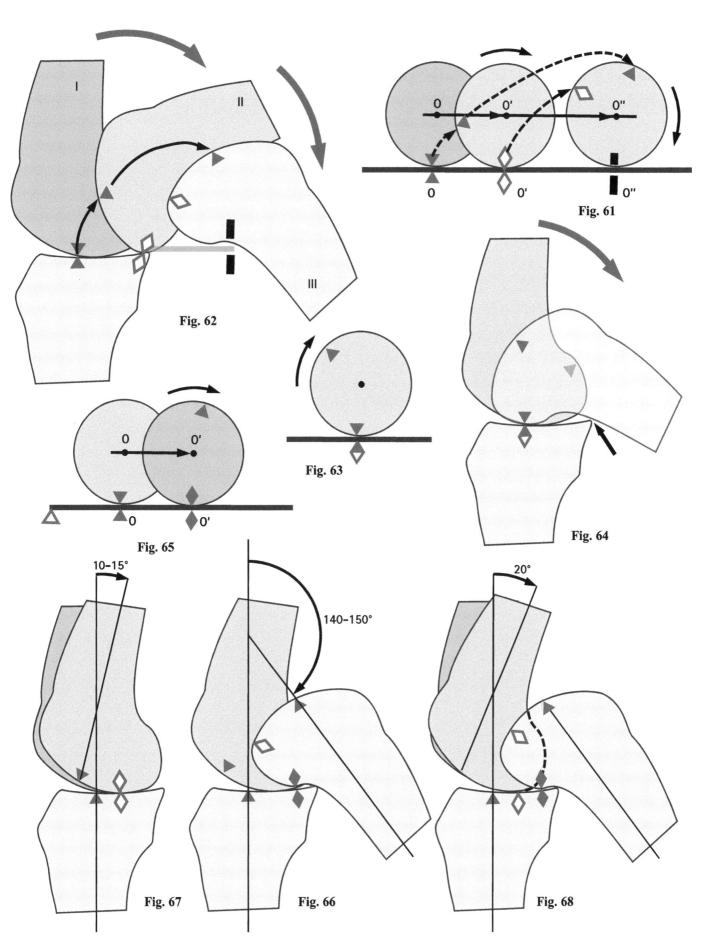

Fig. 62

Fig. 61

Fig. 63

Fig. 65

Fig. 64

Fig. 67

Fig. 66

Fig. 68

10–15°

140–150°

20°

Movements of the femoral condyles on the tibial plateau during axial rotation

It will become clear later why axial rotation can only take place when the knee is flexed. In the **neutral position for axial rotation (Fig. 69)**, with the knee half-flexed, the posterior part of each femoral condyle is in contact with the middle of each tibial articular surface. This is illustrated by the diagram (**Fig. 70**: superior view of the condyles superimposed on the tibial articular surfaces), where the transparent outlines of the condyles lie on top of the darker outlines of the tibial surfaces. The diagram also shows that during flexion the tibial intercondylar eminence moves out of the femoral intercondylar fossa, where it is confined during extension. (This is one of the reasons why axial rotation is checked when the knee is extended).

During lateral rotation of the tibia on the femur (Fig. 71) the lateral condyle moves forwards on the lateral tibial surface, while the medial condyle moves backwards on the medial tibial surface **(Fig. 72)**.

During medial rotation of the tibia on the femur (Fig. 73) the converse is true: the lateral condyle moves backwards and the medial condyle forwards on their corresponding tibial surfaces **(Fig. 74)**. In reality, the anteroposterior movements of the condyles on their corresponding tibial surfaces are not identical:

- the **medial condyle (Fig. 75)** moves relatively little inside the biconcave medial tibial articular surface (1)

- the **lateral condyle (Fig. 76)**, on the other hand, moves nearly twice as much (L) over *the convex lateral tibial surface*. As it moves anteroposteriorly it first 'climbs' up the anterior slope of the convex tibial surface to reach the top of the 'hump' and then goes down on the posterior slope. In this way the condyle changes its 'altitude': (e).

The difference in the slope of the two tibial articular surfaces is reflected in the different configuration of the intercondylar tubercles **(Fig. 77)**. A horizontal section (a) of these tubercles at level xx' shows that the lateral aspect of the lateral tubercle (1) is convex anteroposteriorly like the lateral tibial articular surface, whereas the medial surface of the medial tubercle (m) is concave like the medial tibial articular surface; furthermore, the medial tubercle is clearly higher than the lateral tubercle, as shown by a coronal section (b). Hence, the medial tubercle can act as a buffer for the impacting medial condyle, while the lateral tubercle allows the lateral condyle to move past. As a result, the **real axis of axial rotation** yy' runs not between the two intercondylar tubercles but **through the articular surface of the medial tubercle**, which is the **central pivot of the joint**. The medial shift of this axis from the joint centre is responsible for the greater excursion of the lateral condyle, as shown previously.

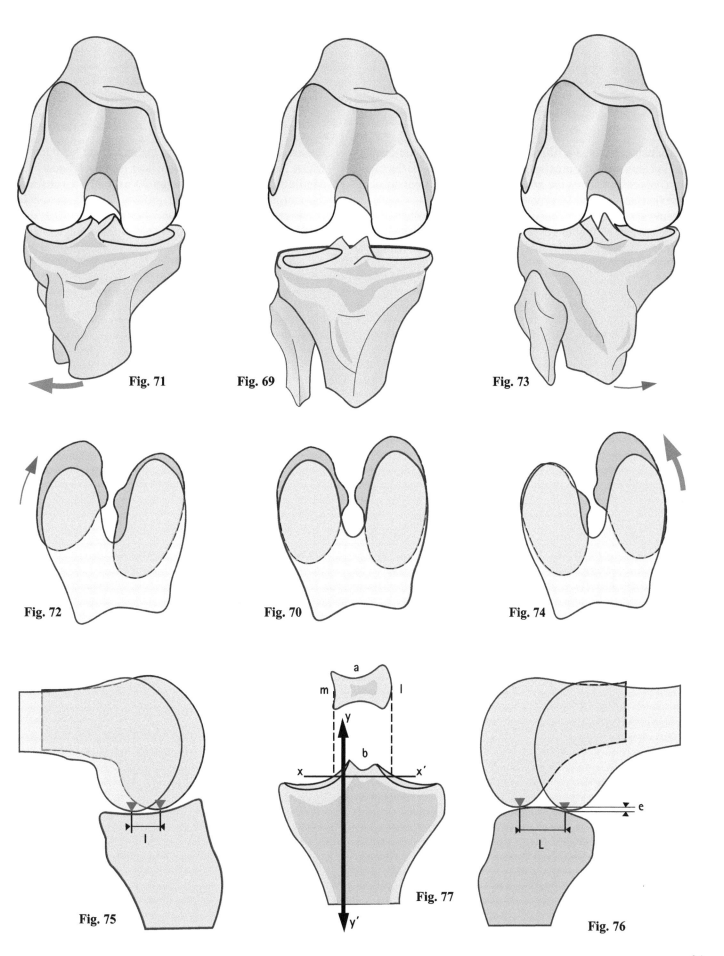

Fig. 71

Fig. 69

Fig. 73

Fig. 72

Fig. 70

Fig. 74

Fig. 75

Fig. 77

Fig. 76

The articular capsule

The articular capsule is a **fibrous sleeve** that invests the distal end of the femur and the proximal end of the tibia, keeps the two bones coapted and forms the non-bony wall of the joint space. Its deep surface is lined by synovium.

The general shape of the capsule (Fig. 78) can be easily understood by comparing it with a cylinder invaginated posteriorly by a generatrix (this movement is illustrated by the arrow), leading to the formation of a sagittal partition that incompletely divides the joint cavity into a *medial and a lateral half.* (The relationship of this partition with the cruciate ligaments will be discussed later; see p. 121.) There is also a window cut out in the anterior surface of the cylinder to receive the **patella.** The upper and lower ends of the cylinder are attached to the femur and tibia, respectively.

The **attachment of the capsule to the tibial plateau is relatively simple (Fig. 79)**. It is inserted (1: green broken line) into the anterior, lateral and medial borders of the tibial articular surfaces. Posteromedially, it blends with the tibial insertion of the posterior cruciate ligament (PCL), and posterolaterally it skirts the lateral tibial articular surface at the level of the posterior intercondylar area before joining the tibial insertion of the posterior cruciate ligament. The capsule does not extend between the two cruciate ligaments (PCL and ACL), and the *interligamentous cleft* (2) is filled by the synovial lining of the ligaments, which can therefore be considered as **thickenings of the articular capsule** in the intercondylar fossa.

The femoral insertion of the capsule is slightly more complex:
- **Anteriorly (Fig. 80**: infero-antero-lateral view of the condyles) it skirts the supratrochlear fossa (7) and forms a deep recess **(Figs 82 and 83)**, i.e. the suprapatellar bursa (5), whose importance will emerge later (see pp. 95 and 103).
- **Medially and laterally (Figs 80 and 81)** it runs along the margins of the trochlear groove, forming the parapatellar recesses (see p. 102), and then along the edges of the cartilage-coated articular surfaces of the condyles, giving rise to the *ramp-like capsular insertions of Chevrier* (8). On the lateral condyle it lies above the *intracapsular insertion of the popliteus tendon* (P), which is therefore intracapsular **(Fig. 80)**.
- **Posteriorly and superiorly (Fig. 81)** it skirts the postero-superior border of the articular surfaces of the condyles just distal to the origins of the medial and lateral heads of the gastrocnemius (G). The capsule therefore lines the deep surfaces of these muscles and separates them from the condylar articular surfaces; in this area the capsule is thickened to form the posterior **condylar plates** (6) (see pp. 114 and 120).
- In the **intercondylar fossa (Figs 82 and 83**: the femur has been cut in the sagittal plane) the capsule is attached to the opposite inner surfaces of the condyles along the articular cartilage and then to the depths of the notch, like a bridge. Its insertion into the inner surface of the medial condyle **(Fig. 82)** *blends with the femoral attachment of the posterior cruciate ligament* (4). Its insertion into the inner surface of the lateral condyle **(Fig. 83)** *blends with the femoral attachment of the anterior cruciate ligament* (3).

Here too the insertion of the cruciate ligaments blends with that of the capsule and reinforces it.

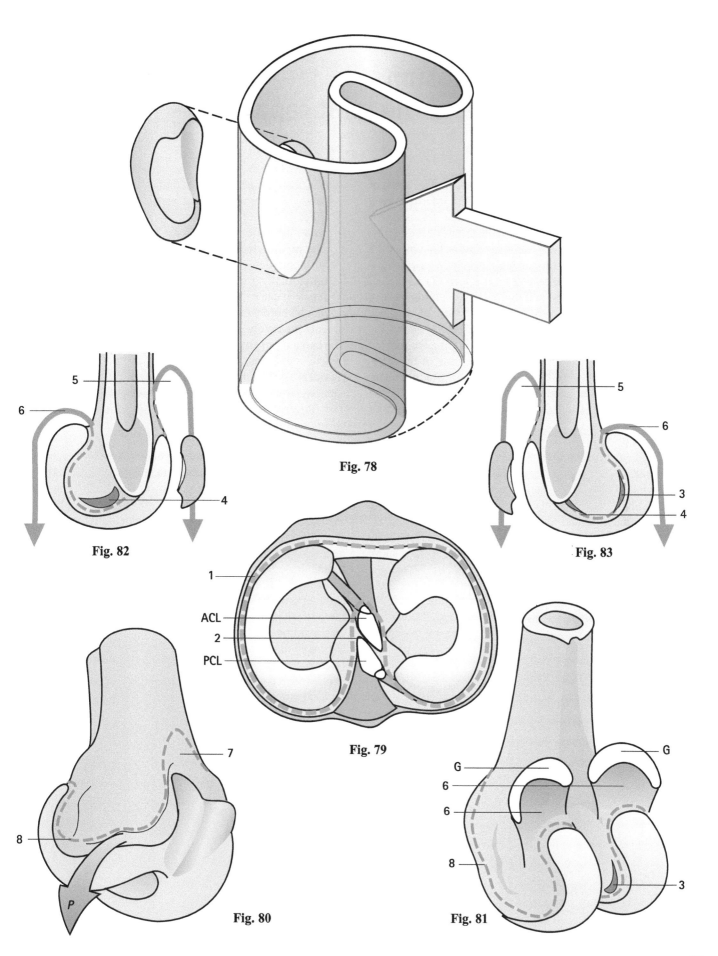

Fig. 78

Fig. 82

Fig. 83

5

6

4

5

6

3

4

Fig. 79

1

ACL

2

PCL

Fig. 80

7

8

P

Fig. 81

G

G

6

6

8

3

93

The ligamentum mucosum, the synovial plicae and the joint capacity

The *dead space*, bounded by the anterior intercondylar fossa of the tibial plateau, the patellar ligament and the inferior aspect of the patellar surface of the femur (**Fig. 84**: posteromedial view of the knee after removal of the medial half of the femur) is filled by a *sizeable piece of adipose tissue*, known as the **infrapatellar fat pad** (1). This pad has the shape of a *quadrangular pyramid*, with its base resting on the deep (2) surface of the patellar ligament (3) and spilling over the anterior part of the anterior intercondylar fossa. An anterior view of the knee opened with the patella tilted downwards (**Fig. 85**) shows the superficial surface of the fat pad (4) attached by a *fibroadipose band* stretching from the patellar apex to the back of the intercondylar fossa (**Figs 84 and 85**), i.e. the **ligamentum mucosum** (5) or the **infrapatellar plica**, which extends bilaterally as the **alar folds** (6) to insert into the lateral margins of the inferior half of the patella. This fat pad acts as a 'fill-in' for the anterior part of the joint: during flexion it is compressed by the patellar ligament and *spreads out on both sides of the patellar apex.*

The ligamentum mucosum is the *vestigial median septum*, which divides the joint into two halves until the 4th month of intrauterine life. In the adult there is normally a *gap* (**Fig. 84**) between the ligamentum mucosum and the median partition formed by the cruciates (arrow I). The lateral and medial halves of the joint communicate via this orifice and via an open space located above the ligamentum mucosum (arrow II) and behind the patella. Sometimes in the adult the median septum persists, and the two halves communicate only above the ligamentum mucosum.

The synovium includes **three plicae or folds** (**Fig. 89**: view of the medial half of the knee split sagittally), which are frequently (85% of knees according to Dupont), but not always, present. They are now well known, thanks to arthroscopy, and include the following:

- The **infrapatellar plica** or **ligamentum mucosum** (5) is an extension of the synovium lining the infrapatellar fat pad (65.5% of cases).
- The **suprapatellar plica** (6), present in 55.5% of cases, forms a partial or complete suprapatellar horizontal parti-

tion that can isolate the suprapatellar bursa from the joint cavity. The communicating bursa can pathologically fill with fluid, i.e. 'water on the knee', forming a fluid-filled swelling above the knee.

- The **mediopatellar plica** (7), seen in 24% of cases, forms an incomplete 'shelf' (in American terminology) running horizontally from the medial border of the patella to the femur. It can cause pain when its free margin rubs against the medial border of the medial condyle. Arthroscopic resection is immediately curative.

The **capacity of the joint cavity** varies under normal and pathological conditions. An intra-articular effusion of synovial fluid (**hydrarthrosis**) or of blood (**haemarthrosis**) can increase its capacity considerably, provided it accumulates progressively. The fluid collects in the *suprapatellar bursa* (Sb) and in the *parapatellar recesses* and also posteriorly in the retrocondylar bursae (Rc) deep to the condylar plates.

The distribution of the intra-articular fluid varies according to *the position of the knee*. **During extension (Fig. 87)**, the retrocondylar bursae are compressed by contraction of the gastrocnemius, and the fluid shifts anteriorly (white arrow) to collect in the suprapatellar bursa and the parapatellar recesses. **During flexion (Fig. 88)** the anterior bursae become compressed by quadriceps contraction, and the fluid is displaced posteriorly (white arrow). Between full flexion and full extension there is a **position of maximal capacity (Fig. 86)**, where intra-articular fluid pressure is *minimal.* Thus, this position of semiflexion is the one taken by patients with a knee effusion, since it is the least painful.

Normally the amount of **synovial fluid** is very small, amounting to a few cubic centimetres, but the movements of flexion-extension ensure that the *articular surfaces are constantly bathed* by fresh synovial fluid and thus assist in the *proper nutrition* of the articular cartilage and above all in the lubrication of the surfaces in contact.

Note in Figure 86 the quadriceps (Q) and the articularis genus (AG) muscle, which braces the suprapatellar bursa.

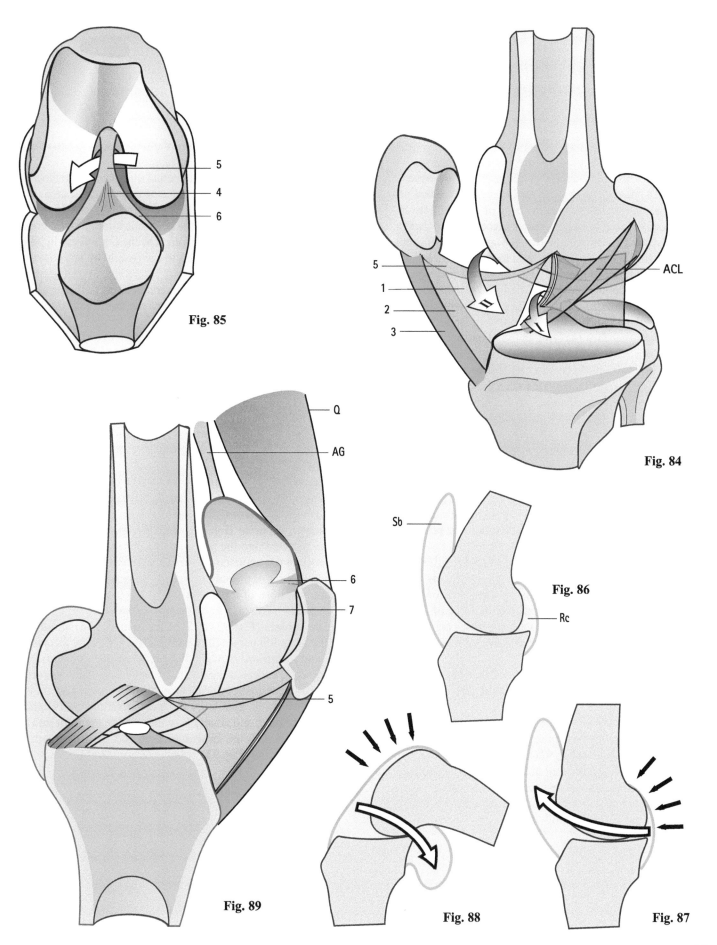

Fig. 85

Fig. 84

Fig. 86

Fig. 89

Fig. 88

Fig. 87

The inter-articular menisci

The lack of congruence of the articular surfaces (see p. 84) is offset by the interposition of **menisci or semilunar cartilages**, whose shapes are easily understood **(Fig. 90)** by the observation that when a sphere (S) is placed on a plane (P) it makes contact only tangentially. To increase the area of contact between the sphere and the plane it will suffice to place between them a ring equal in volume to that bounded by the sphere (S), the plane (P) and the cylinder (C) lying tangential to the sphere. Such a ring (3) (coloured red) has precisely the shape of a meniscus, triangular in cross-section with the following three surfaces:

- *the central or axial surface* (1) in contact with the sphere
- *the peripheral surface* (2) lying on the cylinder
- *the inferior surface* (4) lying in the plane.

A blown-up view of the menisco-ligamentous complex (Fig. 91) shows that the menisci appear to have been 'lifted' above the tibial articular surfaces with the **medial (MM) and the lateral (LM) menisci** lying in the same horizontal plane above the **medial (MAS)** and the **lateral (LAS) tibial articular surfaces**, respectively. Also visible in the diagram are their concave *superior* (1) surfaces in contact with the condyles (not shown here) and their cylindrical *peripheral surfaces* (2), attached to the deep surface of the capsule (represented by the blue colour in the background) but not their fairly flat *inferior surfaces*, which rest on the outer margins of the tibial articular surfaces and are separated by the intercondylar tubercles (3). Here, only the medial tubercle can be seen.

These rings are incomplete at the level of the **intercondylar tubercles** and are shaped therefore like two **crescents**, each with an *anterior horn* and a *posterior horn*. The horns of the lateral meniscus come closer to each other than those of the medial meniscus, so that the lateral meniscus is almost a complete circle *in the shape of an* O, whereas the medial meniscus is semilunate *in the shape of a C* **(Fig. 92)**.

These menisci are not free-floating between the two articular surfaces but have **functionally important attachments.**

- Figure 93 (**coronal section of the knee**) shows the insertion of the capsule (c) into the peripheral surfaces of the menisci, shown in cross-section (in red).
- On the tibial plateau **(Fig. 91)** the anterior and posterior horns of the menisci are secured in the anterior (6) and posterior (7) intercondylar areas respectively, as follows:
  - the anterior horn of the lateral meniscus (4) just in front of the lateral intercondylar tubercle
  - the posterior horn of the lateral meniscus (5) just behind the lateral intercondylar tubercle
  - the anterior horn of the medial meniscus (6) in the anteromedial corner of the anterior intercondylar area
  - the posterior horn of the medial meniscus (7) in the posteromedial corner of the posterior intercondylar area.
- The two anterior horns are joined by the **transverse ligament** (8), which is itself attached to the patella by strands of the infrapatellar fat pad.
- Fibrous bands run from the lateral borders of the patella (P) towards the peripheral borders of the menisci, contributing to the patellar retinacula (9).
- The medial collateral ligament (MCL) is attached by its **most posterior fibres** (2) to the central border of the medial meniscus.
- The lateral collateral ligament (LCL), on the other hand, is separated from its meniscus by the popliteus tendon (Pop), which sends a **fibrous expansion** (10) to the posterior border of the meniscus to form the so-called **posterolateral corner of the knee.** Its relevance in protecting the knee laterally will be discussed later.
- The **semimembranosus tendon** (11) also sends a fibrous expansion to the posterior border of the medial meniscus to form the **posteromedial corner of the knee.**
- Finally, separate fibres of the posterior cruciate ligament are inserted into the posterior horn of the lateral meniscus, forming the **menisco-femoral ligament** (12). There are also a few fibres of the anterior cruciate ligament inserted into the anterior horn of the medial meniscus (see **Fig. 166**, legend 5, p. 119).
- The coronal **(Fig. 93)** and the medial **(Fig. 94)** and the lateral **(Fig. 95)** parasagittal sections illustrate how the *menisci come to intrude between the condylar and tibial articular surfaces*, except at the centre of each tibial articular surface and in the region of the intercondylar tubercles; how they are attached to the patella by the patellar retinacula (9) and to the capsule c; and finally how they divide the joint into two compartments: the **suprameniscal** and the **inframeniscal** compartments **(Fig. 93)**.

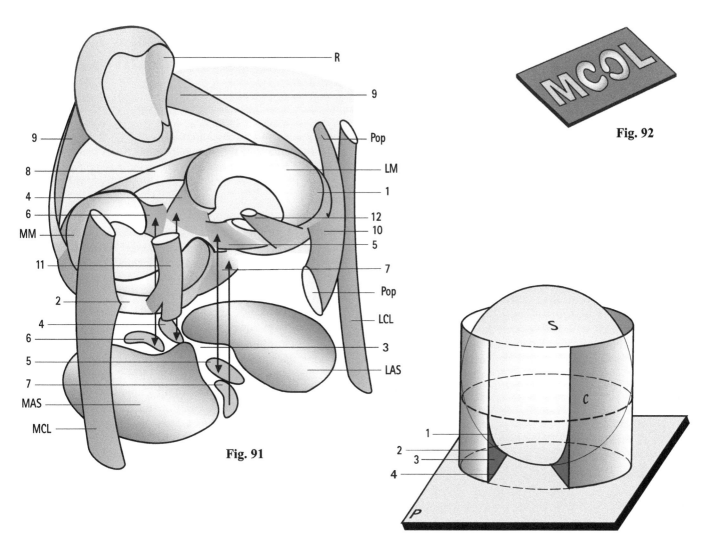

R

9

Pop

LM

1

12

10

5

7

Pop

LCL

3

LAS

9

8

4

6

MM

11

2

4

6

5

7

MAS

MCL

Fig. 91

Fig. 92

S

c

1

2

3

4

P

Fig. 90

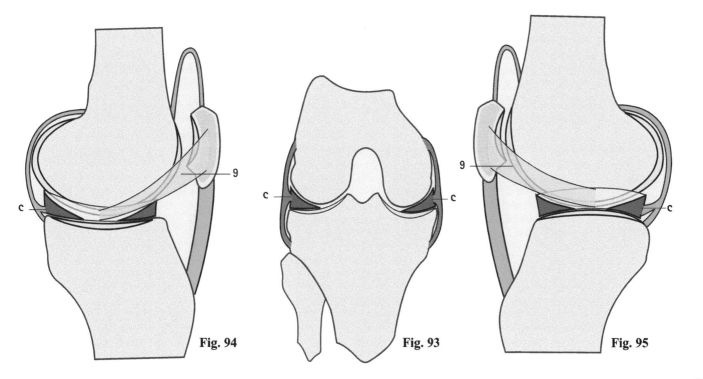

9

c

Fig. 94

c

c

Fig. 93

9

c

Fig. 95

Meniscal displacements during flexion-extension

As already shown (p. 88), the contact point between the femoral and tibial articular surfaces moves posteriorly during flexion and anteriorly during extension. The menisci follow these movements, as is easily demonstrated in an anatomical preparation containing only the ligaments and the menisci. **During extension (Fig. 96**, posteromedial view), the posterior part of each tibial articular surface becomes exposed, *especially* the lateral articular surface (LAS). **During flexion (Fig. 97**, posteromedial view) the medial (MM) and the lateral (LM) menisci come to overlie the posterior part of each tibial articular surface, especially the *lateral meniscus* as it extends down to the posterior aspect of the lateral tibial surface.

Diagrammatic representations from above of the menisci overlying the tibial articular surfaces show that starting from the position of extension **(Fig. 98)**, the menisci already in an anterior location move posteriorly unequally during flexion **(Fig. 99)**, since the lateral meniscus (LM) recedes twice as far as the medial meniscus (MM), with an excursion of 12 mm as against one of 6 mm. It is also clear from these diagrams that while they recede the **menisci become deformed** because the insertions of their horns are **two fixed points**, whereas the rest of their structure is freely mobile. The lateral meniscus undergoes a greater degree of deformation and displacement than the medial meniscus because the horns are attached closer together. The menisci undoubtedly play an important role as elastic couplings for the transmission of compressive forces between femur and tibia (black arrows, **Figs 101 and 102)**. It is worth noting that **during extension** the condyles present their greatest radii of curvature on top of the tibial articular surfaces **(Fig. 100)** and that the menisci are tightly interposed between these two articular surfaces. These two factors promote the transmission of compressive forces during full knee extension. Conversely, **during flexion**, the condyles present their shortest radii of curvature **(Fig. 103)** on top of the tibial articular surfaces, and the menisci maintain only partial contact with the condyles **(Fig. 105)**. These two factors along with slackening of the collateral ligaments (see p. 108) *favour mobility at the expense of stability*.

The mechanisms responsible for these meniscal movements fall into **two groups:** passive and active.

There is only one **passive mechanism** involved in the translational movement of the menisci: the condyles *push the menisci in front of themselves* just as a cherry stone is pushed forward between two fingers. This apparently simplistic mechanism is perfectly obvious on an anatomical preparation where all the connections of the menisci have been severed except for the *attachments of their horns* **(Figs 96 and 97)**. All the surfaces are very slippery, and the meniscal 'wedge' is *expelled* between the condylar 'wheel' and the tibial 'ground' (a very inefficient blocking mechanism).

The **active mechanisms** are numerous:

- **During extension (Figs 101 and 102)**, the menisci are pulled anteriorly by the patellar retinacula (1), which are stretched by forward movement (see p. 103) of the patella as it drags along the transverse ligament. Moreover, the posterior horn of the lateral meniscus **(Fig. 102)** is drawn anteriorly by the tension of the meniscofemoral ligament (2) (see p. 123).
- **During flexion**, the medial meniscus **(Fig. 104)** is pulled posteriorly by the *semimembranosus expansion* (3) attached to its posterior border, while the anterior horn is pulled forward by the *fibres of the anterior cruciate* attached to it (4). The lateral meniscus is pulled posteriorly **(Fig. 105)** by the *popliteal expansion* (5).

The critical role played by the menisci in the transfer of compressive forces between femur and tibia was underestimated until the first patients subjected to 'routine' meniscectomies started to develop premature osteoarthritis compared with non-meniscectomized patients. Considerable progress has followed the advent of arthroscopy. First, it allowed better evaluation of doubtful meniscal lesions seen on arthrography (the false positives), which led to 'routine' meniscectomies. (Menisci were removed to find out if they were abnormal – an illogical approach!). Second, it *led to 'tailored' meniscectomies or partial meniscectomies* with removal of only the damaged segments capable of causing mechanical embarrassment or injury to the articular cartilage. Third, it brought home the lesson that detection of a meniscal lesion is only part of the diagnosis, *since it is often a ligament problem that underlies both the meniscal and the cartilaginous lesions*.

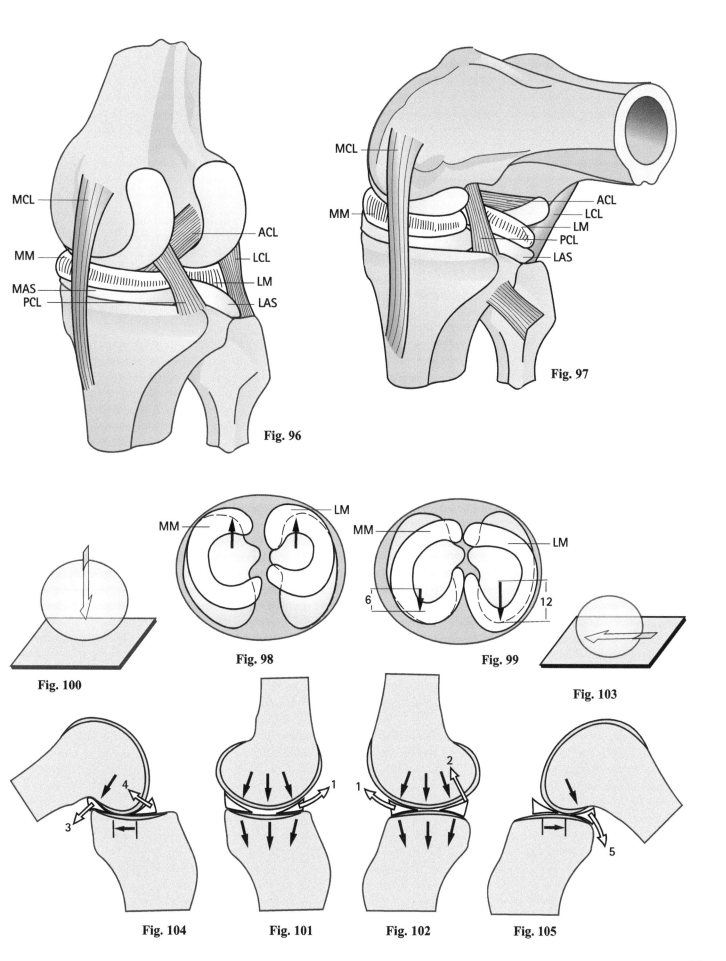

Fig. 96

Fig. 97

Fig. 98

Fig. 99

Fig. 100

Fig. 103

Fig. 104

Fig. 101

Fig. 102

Fig. 105

Meniscal displacements during axial rotation meniscal lesions

During movements of axial rotation, the menisci follow exactly the movements of the condyles on the tibial plateau (see p. 99). **In the neutral position of axial rotation (Fig. 106**: diagrammatic representation of the right tibial plateau) the lateral meniscus (Lm) and the medial meniscus (Mm) are well centred on their corresponding tibial articular surfaces. During rotation the menisci can be seen to move in opposite directions:

- During **lateral rotation (Fig. 107**: the red arrow indicates the rotation of the tibia relative to the femoral condyles) of the tibia on the femur, the lateral meniscus (Lm) is pulled (1) anteriorly on the tibial articular surface, while the medial meniscus (Mm) is pulled posteriorly (2).
- During medial rotation (**Fig. 108**: the arrow indicates the inverse rotation of the tibia), the medial meniscus (MM) advances (3), and the lateral meniscus (LM) recedes (4).

Here again, displacements of the menisci are coupled with their **deformation** around their points of fixation, i.e. the attachment sites of their horns. *The total range of displacement of the lateral meniscus is twice that of the medial meniscus.*

These displacements during axial rotation are *mostly passive* as the menisci are dragged by the condyles, but there is also an active process involved, i.e. *tension in the patellar retinacula* as the patella moves relative to the tibia (see p. 107) and pulls one of the menisci anteriorly.

During knee movements, the menisci can be damaged when they fail to follow the condylar movements on the tibial plateau: they are thus 'caught unawares' in an abnormal position and 'crushed between the anvil and the hammer'. This happens, for instance, during *violent extensions of the knee*, e.g. kicking a football, when one of the menisci does not have time to be pulled forwards **(Fig. 109)** and is *wedged between condyle and tibial articular surface* (double white arrow), more forcefully so since extension applies the tibia to the femur. This mechanism, quite common among soccer players **(Fig. 116)**, is responsible **(Fig. 114) for transverse tears** (a) and **detachments of the anterior horn** (b), which then becomes folded on itself.

The other mechanism responsible for meniscal lesions involves a twist **of the knee (Fig. 110)** due to a combination of a *valgus movement (1)* and a *lateral rotation (2):* the medial meniscus is dragged towards the joint centre below the convex surface of the medial condyle and, as the body tries to correct this twist, the meniscus is caught off guard and trapped between condyle and tibial articular surface, with three probable consequences: (a) **longitudinal fissuring of the meniscus (Fig. 111)**; (b) **total detachment of the meniscus from the capsule (Fig. 112)**; or (c) **complex fissuring of the meniscus (Fig. 113)**. In all these longitudinal lesions, the freely mobile central part of the meniscus can rear itself up into the intercondylar fossa, giving rise to the 'bucket-handle lesion' **(Fig. 111)**. This lesion is very common among soccer players when they fall on a flexed leg and among deep-pit miners **(Fig. 117)**, who have to work crouched between narrow seams of coal.

Another mechanism of meniscal injury **is secondary to rupture of a cruciate ligament**, e.g. the anterior cruciate **(Fig. 115)**. The medial condyle is no longer held back and moves forwards to crush and split the posterior horn of the medial meniscus, which is pulled off its posterior attachment to the capsule or is split horizontally (inset).

As soon as one of the menisci is torn, its damaged part fails to move normally and becomes wedged between the condyle and the tibial articular surface: the knee is then **locked** in a position of flexion, which is more marked the more posterior the meniscal lesion, and *full extension even when passive becomes impossible.*

It is worth noting that because of its avascularity, a damaged meniscus is *unable to form a scar and hence to repair itself.*

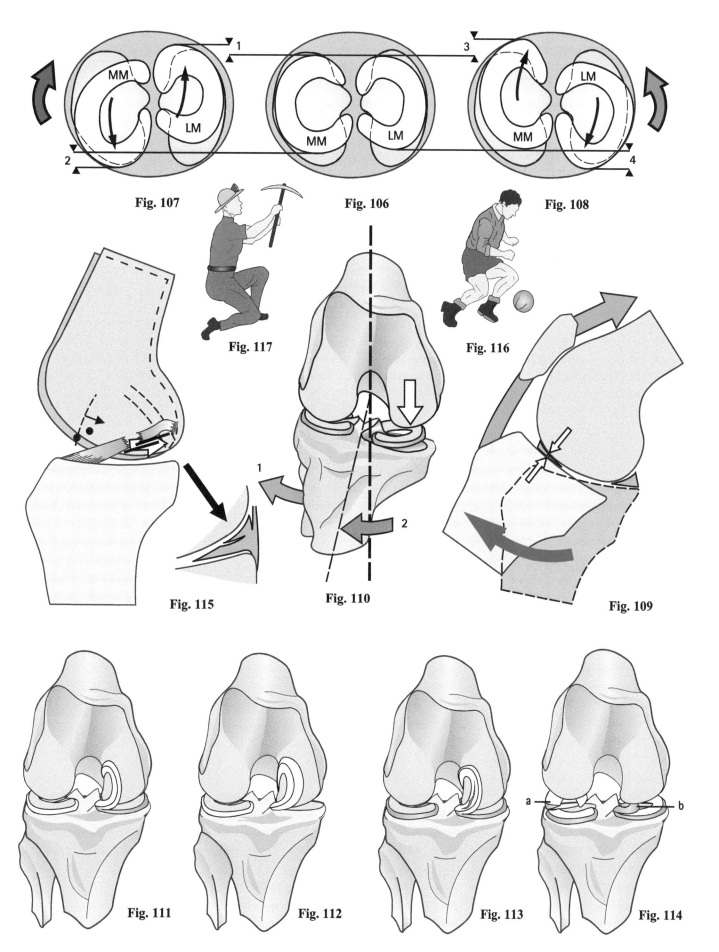

MM

LM

Fig. 107

MM LM

Fig. 106

LM

MM

Fig. 108

Fig. 117

Fig. 116

1

2

Fig. 110

Fig. 115

Fig. 109

Fig. 111

Fig. 112

Fig. 113

a

b

Fig. 114

Patellar displacements relative to the femur

The extensor apparatus of the knee slides on the distal end of the **femur like a cable on a pulley (Fig. 118a)**, except that the femoral trochlea is a fixed pulley **(Fig. 118b)**, which, along with the intercondylar fossa **(Fig. 119)**, effectively forms a deep vertical groove **(Fig. 118b)** for the patella to slide in. Thus the force of the quadriceps, directed obliquely superiorly and slightly laterally, is changed into a strictly vertical force.

The **normal movement of the patella on the femur during flexion** is therefore a vertical translation along the central groove of the femoral trochlea down to the intercondylar fossa **(Fig. 120,** based on radiographs). Thus the patellar excursion is twice that of its length (8 cm) as it rotates around a transverse axis. In effect, its posterior surface, which points directly posteriorly in extension (A), comes to face directly superiorly when, at the end of its excursion (B) in full flexion, it is pressed against the femoral condyles. Therefore the patella undergoes a **circumferential translation.**

This important translation is only possible when the patella **is bound to the femur by attachments of sufficient length.** The articular capsule forms three deep recesses around the patella **(Fig. 120)**, i.e. superiorly, the suprapatellar bursa (SPB) deep to the quadriceps, and on either side the two parapatellar recesses (PPR). When the patella slides under the condyles from A to B these three recesses become unpleated; as a result, the distance XX' can become XX" (i.e. four times as long) because of the *size of the suprapatellar bursa* and the distance YY' can become YY" (i.e. twice as long) because of *the size of the parapatellar recesses.* When inflammatory adhesions develop between the synovial layers of these recesses, they cannot elongate by unpleating, and the **patella remains stuck on the femur.** It cannot slide down its groove, since the distances XX' and YY' cannot be extended. This **capsular shortening** is one of the causes of the post-traumatic or post-infectious stiff knee in extension.

During its 'descent', the patella is *followed by the ligamentum mucosum* **(Fig. 121)**, which moves from position ZZ' to position ZZ", changing its direction by 180°. During its 'ascent' the suprapatellar bursa would become caught between the patella and the femoral trochlea were it not pulled upwards by the **articularis genus muscle (AGM)**, which is the tensor of the suprapatellar bursa and arises from the deep surface of the vastus intermedius.

Normally the patella moves only up and down and not from side to side. It is in effect very strongly applied to its groove **(Fig. 122)** by the quadriceps, the more so as the knee is flexed. At the end of extension **(Fig. 123)**, this appositional force decreases and even tends to be reversed in hyperextension **(Fig. 124)**, causing the patella to *move away from the femoral trochlea.* At this point **(Fig. 125)**, the patella tends to be *pulled laterally* because the quadriceps tendon and the patellar ligament now form an obtuse angle facing laterally. Lateral dislocation of the patella is then only prevented by the lateral cheek of the trochlea, which is distinctly more prominent **(Fig. 126)** than the medial cheek, with a difference of e. If, as part of a congenital malformation **(Fig. 127)**, the lateral cheek is underdeveloped, i.e. is as prominent as or less prominent than the medial cheek, the patella is no longer retained in full extension. This is the mechanism underlying **recurrent dislocation of the patella.**

Both lateral rotation of the tibia under the femur and genu valgum close the angle between the quadriceps tendon and the patellar ligament and thus increase the lateral vector of force that promotes *lateral instability of the patella.* These conditions set the stage for lateral dislocations and subluxations, chondromalacia patellae (softening of the patellar cartilage) and lateral femoropatellar osteoarthritis.

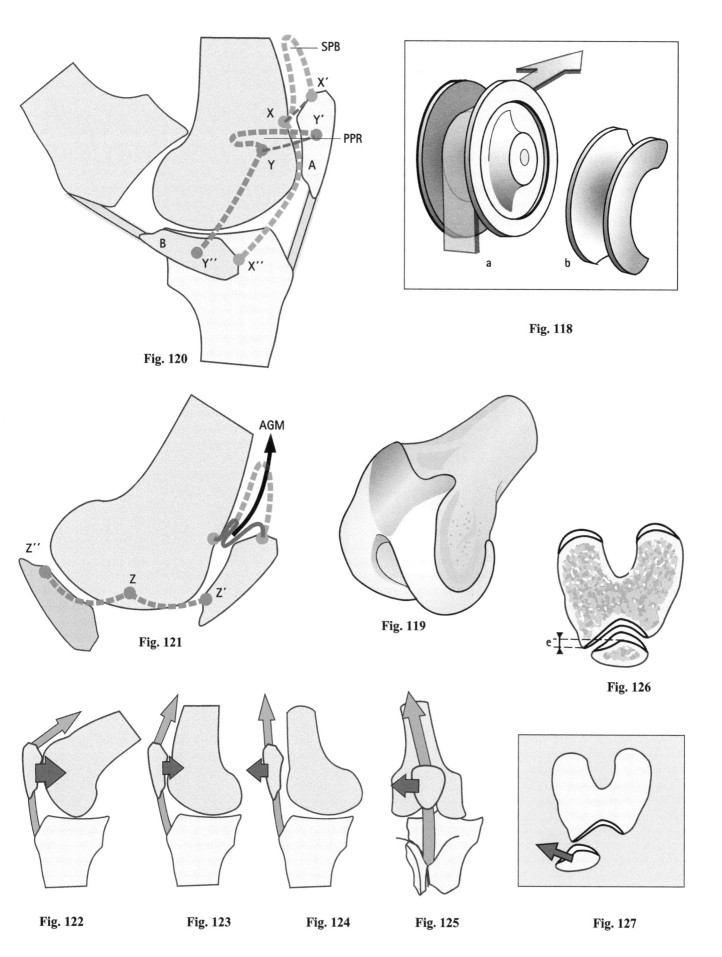

Fig. 118

Fig. 120

Fig. 121

Fig. 119

Fig. 126

Fig. 122

Fig. 123

Fig. 124

Fig. 125

Fig. 127

Femoropatellar relationships

The **posterior surface of the patella (Fig. 128**: posterior view of the right patella), particularly in its medial vertical ridge (1), is coated with **the thickest layer of cartilage** in the whole body (4-5 mm thick). This is due to the considerable pressures (300 kg) exerted on the patella by the contraction of the quadriceps when the knee is flexed, as when going downstairs or rising from the squatting position. Imagine the pressure on the patellae of weightlifters as they lift a weight of 120 kg!

The **median ridge** separates **two biconcave articular facets:**
- the **lateral** (2) articulating with the lateral cheek of the trochlea
- the **medial** (1) articulating with the medial cheek of the trochlea.

The medial facet is subdivided by an ill-defined oblique ridge into a main facet and an accessory or odd facet (4), lying at the superomedial angle of the patella and articulating with the medial edge of the intercondylar fossa *in deep flexion.*

As the patella translates vertically along the trochlea **during flexion (Fig. 129)**, it comes into contact with the trochlea on its inferior part (1) in full extension, on its middle part (2) in 30° flexion and on its superior (3) and superolateral parts in full flexion. It is then possible to determine the *critical angle of flexion* from the topography of cartilaginous lesions and conversely to predict the site of the lesions by determining the *angle of painful flexion.*

Up to now, the features of the femoropatellar joint were studied with the use of *axial* radiographs of the patella or *lateral femoropatellar radiographs* passing through the joint spaces in a row and showing the two patellae with the knee flexed successively at 30° **(Fig. 130)**, 60° **(Fig. 131)** and at 90° **(Fig. 132)** in order to visualize the full height of the joint.

From these femoropatellar radiographs the following observations can be made:
- The **centring of the patella** (especially in the radiograph taken at 30° flexion) can be assessed by the degree of contact between the patellar ridge and the trochlear groove and also by the **overhang of the lateral angle** of the patella relative to the lateral cheek of the trochlear groove. By this procedure the diagnosis of **lateral subluxation** can be made.
- **Thinning of the joint space**, especially laterally, can be evaluated using calipers and comparing it with that of the normal knee. Cartilage erosion can thus be detected in already advanced osteoarthritis.
- **Subchondral eburnation (bone sclerosis)** in the lateral facet of the patella indicating the presence of severe overloading.
- **Lateral displacement of the tibial tuberosity**, relative to the trochlear groove, can only be seen in radiographs taken at 30° and 60° knee flexion and indicates *lateral rotation* of the tibia under the femur associated with subluxations and severe lateral overloading.

Nowadays, with the CT scan and MRI the femoropatellar joint can be viewed with the knee fully extended or even hyperextended, which was impossible to do radiographically. These scans demonstrate lateral subluxation of the patella in positions where the appositional force is nil or even negative, and thus allow the detection of **minor degrees of femoropatellar instability.**

Arthroscopy, now an essential investigative procedure, detects *cartilaginous lesions* in the femur and the patella undetectable on axial radiography as well as *dynamic imbalances* in the joint.

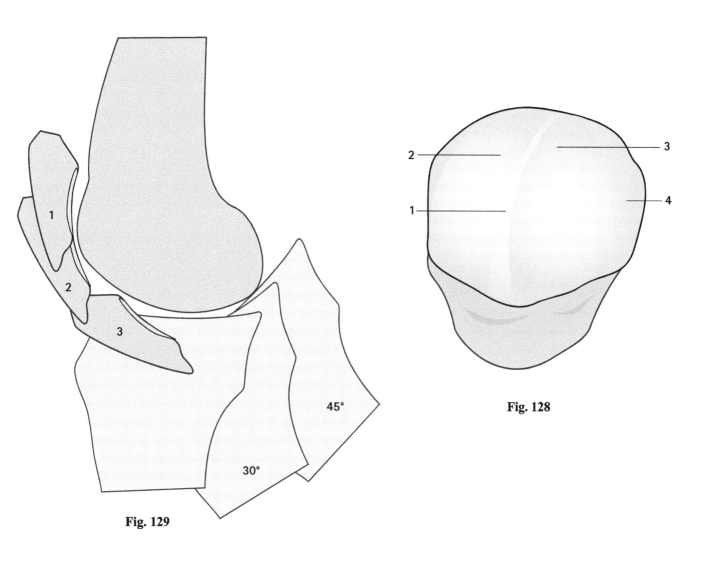

Fig. 128

Fig. 129

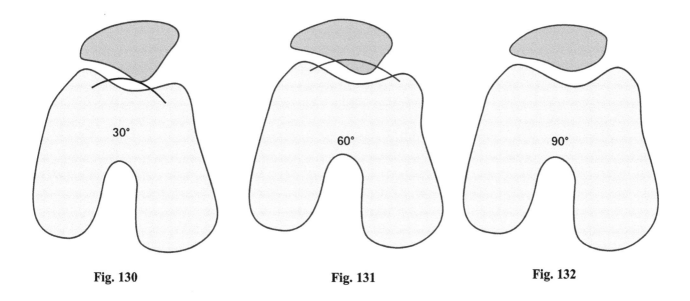

Fig. 130

Fig. 131

Fig. 132

Patellar movements relative to the tibia

One could imagine the patella welded to the tibia like an **olecranon process (Fig. 133)** at the elbow. This arrangement would prevent all patellar movements relative to the tibia and would notably curtail its mobility and even preclude any axial rotation. In fact, there are **two types of patellar movements relative to the tibia**, one type during flexion-extension and the other during axial rotation.

During flexion-extension (Fig. 134), the patella *moves in a sagittal plane.* Starting **from its position in extension A**, it recedes along the arc of a circle with its *centre at the tibial tuberosity* O and its *radius equal to the length of the patellar ligament.* During this movement, it has tilted on itself by an angle of about 35°, so that its posterior surface, which faced posteriorly initially, now looks posteriorly and inferiorly in **extreme flexion (B).** Thus it has also undergone *axial rotation* or *circumferential translation* with respect to the tibia. This posterior movement of the patella is the result of the following two mechanisms:

- posterior displacement D of the point of contact between the condyles and the tibial plateau
- shortening by r of the distance R between the patella and the axis of flexion-extension (+).

During movements of axial rotation (Figs 135-137) the patellar displacements relative to the tibia occur *in a coronal plane.* In the **neutral position of rotation (Fig. 135)** the patellar ligament runs a slightly oblique course inferiorly and laterally. During **medial rotation (Fig. 136)**, the femur is laterally rotated with respect to the tibia (assumed to be fixed for demonstration purposes), drags the patella *laterally*, while the patellar ligament now runs *obliquely inferiorly and medially.* **During lateral rotation (Fig. 137)**, the opposite movements take place: the femur *drags the patella medially* and the patellar ligament now runs *inferiorly and laterally* with a greater obliquity than in the neutral position.

Patellar displacements relative to the tibia are therefore indispensable for movements of both flexion-extension and axial rotation.

We have demonstrated using a mechanical model (see Model 2 at the end of the volume) that the patella is responsible for moulding the shape of the femoral trochlea and the anterior aspects of the condyles. During its movements, the patella is in effect *attached to the tibia by the patellar ligament and to the femur by the patellar retinacula* (see next page). During knee flexion the condyles move on the tibial plateau, and the posterior patellar surface is dragged by its ligamentous attachments along a surface geometrically equivalent to the anterior profiles of the condyles, which correspond to the curve encompassing the successive positions of the posterior patellar surface. These profiles are moulded essentially by the mechanical attachments of the patella and their disposition, just as the posterior profiles of these condyles are shaped by the cruciate ligament.

We have seen (p. 86) how the condylotrochlear profile is moulded by the tibia and the patella, which are attached to the femur by the cruciate ligaments and by the patellar ligament and retinacula, respectively.

Certain operations *transferring the tibial tuberosity anteriorly* (Maquet) or *medially* (Elmslie) alter the relationships between patella and femoral trochlea, in particular the force vector promoting articular coaptation and that promoting lateral subluxation. Hence their potential value in the treatment of patellar syndromes.

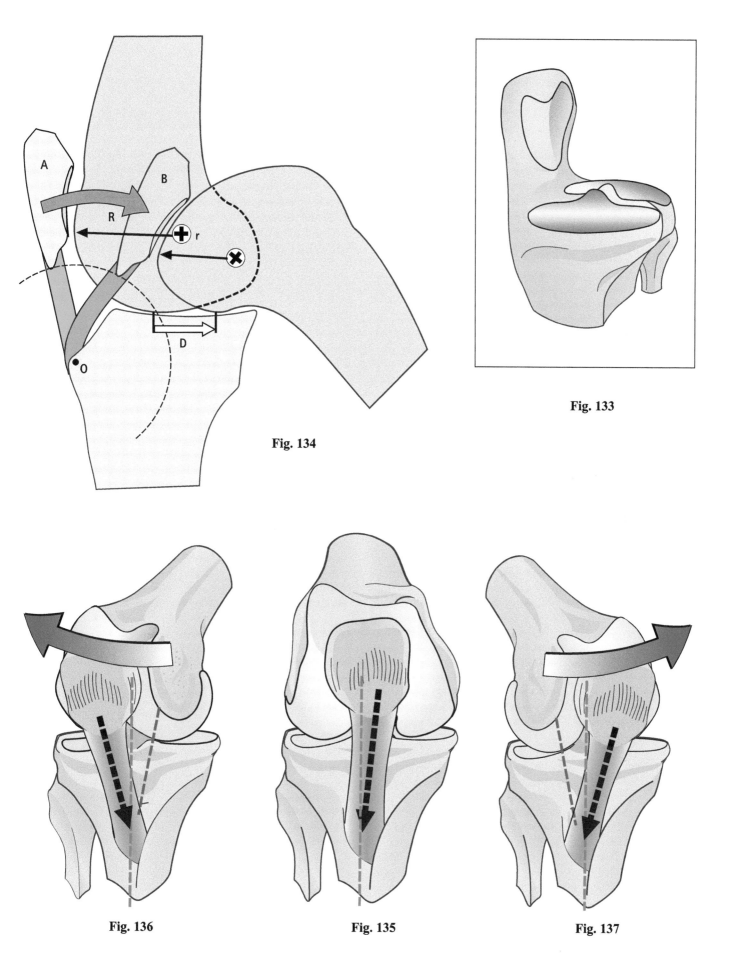

Fig. 133

Fig. 134

Fig. 136

Fig. 135

Fig. 137

The collateral ligaments of the knee

Knee joint stability depends on two sets of powerful ligaments, i.e. the cruciates and the collateral ligaments.

The collateral ligaments reinforce the articular capsule *medially and laterally* and secure the **transverse stability of the joint during extension.**

The **medial collateral ligament (Fig. 138)** runs from the subcutaneous aspect of the medial condyle to the upper end of the tibia (MCL):

- Its femoral insertion lies on the posterosuperior aspect of the medial condyle, posterior and superior to the line joining the centres of curvature (XX') of the condyle (see p. 85).
- Its tibial insertion lies posterior to the insertions of the anserine muscles (see p. 113) on the medial surface of the tibia.
- It runs an oblique course inferiorly and anteriorly, i.e. in a direction that intersects in space that of the lateral collateral ligament (arrow A).

The **lateral collateral ligament (Fig. 139)** stretches from the lateral surface of the lateral condyle to the head of the fibula (LCL):

- Its *femoral insertion* lies *superior and anterior* to the line joining the centres of curvature yy' of the lateral condyle (see p. 85).
- Its *fibular insertion* lies anterior to the fibular styloid process deep to the insertion of the biceps femoris.
- It is *distinct from the capsule* along its entire course.
- It is separated from the lateral surface of the lateral meniscus by the popliteus tendon, which contributes to the formation of the posterolateral corner (see **Fig. 267**, p. 155).
- It runs *obliquely inferiorly and posteriorly*, i.e. in a direction that *intersects in space that of the medial collateral ligament* (arrow B).

Both diagrams **(Figs 138 and 139)** show the **meniscopatellar ligaments** (1 and 2) and the **patellar retinacula** (3 and 4), which keep the patella pressed against the femoral trochlea. The collateral ligaments are **stretched during extension (Figs 140 and 142)** and **slackened during flexion (Figs 141 and 143).** Figures 140 and 141 show the difference (d) in the length of the medial collateral ligament when the knee is extended or flexed, as well as the slight increase in the obliquity of its course posteriorly and inferiorly. Figures 142 and 143 show the difference in length (e) of the lateral collateral ligament and its change in direction from oblique inferiorly and posteriorly to more vertical.

The change in tension of these ligaments can easily be explained by a **wedge mechanism** and illustrated by a mechanical model **(Fig. 144)**. A wedge C slides from **position 1 to position 2** on a board B, and it fits into a strap (ab) attached to the board B at a. When the wedge C slides from 1 to 2, the strap (taken to be *elastic*) is stretched to a new length of ab', and the difference in length **e** corresponds to the difference in thickness of the wedge between points 1 and 2 and represents the *degree of stretching* of the strap, i.e. of the ligaments.

In the knee, as extension proceeds, each femoral condyle slides like a wedge between the tibial plateau and the condylar attachment of its corresponding collateral ligament: the condyle behaves like a wedge because its *radius of curvature increases regularly posteriorly and anteriorly*, while the collateral ligaments are attached to the concavity of the line joining the centres of curvature of the condyles. Flexion at 30° relaxes the collateral ligaments and is the position of immobilization following surgical repair of these ligaments.

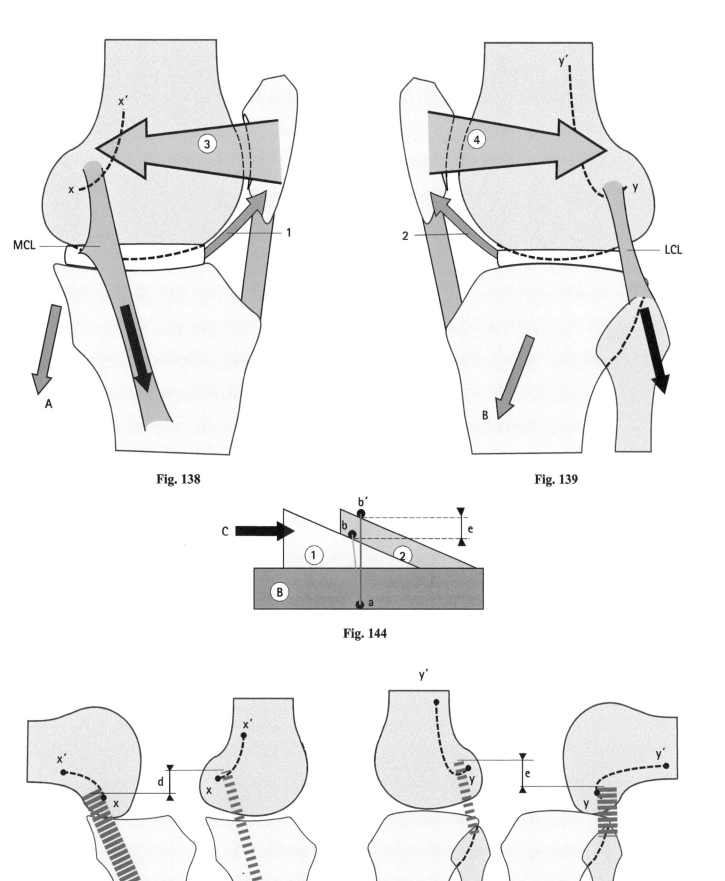

Fig. 138

MCL

1

Fig. 139

2

LCL

Fig. 144

Fig. 141   **Fig. 140**   **Fig. 142**   **Fig. 143**

Transverse stability of the knee

The knee is subjected to considerable varus and valgus mechanical stresses, which are reflected in the **trabecular structure of the bony extremities** (**Fig. 145**, coronal section of the knee). As in the upper end of the femur, **various bony trabecular systems** correspond to *these lines of force:*

- The **distal end of the femur** contains two *sets of trabeculae.* The first set runs from the medial cortex and fans out into the ipsilateral condyle, as the compression-resisting trabeculae, and into the contralateral condyle as the traction-resisting trabeculae. The second set runs from the lateral cortex and fans out in a symmetrically similar fashion to the first set. *Horizontal trabeculae* also unite the condyles.
- The **proximal end of the tibia** has a similar trabecular structure with two *oblique systems* starting from its lateral and medial cortices and fanning out, respectively below the ipsilateral tibial articular surface as compression-resisting trabeculae and the contralateral articular surface as traction-resisting trabeculae. The articular surfaces are joined by horizontal trabeculae.

The physiological valgus (**Fig. 146**: the knee viewed from in front) corresponds to the inclination of the femoral axis as it runs inferiorly and medially. The force (F) applied to the upper end of the tibia by the femur is not strictly vertical and can be resolved into a *vertical component* v and a *transverse component* t, which acts horizontally and medially. By pulling the joint medially, this transverse component t *tends to exaggerate the valgus* and to cause the *joint space to gap medially by an angle of* a. **Such a dislocation is normally prevented by the medial ligamentous system.**

The angle of valgus is critical for the **transverse stability of the knee.** The strength of the transverse component t is directly proportional to the angle of valgus (**Fig. 147**: diagrammatic decomposition of forces according to the angle of valgus) as follows:

- The physiological angle of valgus is 170° (blue lines) and corresponds to a transverse component t1.
- If the valgus becomes pathological (e.g. angle = 160°), the direction of the force F2 produces a transverse component t2 twice that associated with the physiological valgus (angle = 170°). Hence, the more marked the pathological genu valgum, the *more it stretches the medial ligaments and the greater its tendency to increase in severity.*

Traumatic injuries involving the medial and lateral aspects of the knee will cause fractures of the proximal end of the tibia. If the traumatic injury involves the **medial aspect of the knee (Fig. 148)**, it tends to straighten the physiological valgus and produces first an **avulsion fracture of the medial tibial plateau** (1) and then, if the disruptive force is still unspent, a **rupture of the lateral collateral ligament** (2). If the ligament snaps at the outset, there is no fracture of the tibial plateau.

When the traumatic injury involves the **lateral aspect of the knee (Fig. 149)**, e.g. in the car bumper injury, the *lateral femoral condyle is displaced slightly medially* and then *sinks into the lateral tibial plateau* and eventually shatters its lateral cortex. This combination produces a **mixed type of fracture** or the **impaction (i)-dislocation (d) fracture** of the lateral part of the tibial plateau.

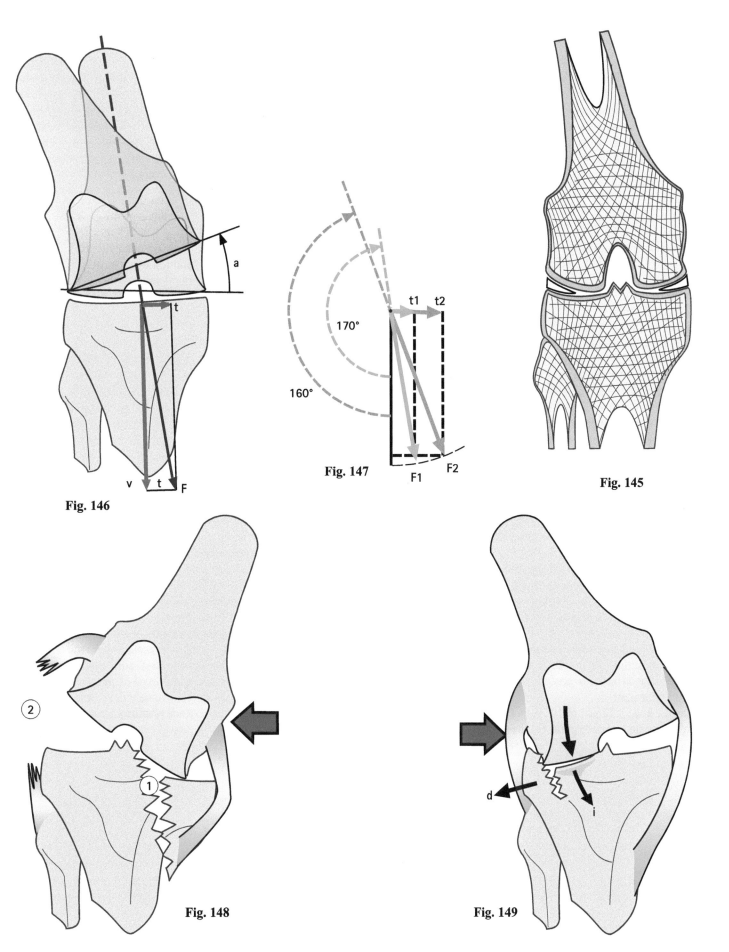

Fig. 146

Fig. 147

Fig. 145

Fig. 148

Fig. 149

111

Transverse stability of the knee (*continued*)

During walking and running the knee is continuously subjected to transverse stresses. In some postures the body is in a **state of medial imbalance relative to the supporting knee**, increasing the physiological valgus and opening out the joint space medially. If the transverse force is too strong, the medial collateral ligament will snap **(Fig. 151)**, leading to a **severe* sprain of the medial collateral ligament** associated with gapping of the joint space (a) medially. This statement should be qualified by stressing that a severe sprain is never the result of a simple state of imbalance but requires also a **violent blow to the knee.**

Conversely, when the body is in a **state of lateral imbalance relative to the supporting knee (Fig. 152)**, the physiological valgus is decreased. If a violent force is applied to the medial aspect of the knee, the lateral collateral ligament can be torn as a result **(Fig. 153)**, producing the **severe sprain of the lateral collateral ligament** associated with lateral gapping of the joint space (b).

When the knee is severely sprained, **valgus or varus movements** can be shown to occur around an anteroposterior axis. For their detection, the knee must be kept completely extended or slightly flexed, and they must be *compared with those occurring in the other knee, considered to be normal.*

When the **knee is extended (Fig. 155)** or even hyper-extended, since the sheer weight of the thigh tends to cause hyperextension, moving the knee from side to side with both hands will reveal the following:

- a **movement laterally** in the **valgus** direction. This indicates **combined rupture of the medial collateral ligament (Fig. 151)** and of the fibroligamentous structures lying posteriorly, i.e. the medial condylar plate and the posteromedial corner
- a **movement medially** in the **varus** direction. This indicates rupture of the lateral collateral ligament and of the fibroligamentous structures posteriorly, i.e. essentially the lateral condylar plate.

When the knee is **flexed at 10° (Fig. 156)**, valgus or varus movements indicate isolated rupture of the medial collateral ligament (MCL) or of the lateral collateral ligament (LCL), since the condylar plates are slackened in very early flexion. It is impossible to be certain in what position a radiograph was taken, and so one cannot rely diagnostically on the presence of a gapping joint space medially in a forced valgus position or laterally in a forced varus position.

In reality, it is very difficult to obtain adequate muscular relaxation for a meaningful examination of a painful knee and it is imperative to do so under general anaesthesia.

A severe sprain of the knee impairs the stability of the joint. In fact, when one collateral ligament is torn, the knee cannot resist the transverse stresses to which it is continually subjected **(Figs 151 and 153)**.

When violent transverse stresses are applied during running and walking, the collateral ligaments are not the only structures able to stabilize the knee; they are assisted by the muscles, which constitute veritable **active articular ligaments** and thus play a vital role in securing the stability of the knee **(Fig. 154)**.

The *lateral collateral ligament* (LCL) is strongly assisted by the *iliotibial tract* (1), which is tightened by the tensor fasciae latae, as shown in Figure 152.

The *medial collateral ligament* (MCL) is likewise assisted by the **anserine muscles**, i.e. the sartorius (2), the semitendinosus (3) and the gracilis (4). The contracting sartorius is shown in **Fig. 150**.

The collateral ligaments are therefore reinforced by thick tendons. They are also assisted powerfully by the **quadriceps** with its *straight (S) and its cruciate (C) expansions* forming a **predominantly fibrous canopy** for the anterior aspect of the joint. The straight fibres prevent ipsilateral gapping of the joint space, while the cruciate fibres prevent its contralateral gapping. Therefore each vastus muscle, by virtue of its two types of expansions, influences knee stability both medially and laterally. This highlights the *significance of an intact quadriceps* in ensuring knee stability and conversely the deleterious effects of an atrophic quadriceps on knee posture at rest, e.g. '**the knee that gives way**'.

---

* Severe means rupture of the ligament, whereas in a simple sprain the ligament is overstretched.

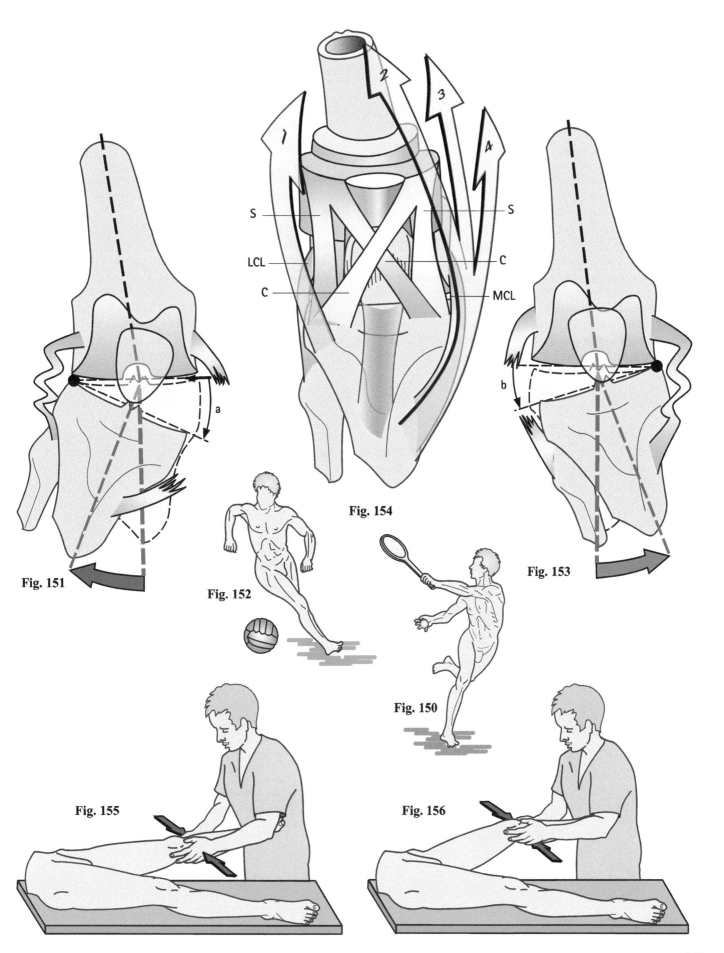

Fig. 151

Fig. 152

Fig. 150

Fig. 154

Fig. 153

Fig. 155

Fig. 156

S

LCL

C

S

C

MCL

a

b

1

2

3

4

Anteroposterior stability of the knee

The mechanism of knee stabilization is completely different depending on whether it is very slightly flexed or hyperextended. **When the knee is straight and very slightly flexed (Fig. 157)**, the force exerted by the body weight passes posterior to the flexion-extension axis of the knee and tends to flex the knee further unless prevented by isometric contraction of the quadriceps (red arrow). Therefore *in this position the quadriceps are essential to maintain the erect posture.*

Conversely, as the knee is **hyperextended (Fig. 158)**, the natural tendency for this hyperextension to increase is soon checked by the capsular and other ligaments acting posteriorly (in green); the erect posture can thus be maintained *without the quadriceps*, i.e. in the **locked position**. This explains why, when the *quadriceps is paralysed*, the patient exaggerates a genu recurvatum to be able to stand and even to walk.

With the knee hyperextended (Fig. 159) the axis of the thigh runs an oblique course inferiorly and posteriorly, and the active force f can be resolved into a vertical vector v transmitting the body weight to the leg and a *horizontal vector h*, which is directed *posteriorly* and so tends to *exaggerate the hyperextension*. The more oblique posteriorly is the direction of the force, the greater is the vector h and the more strongly recruited are the posterior fibrous layers of the knee. Therefore a genu recurvatum, if too severe, will eventually overstretch the ligaments and *increase its own severity.*

Although knee hyperextension is not checked by bony impact, as with the olecranon at the elbow, it is still **very efficiently checked**, as illustrated by this acrobatic figure **(Fig. 160)**, where *the full weight of the female partner tends to dislocate her left knee*, but without success.

Knee hyperextension is checked mostly by the **capsule and its related ligaments** and also secondarily by **muscle action**. The ligaments involved include the collateral ligaments (7-8) and the posterior cruciate ligament (9) **(Fig. 162)**.

The **posterior aspect of the articular capsule (Fig. 161)** is reinforced by powerful fibrous bands. On either side, opposite the condyles the capsule is thickened to form the **condylar plates** (1), which give attachment to the gastrocnemius on their posterior surfaces. **Laterally**, a fan-shaped fibrous ligament radiates from the fibular styloid process, i.e. the **arcuate ligament of the knee** with its *two bundles*:

- the *lateral bundle* or the short lateral ligament of Valois, whose fibres terminate on the lateral condylar plate (3) and the sesamoid bone or *fabella* (3) located in the tendon of the lateral head of the gastrocnemius
- the *medial bundle* (2) runs medially, and its lowest fibres form the **arcuate popliteal ligament** (4), which straddles the *popliteus tendon* (red arrow) entering the joint and thus forms the superior margin of the point of entrance of the tendon on its way through the capsule.

Medially, the fibrous capsule is strengthened by the **oblique popliteal ligament** (5), which is formed by the recurrent fibres emanating from the lateral border of the semimembranosus tendon (6) and runs superiorly and laterally to be inserted *into the lateral condylar plate and the fabella*, when present.

All these fibroligamentous structures on the posterior aspect of the joint are stretched during hyperextension **(Fig. 162)**, especially the **condylar plates.** We have already seen that the lateral collateral ligament (7) and the medial collateral ligament (8, seen as transparent) are stretched during extension. The posterior cruciate ligament (9) is also stretched during extension. It is easy to observe that the *upper attachments* of these ligaments A, B and C rotate anteriorly around a centre O during hyperextension. Recent studies, however, have shown that the **anterior cruciate ligament** (not shown here) is the most stretched ligament in this position.

Finally the flexor muscles **(Fig. 163)** are the active checks of extension, i.e. the **anserine muscles** (gracilis 10, semitendinosus 13 and semimembranosus 14), which course behind the medial condyle, and the biceps femoris (11) as well as the gastrocnemius (12), also called the triceps surae, provided it is already stretched by ankle joint flexion.

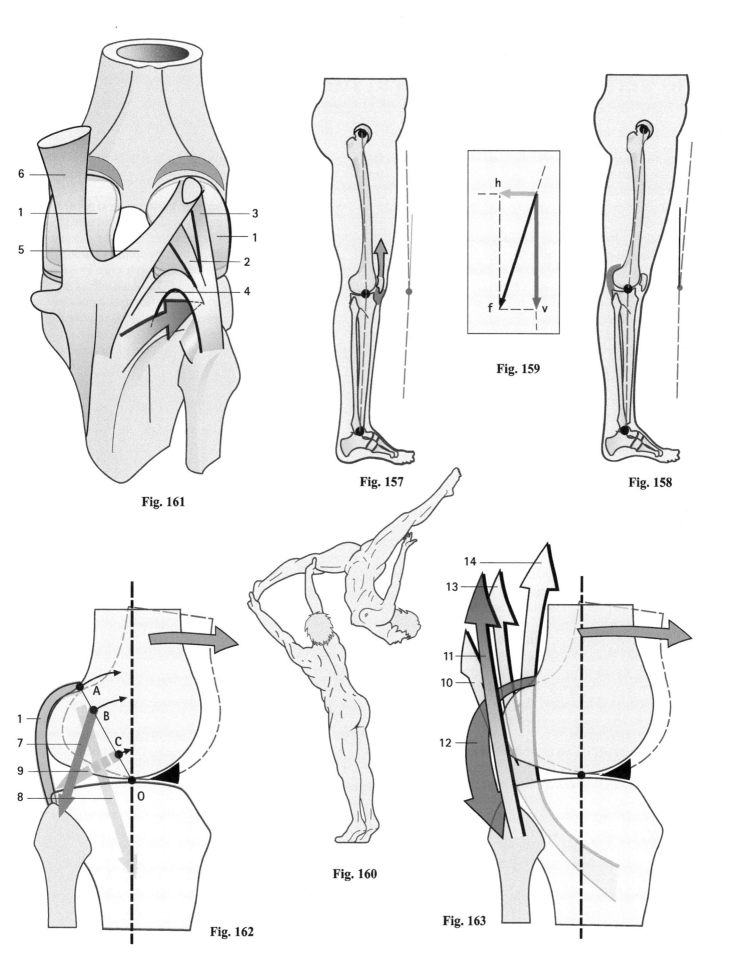

Fig. 161

Fig. 157

Fig. 159

Fig. 158

Fig. 160

Fig. 162

Fig. 163

The peri-articular defence system of the knee

The capsule and its various related ligaments constitute an integrated and coherent system, i.e. the peri-articular defence system of the knee **(Fig. 164)**.

This transverse section of the knee through the joint space shows the following:

- the capsular insertion (1 green dashed line)
- medially, the **medial tibial articular surface** (2) with the medial intercondylar tubercle (3), the **anterior horn** (4) and the **posterior horn** (5) of the **medial meniscus**
- laterally, the **lateral tibial articular surface** (6) with the lateral intercondylar tubercle (7) and the **lateral meniscus** (8 and 9) united to the medial meniscus by the **transverse ligament** (10)
- anteriorly, the **patella** (11), overhanging the anterior tibial tuberosity (12) and attached to the menisci by the **medial** (13) **and lateral** (14) **menisco-patellar ligaments**, and the anterior insertion of the **anterior cruciate ligament** (15) with its **expansion** (16) to the anterior horn of the anterior meniscus
- posteriorly, the posterior insertion of the **posterior cruciate ligament** (17) with the **menisco-femoral band of Wrisberg** (18).

The peri-articular defence system of the knee comprises **three major components**: the medial collateral ligament, the lateral collateral ligament and the posterior capsuloligamentous complex.

- The **medial collateral ligament** (19) can sustain (according to Bonnel) a force of 115 kg/cm² and an elongation of 12.5% before rupture.
- The **lateral collateral ligament** (20) can sustain a force of 276 kg/cm² and an elongation of 19% before rupture. It is unexpectedly both more resistant and more elastic than the medial ligament.
- The **posterior capsulo-ligamentous complex** consists of the medial condylar plate (21), the lateral condylar plate (22) with its sesamoid or fabella (23) and additional reinforcements, i.e. the oblique popliteal ligament (24) and the arcuate popliteal ligament (25).

There are also **four accessory fibrotendinous sheets** of unequal strength and importance:

- The **posteromedial layer or the posteromedial corner** is the most important. Bonnel calls it the fibrotendinous nucleus, which certainly applies to the posteromedial fibres but not to its other constituents. G. Bousquet calls it the posteromedial corner, which is more in keeping with a surgical than an anatomical concept. It lies posterior to the medial collateral ligament and consists of:
  - the most posterior fibres of the medial collateral ligament (26)
  - the medial border of the medial condylar plate (27)
  - two expansions (29-30) of the semimembranosus (28), i.e. its **reflected bundle** (29) skirting the medial margin

of the tibial articular facet and the **meniscal expansion** (30), which is inserted into the posterior margin of the medial meniscus.

- The **posterolateral layer or posterolateral corner** is clearly less strong than the posteromedial layer because at this point the lateral meniscus is separated from the capsule and the lateral collateral ligament by the **popliteus tendon** (31) soon after its origin from the lateral condyle (32). This tendon also sends a **meniscal expansion** (33), which tethers the posterior part of the lateral meniscus. The fibrotendinous sheet is reinforced by the **short process of the lateral collateral ligament** (20) and the lateral margin of the lateral condylar plate.
- The **anterolateral layer or the anterolateral corner** is made up of the **iliotibial tract** (35), which sends an **expansion** (36) to the lateral border of the patella and of the straight and cruciate expansions of the quadriceps tendon (37).
- The **anteromedial layer or the anteromedial corner** consists of the direct and cruciate fibres of the quadriceps tendon (38), reinforced by the expansion (39) of the **sartorius tendon** (41) attached to the medial border of the patella.

The **peri-articular muscles** also contribute to the defence system of the knee. By contracting in a manner perfectly synchronized during a particular movement and *preconditioned by the cerebral cortex*, they counter the mechanical distortions of the joint and provide an indispensable assistance to the ligaments, which can only react passively. The most important of these muscles is the **quadriceps**, which is essential for knee-joint stability. By its strength and its exquisite coordination it is able, up to a point, to compensate for ligamentous failure. For any surgical operation to succeed, the quadriceps must be in good physical condition. Since it atrophies quickly and is slow in recovery, it deserves special attention from surgeons and physiotherapists.

Laterally lies the **iliotibial tract** (35), which should be considered as the terminal tendon of the gluteal 'deltoid'. Posteromedially lie the semimembranosus (28) and the anserine muscles, i.e. the sartorius (41), the gracilis (42) and the semitendinosus (43). Posterolaterally, there are two muscles: the popliteus (31), whose peculiar physiology will be discussed later, and the biceps femoris (44), whose strong tendon is inserted into the fibular head (45) and reinforces the lateral collateral ligament (20).

Finally, posteriorly lies the gastrocnemius, arising from the femoral condyles and the condylar plates. The tendon of origin of its medial head (46) crosses the semimembranosus tendon with an intervening **bursa** (the semimembranosus bursa), which is often connected with the joint cavity. The tendon of origin of its lateral head (47) also crosses the biceps tendon, but there is no intervening bursa. The knee is encased within an **aponeurotic fascia** (49).

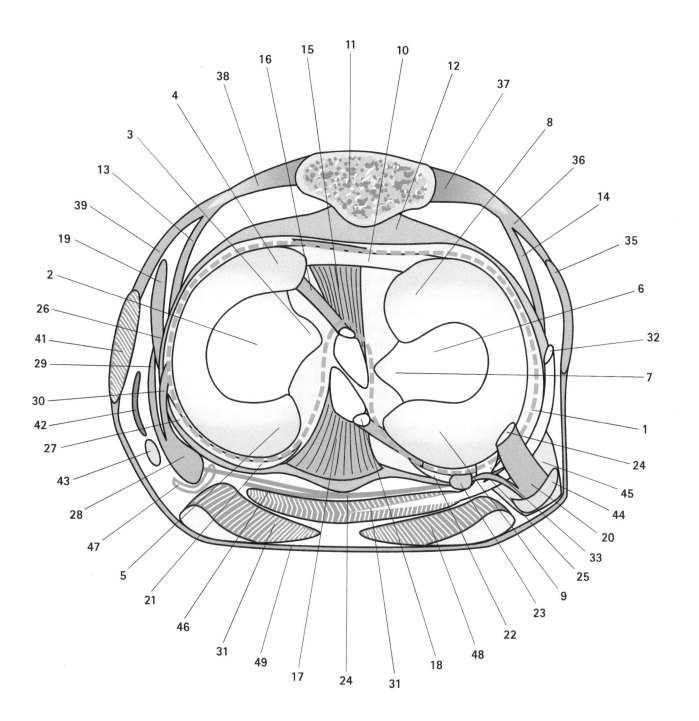

Fig. 164

117

The cruciate ligaments of the knee

When the joint is open anteriorly (**Fig. 165**, inspired by Rouvière) it becomes obvious that the **cruciate ligaments lie in the very centre of the joint**, being mostly contained within the intercondylar fossa.

The first to be seen is the **anterior cruciate ligament** (1), which is attached to the *tibial anterior intercondylar area* along the edge of the medial articular facet (12) and between the insertion of the *anterior horn of the medial meniscus* (7) medially and *that of the lateral meniscus* laterally (8) (see also **Fig. 79**, p. 93). It runs obliquely and laterally and is attached (**Fig. 167**, inspired by Rouvière) to the medial aspect of the lateral femoral condyle (1) along a narrow posteriorly located strip, which runs vertically above and along the edge of the articular cartilage (see **Figs 81 and 83**, p. 93).

It consists of *three bands*:
- the **anteromedial band** the largest, most superficial and most prone to injury
- the **posteromedial band**, which is concealed by the former and remains intact when the ligament is partially torn
- the **intermediate band.**

Taken as a whole, the ligament is *twisted on itself*, since its most anterior tibial fibres are inserted into the femur the most anteriorly and interiorly, while its most posterior tibial fibres are inserted the most superiorly on the femur. As a result, *its fibres are not all of the same length*. According to F. Bonnel, their mean lengths range from 1.85 to 3.35 cm, i.e. a great variation in length depending on their location with the result that they are not stretched at the same time.

The **posterior cruciate ligament** (2) lies deep in the intercondylar fossa *behind the anterior cruciate ligament* (**Fig. 165**). It is attached (**Fig. 166**) to the most posterior part (6) of the posterior intercondylar area, and even (**Figs 167 and 168**, inspired by Rouvière) to the posterior border of the tibial plateau (see also **Fig. 79**, p. 93); hence its tibial insertion is located well posterior to the attachments of the posterior horns of the lateral meniscus (9) and of the medial meniscus (10). The ligament *runs obliquely medially, anteriorly and superiorly* (**Fig. 168**: knee flexed at 90°) to be inserted along the articular surface (2) deep in the femoral intercondylar fossa (**Fig. 169**, inspired by Rouvière) and also (**Fig. 168**) horizontally into the lower margin of the lateral surface of the medial condyle along the articular surface (see also **Fig. 79**, p. 93). It comprises *three bands*:
- the **posterolateral** band, inserted the most posteriorly into the tibia and the most laterally into the femur
- the **anteromedial band**, inserted the most anteriorly into the tibia and the most medially into the femur
- the **menisco-femoral ligament** (3), which is attached to the posterior horn of the lateral meniscus (**Figs 166 and 167**) and very soon afterwards runs along the anterior surface of the body of the main ligament (2) before gaining a common insertion into the lateral surface of the medial condyle. Occasionally a similar ligament is present in relation to the medial meniscus (**Fig. 166**): a few fibres (5) of the anterior cruciate are inserted into the anterior horn of the medial meniscus close to the insertion of the transverse ligament (11).

The cruciates are in contact with each other (**Fig. 169**: the cruciates have been sectioned near their femoral insertion) along their axial borders, with the anterior (1) running lateral to the posterior (2) ligament. They do not lie free in the joint cavity but are lined by **synovium** (4). They have important relationships with the capsule, which will be discussed on the next page. They slide one against the other along their axial margins during knee movements.

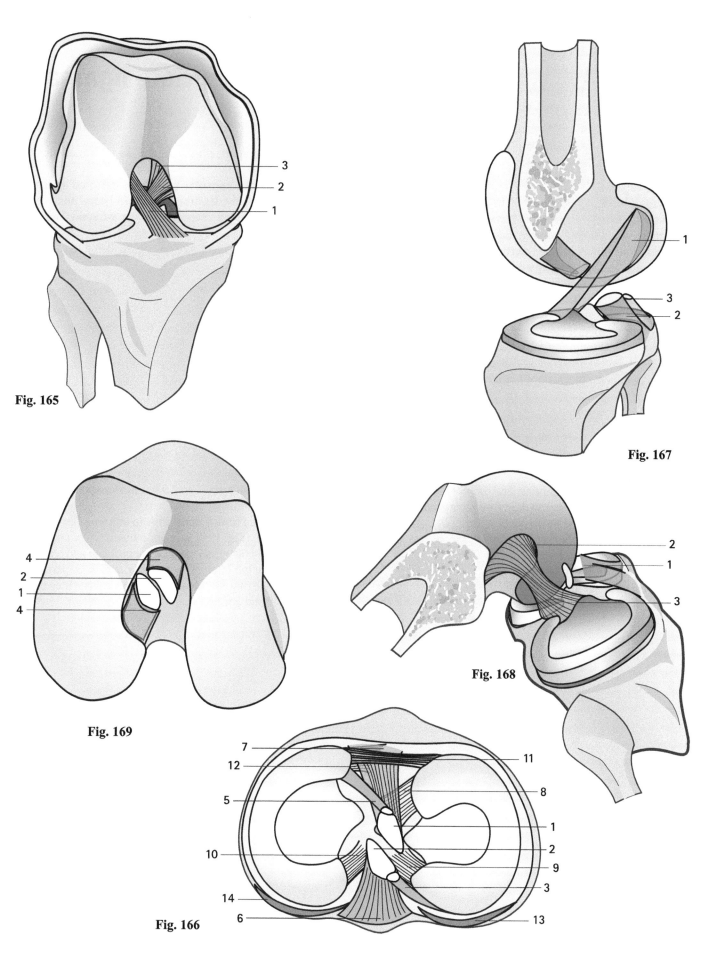

Fig. 165

Fig. 167

Fig. 169

Fig. 168

Fig. 166

119

Relations between the capsule and the cruciate ligaments

The cruciates are so intimately related to the capsule that they can be considered as actual thickenings, and thus as integral parts, of the capsule. We have seen **(Fig. 78**, p. 93) how the capsule dips into the intercondylar fossa to form a double-layered partition along the axis of the joint. It was said earlier, as a first approximation for the sake of convenience, that the tibial insertion of the capsule excluded the insertions of the cruciates from the joint cavity. In fact, **the capsular insertion runs through the cruciate insertions** in such a way that the capsular thickenings formed by the cruciates stand out on the outer surface of the capsule, i.e. between the two layers of the double partition. Figure 171 (posteromedial view, after removal of the medial condyle and partial sectioning of the capsule) shows the **anterior cruciate ligament** clearly 'plastered' against the lateral layer of the capsular partition (the posterior cruciate is not shown in the diagram). Also seen anteriorly are the suprapatellar bursa and the concavity for the patella.

Figure 172 (posteromedial view, after removal of the medial condyle and partial resection of the capsule) shows the **posterior cruciate ligament** 'plastered' against the medial layer of the capsular partition.

Note that all the fibres of the cruciates do not have the same length or the same direction and therefore are not shortened at the same time during knee movements (see p. 124).

These diagrams also illustrate the **condylar plates** partly resected at the level of the lateral condyle **(Fig. 171)** and of the medial condyle **(Fig. 172)**.

A **vertico-coronal section (Fig. 170)**, taken through the posterior parts of the condyles after the femur and tibia have been artificially pulled apart, illustrates the 'compartmentalization' of the joint cavity:

- *In the middle* the **capsular partition**, indented by the cruciate ligaments, divides the cavity into a lateral and a medial half and is extended anteriorly by the infrapatellar fat pad (see p. 94).
- *Each half of the joint cavity* is in turn divided into two storeys by the meniscus, i.e. the upper or **suprameniscal** storey corresponding to the femoromeniscal joint space and the lower or **submeniscal** storey corresponding to the tibiomeniscal joint space.

It is the presence of the cruciate ligaments that profoundly alters the structure of this hinge (trochlear) joint. The term *bicondylar joint* here is meaningless mechanically speaking because, if the two condyles were united, they would form a trochlea. The anterior cruciate **(Fig. 173)** from its initial neutral position (1) starts *by lying down horizontally* (2) on the tibial plateau during flexion to 45-50° and then climbs to its highest point (3) during extreme flexion. On its way down it lodges itself in the groove as if it had 'sawn' through the intercondylar eminence between the intercondylar tubercles like a bread-knife **(Fig. 174**: diagrammatic representation of the bread-knife separating the two intercondylar tubercles).

As the knee moves from extension A to extreme flexion B, the posterior cruciate **(Fig. 175)** 'sweeps' a much wider sector (over an angle of nearly 60°) than the anterior cruciate and 'carves' in the femoral bone the intercondylar fossa, which 'separates' the two cheeks of the physiological and theoretical trochlea formed by the two femoral condyles.

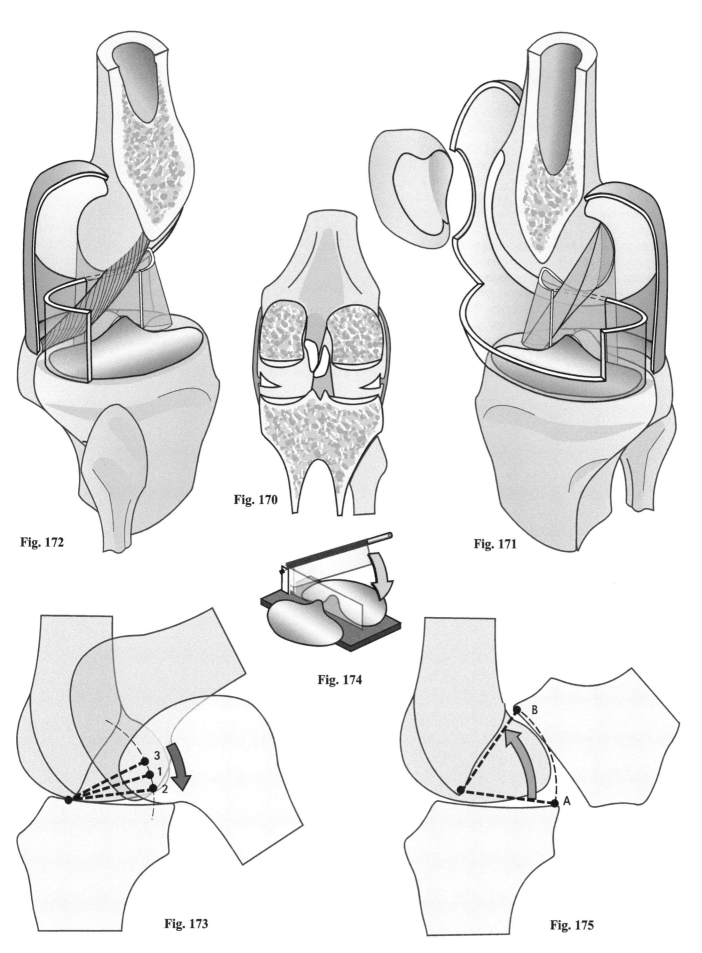

Fig. 170

Fig. 172

Fig. 171

Fig. 174

Fig. 173

Fig. 175

The direction of the cruciate ligaments

The posterolateral view in perspective **(Fig. 176)** shows the *stretched* cruciates **crossing each other in space.** In the **sagittal plane (Fig. 177**: medial view of the lateral condyle), they clearly cross each other with the anterior cruciate (ACL) running obliquely superiorly and posteriorly and the posterior cruciate (PCL) running obliquely superiorly and anteriorly.

If these ligaments are dissected out they can be seen to cross each other *during* both extension **(Fig. 178)** and flexion **(Fig. 179)** and to slide one against the other on their axial surfaces. Their directions also **cross each other in the coronal plane (Fig. 180,** posterior view) since their tibial insertions (black dots) are lined up along the anteroposterior axis (arrow S) and their femoral insertions are 1.7 cm apart. As a result, the posterior cruciate runs *obliquely, superiorly and medially*, while the anterior cruciate runs *obliquely, superiorly and laterally*.

By contrast, in the horizontal plane (see **Fig. 205**, p. 131) they are parallel to each other in space and are in contact along their axial borders, but each one also **crosses the ipsilateral collateral ligament*.** Thus the anterior or anterolateral cruciate crosses the *lateral collateral ligament* (LCL) **(Fig. 181,** lateral view) and the posterior or posteromedial cruciate crosses the *medial collateral ligament* (MCL) **(Fig. 182,** medial view). Therefore the obliquity of these four ligaments *alternates regularly* when they are viewed in sequence lateromedially or vice versa **(Fig. 183**: diagrammatic representation of the four ligaments in relation to the tibial plateau.)

The cruciates also **have different inclinations:** *with the knee extended* **(Fig. 177)** the anterior ligament (ACL) is *more vertical*, while the posterior cruciate (PCL) is *more horizontal*. The same applies to the general direction of their sites of femoral insertion (shown as transparent): that of the posterior cruciate is *horizontal* **b** and that of the anterior cruciate is *vertical* **a.**

As the knee is flexed **(Fig. 184**: the lateral condyle viewed from inside), the posterior cruciate (PCL), which was horizontal in extension, rears itself up to the vertical position **(Fig. 179)** and sweeps a 60° angle relative to the tibia, while the anterior cruciate (ACL) is raised only very slightly (red arrow).

The length ratio of the cruciates *shows individual variations*, but, just like the distances between their tibial and femoral insertions, it is **typical of each knee**, since it is one of the determinants of the condylar profiles, as demonstrated earlier.

---

* The author views the anterior cruciate as the anterolateral cruciate and the posterior cruciate as the posteromedial cruciate.

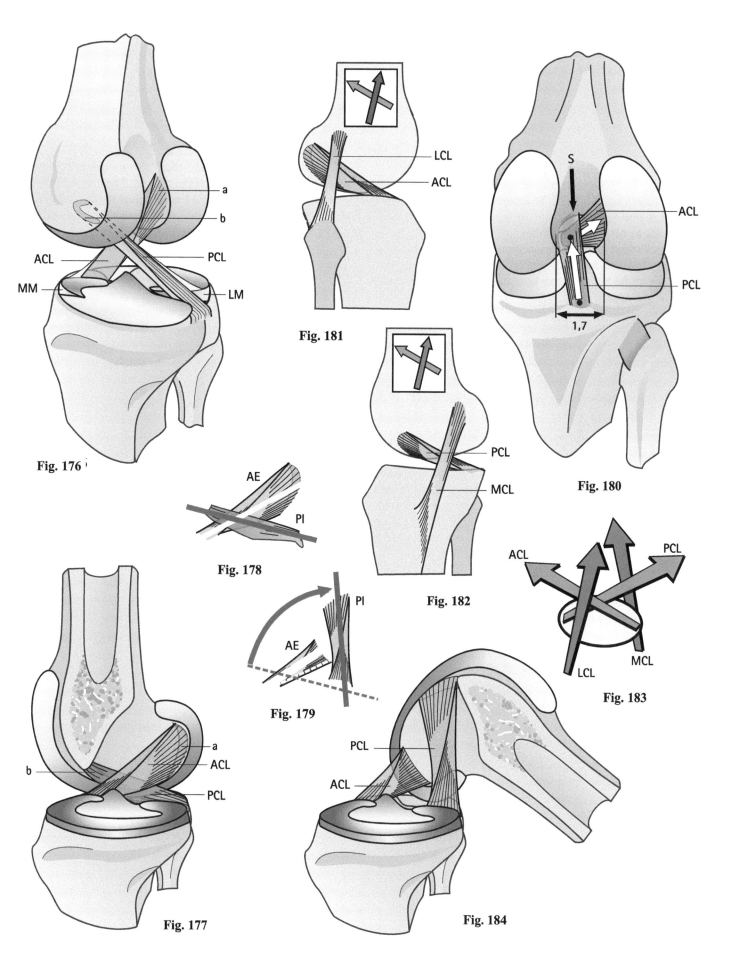

Fig. 176

Fig. 177

Fig. 178

Fig. 179

Fig. 180

Fig. 181

Fig. 182

Fig. 183

Fig. 184

The mechanical role of the cruciate ligaments

It is customary to reduce the cruciates to linear cords with almost dot-like insertions. This first approximation has the advantage of revealing the general actions of ligaments but fails to bring out their functional subtleties. To achieve this, three factors need to be taken into account:

1. The thickness of the ligament
The thickness and volume of a ligament are directly proportional to its resistance and inversely proportional to its elasticity, since each fibre of the ligament can be considered as an elementary spring of low elasticity.

2. The structure of the ligament
Because of the size of its insertions, the fibres of a ligament are *not all of the same length*, with the important consequence that the fibres are not all recruited at the same time. As with muscle fibres, there is fibre recruitment during the movements themselves and, as a result, the resistance and elasticity of the ligament are variable.

3. The size and direction of its insertions
Furthermore, the fibres are not all parallel to one another but are often arranged in planes that are twisted on themselves and 'warped' because their lines of insertion are not parallel to one another but are often oblique or perpendicular to one another in space. Also the relative orientation of the insertions varies during movements, contributing to differential recruitment of the fibres and modifying the overall direction of action of the ligaments. This variation in the orienting action of the ligament occurs not only in the sagittal plane but also *in all the three planes of space*, accounting perfectly for **their complex and concurrent actions on the anteroposterior, transverse and rotational stability of the knee.**

Thus, the geometry of the cruciate ligaments, as shown previously, determines the *condylotrochlear profile* in the sagittal plane as well as in the other planes of space.

Globally, the cruciates ensure the **anteroposterior stability** of the knee and allow **hinge-like movements** to occur while keeping the articular surfaces in contact. Their role can be illustrated by an easily constructed **mechanical model (Fig. 185**: the model shown in cross-section). Two planks A and B are joined by two strips of paper **ab** and **cd** linking their opposite ends, so that they can move with respect to each other about *two hinges*. Hinge **a** and hinge **b** coincide with points **c** and **d**, respectively, but they *cannot slide on each other.*

The cruciates are anatomically and functionally similar, except that instead of two hinges, there is a series of hinges lined up along the curve of the condyle. As in the model, **anteroposterior sliding is impossible.**

To continue with the model, the cruciates are represented by two straight lines with the ACL and the PCL corresponding to **ab** and **cd**, respectively in Figures 186 and 188. Figures 187 and 189 show the outermost and the middle fibres of the ligaments and their sites of insertion.

Starting from the straight position **(Fig. 186)** or from slight flexion at 30° **(Fig. 187)**, when the cruciates are taut to the same degree, flexion tilts the '**femoral plank' cb*** **(Fig. 188)** while the anterior cruciate **cd** *rears itself up* and the posterior cruciate **ab** *becomes horizontal*. The more detailed diagram (**Fig. 189**: in flexion at 60°) shows upward and downward displacements of the sites of insertion of the ACL (red) and of the PCL (green), respectively. Yet an accurate study to be done is of the successive stretching of the elementary fibres of each cruciate during movements, since it is clear that they are stretched to a variable degree depending on their positions within the ligament (**Fig. 190**: diagram in space of the fibres of PCL).

---

* The linear space between the insertions of the two cruciate ligaments.

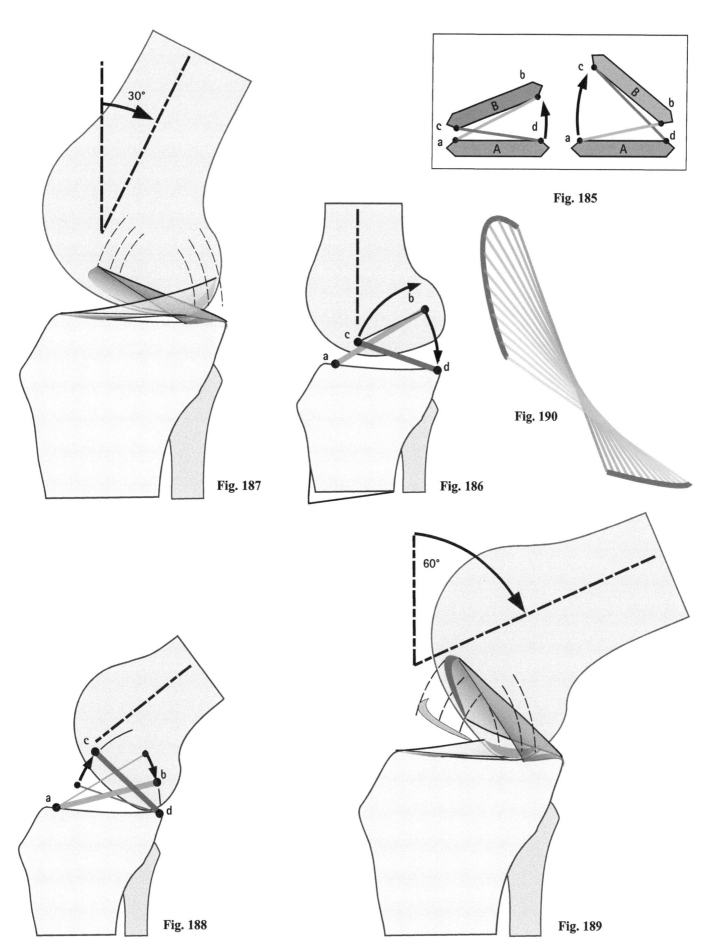

Fig. 185

Fig. 187

Fig. 186

Fig. 190

Fig. 188

Fig. 189

The mechanical role of the cruciate ligaments (continued)

As **flexion** increases to 90° **(Fig. 191)** and then to 120° **(Fig. 192)** the posterior cruciate (PCL) *rears itself up to the vertical position* and is proportionately more tensed than the anterior cruciate (ACL). The more detailed diagram **(Fig. 193)** shows that the middle and inferior fibres of the ACL are slackened (−), and only its anterosuperior fibres are tensed (+), whereas the posterosuperior fibres of the PCL are slightly slackened (−), and its anterosuperior fibres are tensed (+). The posterior cruciate is tensed in flexion.

During **extension** and **hyperextension (Fig. 194)** from the initial position **(Figs 195 and 196)**, all the fibres of anterior cruciate are tightened (+), whereas only the posterosuperior fibres of the posterior cruciate are tightened (+). Furthermore, during hyperextension **(Fig. 197)**, the floor of the intercondylar fossa (c) comes to press against the anterior cruciate and *stretches* it in the manner of the chord of an arc. Thus the anterior cruciate is tensed during extension and *becomes one of the checks on hyperextension*.

Bonnel has recently confirmed the notion, first enunciated by Strasser (1917) on the basis of a mechanical model, that the anterior cruciate and the posterior cruciate are tensed during extension and flexion, respectively. A more refined mechanical analysis, however, has shown that Roud (1913) was also right in believing that **some of the fibres of the cruciates are always under tension** because of their unequal lengths. As is often the case in biomechanics, *two apparently contradictory ideas can be correct at the same time without being mutually exclusive.*

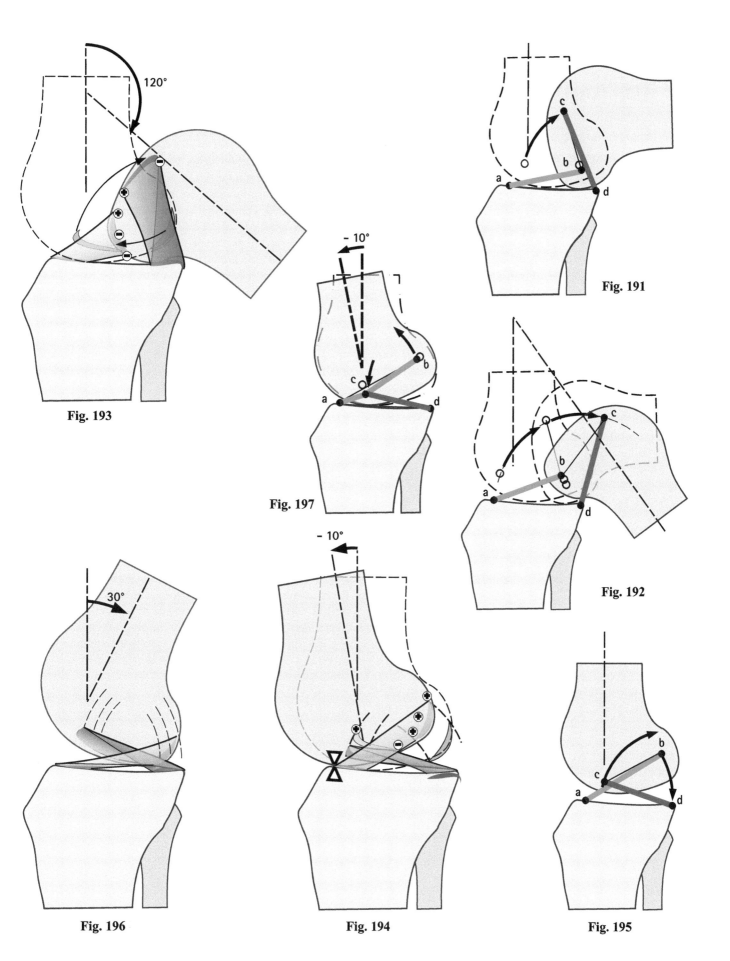

Fig. 193

Fig. 197

Fig. 191

Fig. 192

Fig. 196

Fig. 194

Fig. 195

127

The mechanical role of the cruciate ligaments (*final*)

Condylar movements on the tibial plateau include rolling and sliding (see p. 88). It is easy to imagine these rolling movements, but how can gliding occur in such a loosely interlocked joint as the knee? **Muscles play an active role: the extensors** pull the tibia anteriorly under the femur during extension, and conversely the **flexors** cause the tibial plateau to slide posteriorly during flexion. But, when these movements are studied on a cadaver, **passive factors**, especially the cruciates, appear to predominate. It is the cruciates that pull back the femoral condyles and cause them to slide on the tibial plateau in a direction opposite to their rolling motion.

Starting **(Fig. 198)** from the position of extension (I), if the condyle rolled without sliding it should recede to position II, and the femoral insertion **b** of the anterior cruciate **ab** should hit **b**"after a supposed displacement equal to **bb'**. Such a displacement, illustrated in Figure 62 on p. 89, would damage the posterior horn of the medal meniscus. Now point **b** can only move along a circle with centre **a** and radius **ab** (the ligament being taken as inelastic); thus the real path of **b** does not lead to **bb"** but to **bb'**, which corresponds to position III of the condyle lying more anterior than position I by a distance of **e**. During flexion, the anterior cruciate is called into action and pulls back the condyle anteriorly. It can be said therefore that **during flexion, the anterior cruciate is responsible for the forward sliding of the condyle,** coupled with its backward rolling.

The **role of the posterior cruciate** during extension is similarly demonstrated in Figure 199. As it rolls from position I to position II the condyle is *pulled back posteriorly* by the posterior cruciate **cd**, and its femoral insertion **c** travels not to **cc'** but to **cc"** along a circle with centre **d** and radius **dc**. Hence the condyle slides posteriorly for a distance of **n** to reach position III. **During extension, the posterior cruciate is responsible for the backward sliding of the condyle** coupled with its forward rolling.

These observations can also be demonstrated using the mechanical model (see Model 3 at the end of this volume), which illustrates the alternating tension in the cruciates represented by elastic bands.

Drawer movements are **abnormal anteroposterior movements of the tibia under the femur** and can be looked for in two positions:

1. with knee flexed at 90°
2. with knee in full extension.

With knee flexed at 90° (Fig. 202): the patient lies supine on a plinth, and the examiner flexes the knee in question to 90° with the foot lying on the table. He then immobilizes the patient's foot by partially sitting on it and, **with the palms of his hands,** grasps the upper part of the leg. He then pulls the leg *anteriorly towards himself or posteriorly away from himself as* he looks **for an anterior or a posterior drawer movement,** respectively. He must perform this examination with the patient's foot in the neutral position of rotation to demonstrate a *direct drawer movement,* with the patient's foot in lateral rotation to demonstrate a *drawer movement in lateral rotation* and with the patient's foot in medial rotation to demonstrate a *drawer movement in medial rotation.* This terminology is preferable to the label of 'lateral or medial rotational drawer movement', which implies that rotation occurs during the drawer movement.

The **posterior drawer movement (Fig. 200)** is elicited by the **posterior** (red arrow) displacement of the tibia under the femur; it is the result of **a rupture of the posterior cruciate** (black arrow). Hence the mnemonic: posterior drawer = posterior cruciate.

The **anterior drawer movement (Fig. 201)** is elicited by **anterior** (green arrow) displacement of the tibia under the femur; it is the result of a **rupture of the anterior cruciate.** Hence the mnemonic: anterior drawer movement = anterior cruciate.

With the **patient's knee extended,** the examiner supports the posterior aspect of the patient's thigh with one hand **(Fig. 202),** while the other hand holds the upper end of the leg and tries to move it anteroposteriorly or posteroanteriorly (the **Lachmann-Trillat test).** Any anterior movement (the so-called anterior Lachmann) is proof of *rupture of the anterior cruciate* coupled in particular with rupture of the posterolateral corner (according to Bousquet). This test is **difficult to perform** because of the small range of movement involved.

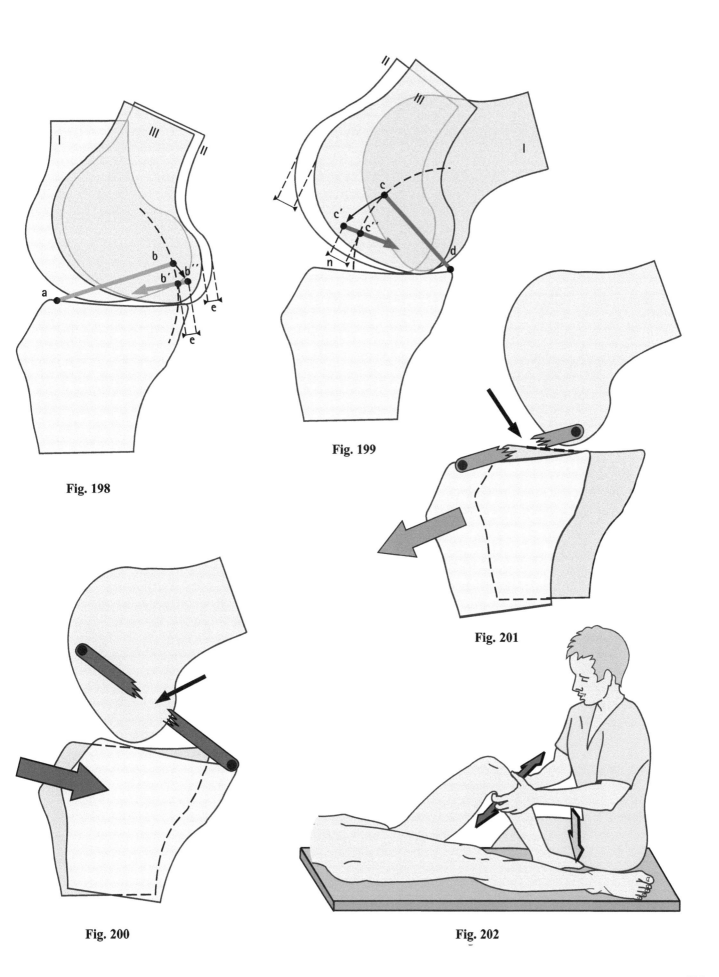

Fig. 198

Fig. 199

Fig. 200

Fig. 201

Fig. 202

Rotational stability of the extended knee

We already know that axial rotation can occur only when the knee is flexed. On the other hand, **with the knee in full extension, axial rotation is impossible**, since it is **inhibited by the taut collateral and cruciate ligaments.**

When **the knee is in the neutral position for axial rotation (Fig. 203**: frontal view of the articular surfaces separated by making the ligaments artificially elastic), the ligaments clearly cross each other in space and the obliquity of the dissected ligaments is quite obvious **(Fig. 204)**. In the **horizontal plane**, however **(Fig. 205**: superior view with the condyles shown as transparent), the two cruciates are parallel to and in contact with each other.

During **medial rotation of the tibia under the femur (Fig. 206**, frontal view) the ligaments are clearly *more acutely crossed in the coronal plane* **(Fig. 207)**, while in the *horizontal plane* **(Fig. 208**, superior view) their inner borders come to touch each other. Thus they wrap themselves around each other and tense each other up like the bands of a tourniquet and **quickly check any medial rotation.**

During lateral rotation of the tibia under the femur (Fig. 209, anterior view) the cruciates tend to become parallel in the *coronal plane* **(Fig. 210)**, whereas in the *horizontal plane* **(Fig. 211**, superior view) their inner borders tend to lose contact with each other, thereby relaxing the 'tourniquet'. Thus **tightening of the cruciates plays no part in checking lateral rotation.**

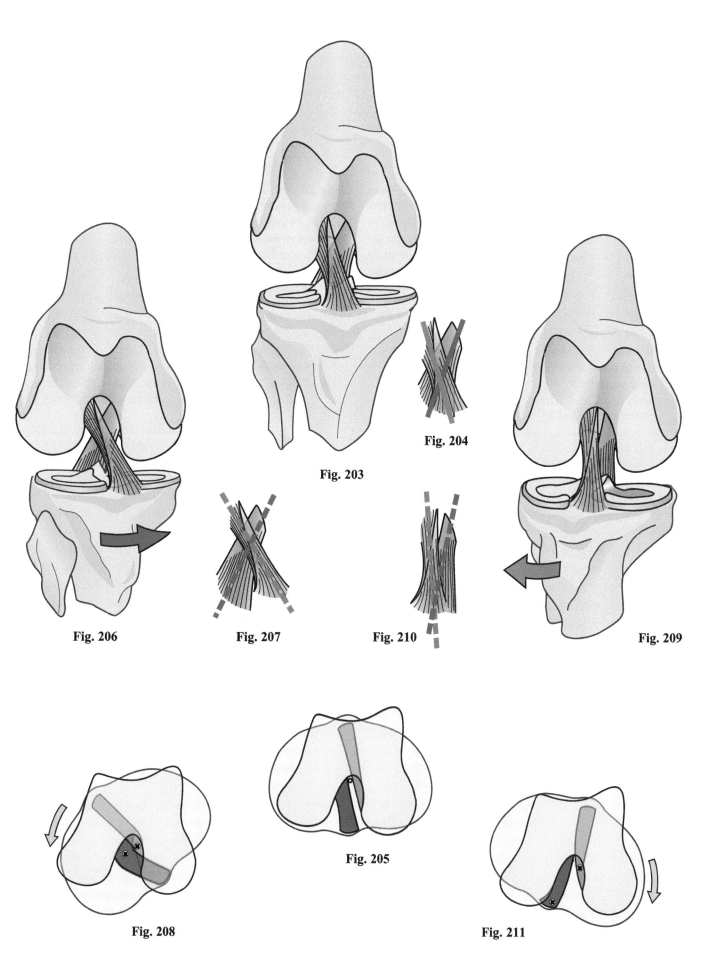

Fig. 203

Fig. 204

Fig. 205

Fig. 206

Fig. 207

Fig. 208

Fig. 209

Fig. 210

Fig. 211

Rotational stability of the extended knee (*continued*)

How will the rotational stability of the knee in the straight position be affected by forced rotation of the tibia under the femur? With the knee in full extension, **forced medial rotation of the tibia under the femur (Fig. 212**: more detailed superior view with the femoral condyles shown as transparent) occurs not around a centre located in the intercondylar fossa between the tibial intercondylar tubercles but around a real centre (marked by a cross) corresponding to the medial border of the medial intercondylar tubercle.

At the same time, since this centre of rotation (marked by a cross, **Fig. 212**) does not coincide with the joint centre (white circle), this off-centre movement slackens (–) the *posterior cruciate* (**in red**) and *tightens* (+) *the anterior cruciate* (**in green**), as well as its expansion to the anterior horn of the medial meniscus, which is then pulled posteriorly.

The ligaments touch each other more and more (**Fig. 213**: view of the ligaments after dissection) and cross each other more and more acutely. If this movement were to go on (**Fig. 214**: the tibia has been *artificially medially rotated* by 180°), the ligaments would be wrapped around each other and become shorter, pulling the femur and tibia closer together (black arrows). This is exactly what happens in reality: the wrapping of the cruciates around each other brings the femur and tibia closer together and **checks medial rotation**. Medial rotation tightens the anterior cruciate and relaxes the posterior cruciate. **The cruciate ligaments inhibit medial rotation when the knee is extended.**

Conversely, with the knee still fully extended, **forced lateral rotation of the tibia under the femur (Fig. 215**: superior view, condyles transparent) produces tibial rotation around a real centre (marked by a cross), and this off-centre movement *tenses (+) the posterior cruciate* (in red) and *slackens the anterior*

(–) cruciate (in green). The ligaments tend to become parallel to each other (**Fig. 216**) and if this movement of lateral rotation (**Fig. 217**: 90° rotation only) were to go on, the ligaments would become parallel, allowing the articular surfaces to move apart slightly (black arrows). **The cruciates do not check lateral rotation when the knee is extended.**

Slocum and Larson studied in detail the rotational stability of the flexed knee in athletes, in particular soccer players. A soccer player violently rotates his supporting knee laterally when he turns away from that knee. The important involvement of the medial articular capsule was demonstrated as follows:

- Its anterior third is very prone to rupture if the knee flexed at 90° is exposed to a valgus-lateral rotation trauma
- Its posterior third is vulnerable when the knee is extended
- Its middle third, blending with the deep fibres of the medial collateral ligament, ruptures when the trauma involves a knee flexed between 30° and 90°
- In addition, if the knee is flexed at 90° or more, the anterior cruciate starts to slacken during the first 15-20° of lateral rotation and then tenses up. If lateral rotation proceeds, the ligament can be torn as it wraps itself around the medial surface of the lateral condyle
- Finally, through its capsular connections to the tibia, the posterior part of the medial meniscus can by itself prevent lateral rotation of the flexed knee.

In summary, **exposure of the flexed knee to a valgus-lateral rotation trauma** can have the following consequences in succession as the severity of the injury increases:

- rupture of the medial collateral ligament, first its deep fibres and later its superficial fibres
- rupture of the anterior cruciate
- detachment of the medial meniscus.

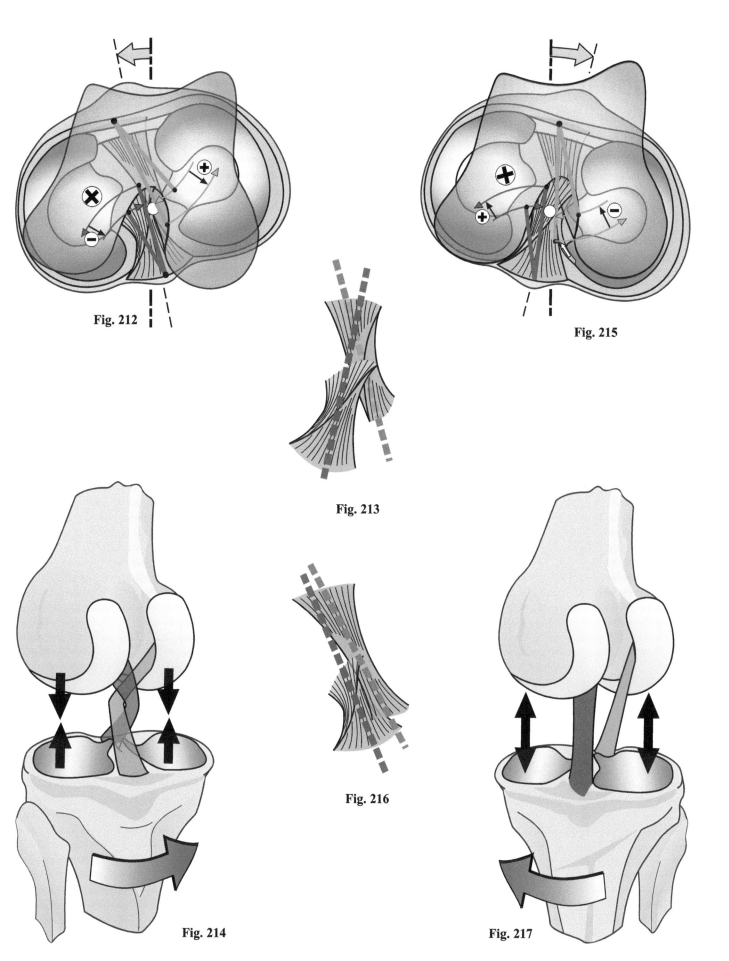

Fig. 212

Fig. 213

Fig. 214

Fig. 215

Fig. 216

Fig. 217

Rotational stability of the extended knee (*continued*)

The role of the collateral ligaments in securing the rotational stability of the knee can be explained by their symmetry.

In the **null rotation** position (**Fig. 218**, superior view, condyles transparent) the obliquity of the lateral collateral ligament as it runs inferiorly and anteriorly and that of the medial collateral ligament as it runs inferiorly and posteriorly causes them to *coil round the upper extremity of the tibia.*

Medial rotation (Fig. 219) prevents this coiling movement, and the obliquity of these ligaments decreases as they tend to *become parallel* (**Fig. 220**: posteromedial view with the articular surfaces 'separated'). As the coiling decreases, the articular surfaces are *less strongly coapted* by the collateral ligaments, while they are *more strongly coapted by the cruciates.* **Thus the 'play' permitted by relaxation of the collateral ligaments is offset by the tension in the cruciates.**

Conversely, **lateral rotation (Fig. 221)** increases the coiling, which brings the articular surfaces closer together (**Fig. 222**, posteromedial view) and limits their movements while the *cruciates are slackened.*

On the whole, it can be said that the collateral ligaments check lateral rotation and the cruciates check medial rotation. Therefore **the rotational stability of the extended knee is ensured by the collateral ligaments during lateral rotation and by the cruciates during medial rotation.**

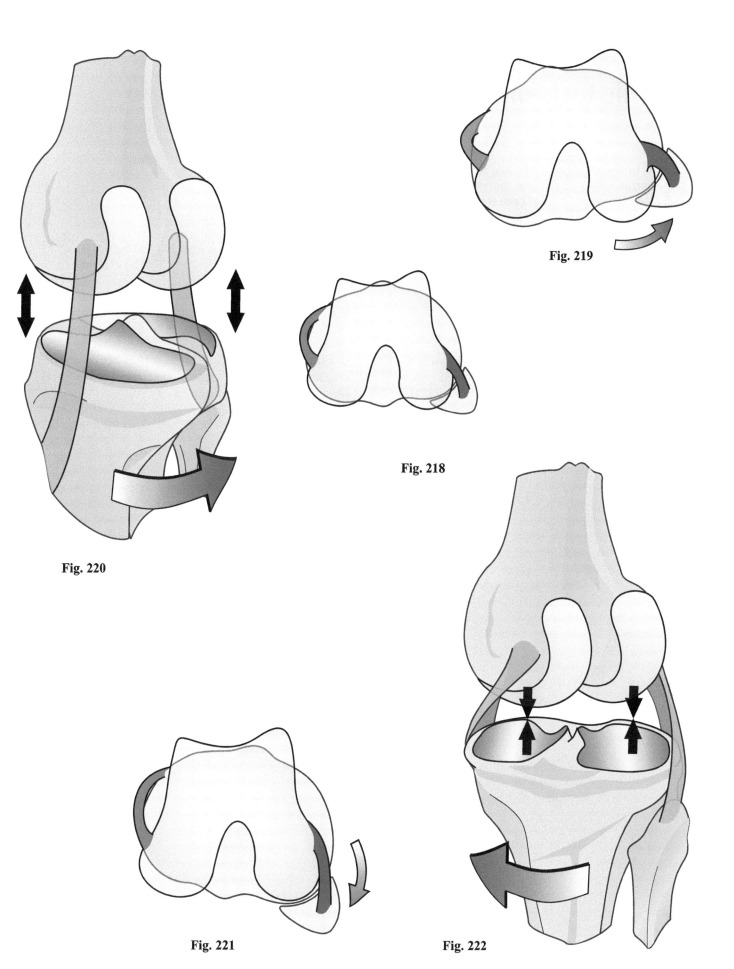

Fig. 219

Fig. 218

Fig. 220

Fig. 221

Fig. 222

Dynamic tests of the knee during medial rotation

In addition to the static tests of knee stability looking for **abnormal varus-valgus and drawer movements**, there are now well-established **dynamic tests of knee stability** (or instability) that aim at revealing *an abnormal movement occurring during the very performance of a test movement*. These dynamic tests of instability are so numerous (each school of knee surgery presents a new one at every congress) that they need to be classified with emphasis on the most important ones. Practically speaking they fall into two groups:

• Tests combining valgus and medial rotation
• Tests combining valgus and lateral rotation.

The first group includes the following:

The **lateral pivot shift test or the MacIntosh test** is the *best known and the most widely used*. It is performed on a patient lying supine **(Fig. 223)** or at an angle of 45° **(Fig. 224)**. In the first case the examiner places one hand on the plantar aspect of the foot to support it and to rotate it forcibly medially, while the sheer weight of the limb accentuates the valgus at the knee. In the second case, the examiner grasps the foot at the instep by passing under the ankle with one hand and extends his own wrist in order to rotate the foot medially. The starting position of the knee is in extension **(Fig. 223)**, and the examiner's free hand pushes the knee anteriorly to initiate flexion and inferiorly to accentuate the valgus at the knee. During this movement of flexion **(Fig. 224)**, the examiner feels some resistance initially, but at about 25-30° flexion there is a sudden *unlocking* so that he feels and sees the lateral femoral condyle literally jump in front of the lateral tibial plateau.

A positive MacIntosh test associated with a lateral jerk during medial rotation indicates a **rupture of the anterior cruciate.**

In fact, since the anterior cruciate checks medial rotation of the extended knee when medially rotated (MR) **(Fig. 225)**, *the lateral femoral condyle shifts into a position of posterior subluxation* (PSL) on the *posterior downslope* (1) of the convexity of the lateral tibial articular surface and is held in that position by the tension in the *fascia lata* (FL) and the valgus, which keep the femur and tibia tightly apposed. The condyle stays put in the position of posterior subluxation as long as the fascia lata lies anterior to the convexity of the tibial articular surface, but beyond this point, *as occurs with increasing flexion* **(Fig. 226)**, the condyle passes over the apex of the convexity (A) and is arrested *anteriorly* (2) on the anterior border of the tibial articular surface, where it is held in check **(Fig. 226)** by the posterior cruciate (in pink). **Importantly, the patient also observes this jerky movement (J) spontaneously.**

The Jerk Test of Hughston is the converse of the MacIntosh test. It is performed with the patient lying supine **(Fig. 227)** or at an intermediate angle of 45° **(Fig. 228)**, and with the examiner using his hands in a similar manner. The difference is that the starting position is at 35-40° flexion when the knee is moved back into the position of extension, while the examiner rotates the foot medially and accentuates the valgus. Thus, the lateral femoral condyle **(Fig. 225)** starts from its 'advanced' position (stippled) in contact with the anterior border of the lateral tibial surface (2) and then abruptly 'jumps' (1) into the position of posterior subluxation, since it is no longer retained by the anterior cruciate as extension progresses. **A positive Jerk Test also indicates rupture of the anterior cruciate.**

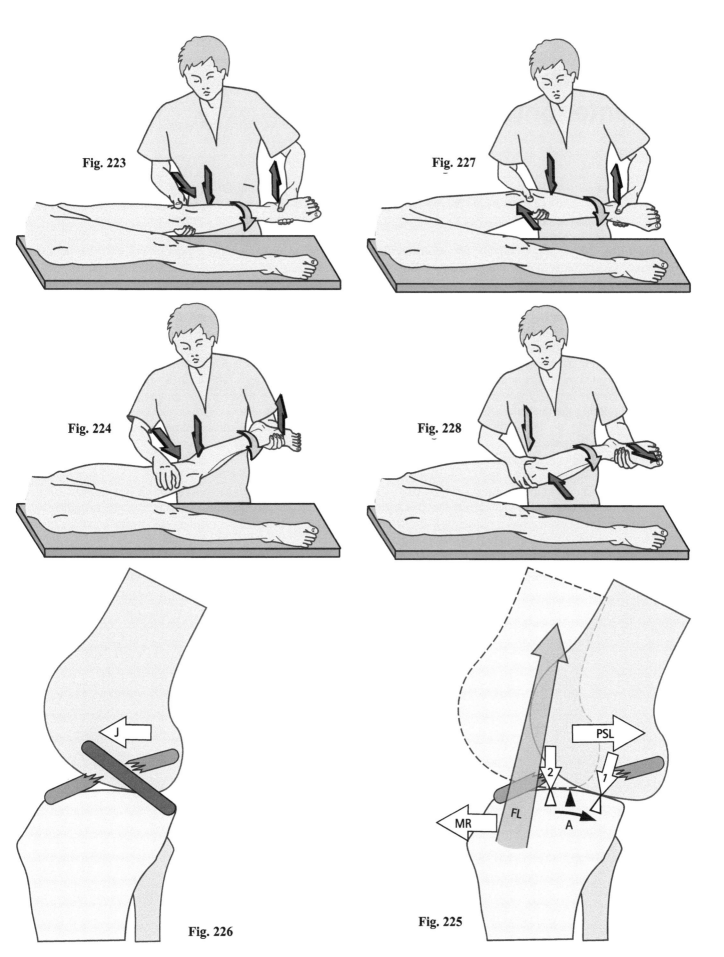

Fig. 223

Fig. 227

Fig. 224

Fig. 228

Fig. 226

Fig. 225

Dynamic tests for rupture of the anterior cruciate ligament

Although the MacIntosh and Hughston tests are the most frequently used, being the easiest to perform and the most reliable, they are not the only ones to reveal rupture of the anterior cruciate. There are three other tests:

The **Losee test (Fig. 229)** is performed with the patient supine. With one hand the examiner supports the heel with the *knee flexed at 30°*, and with the other hand he grasps the anterior surface of the knee with his thumb gripping the fibular head. At the same time, his first hand *rotates the knee laterally*, thus preventing any posterior subluxation of the lateral femoral condyle, while the other hand *exaggerates the valgus*. He then *extends the knee* while *reducing the degree of lateral rotation of the knee*. (This combination of movements is critical for the test to be positive.) As the knee is being fully extended, the thumb of the examiner's hand holding the knee pushes the fibula anteriorly. The test is **positive** when the proximal articular surface *jerks anteriorly* at the end of extension.

The **Noyes test (Fig. 230)** or the **Flexion Rotation Drawer test** is also performed on a supine patient with knee flexed at 20-30° and in null rotation. The examiner's hands serve only to support the leg, and the sheer weight of the thigh causes **posterior subluxation** of the lateral condyle (two red arrows) and lateral rotation of the femur. It is possible to reduce this subluxation by pushing the upper tibial extremity posteriorly (yellow arrow), as when one is looking for a posterior drawer movement (hence, the Anglo-Saxon label for the test), which is another indicator of rupture of the anterior cruciate.

The **Slocum test (Fig. 231)** is performed on a supine patient half-turned away from the examiner with the limb lying on the board. Thus, with the knee extended, the sheer weight of the limb *automatically causes it to adopt the valgus-medial rotation position*. The fact that the limb does not have to be supported is useful when dealing with heavy patients. With one hand lying on either side of the knee joint, the examiner flexes the knee progressively while accentuating the valgus. As in the MacIntosh test, a *sudden jerk is felt at 30-40° flexion*, and a *jerk in the opposite direction is felt* when the knee is extended, as in the Hughston test. A positive Slocum test indicates **rupture of the anterior cruciate.**

These five tests are quite important indicators of rupture of the anterior cruciate, but they can be *unreliable* under two conditions:

- In young girls with joint hyperlaxity, they can be positive in the absence of ligamentous rupture; hence the *need to examine the other knee*, which may also turn out to be unduly lax.
- After a severe injury to the posteromedial corner of the knee, the lateral condyle is no longer checked by the valgus, and the demonstration of the jerk can be difficult.

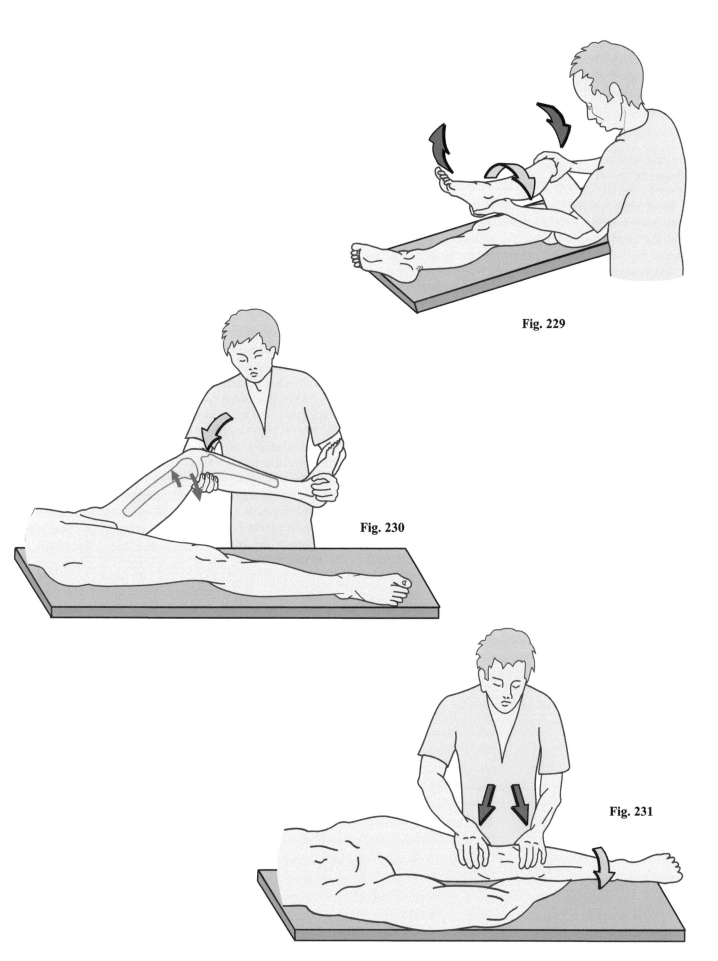

Fig. 229

Fig. 230

Fig. 231

Dynamic tests of the knee during lateral rotation

Knee examination would be incomplete without the **dynamic tests during lateral rotation**, which look for a lateral jerk when the knee is laterally rotated.

The **Pivot Shift Reverse test or the test in lateral rotation-valgus-extension (Fig. 232)** is performed like the MacIntosh test, except that lateral rotation replaces medial rotation of the leg, produced by the examiner's hand supporting the foot. Starting from the position of flexion at 60-90°, progressive extension, combined with pressure constantly applied to the lateral surface of the knee, leads to the appearance at –30° extension **(Fig. 233)** of a *sudden jerk of the lateral femoral condyle* towards the posterior downslope of the lateral tibial articular surface.

When the *laterally rotated knee is flexed* **(Fig. 235)**, the lateral condyle, no longer held back by the tension in the posterior cruciate (in red) during lateral rotation (LR), undergoes anterior subluxation (ASL) on the anterior downslope of the convex surface of the lateral tibial surface (arrow 1). With progressive knee extension **(Fig. 234)** the *iliotibial tract* (ITT) moves anterior to the point of contact between femoral condyle and tibial articular surface; as a result, the lateral condyle is pulled back posteriorly **(Fig. 235)** into its normal position (dashed line) and abruptly crosses the apex of the convex lateral tibial articular surface (A) to land (arrow 2) on its sloping posterior surface. The jerk, which can be felt by the patient whenever the knee becomes unstable and by the examiner during the procedure, is caused by the *sudden reduction of the anterior dislocation of the lateral condyle*, which can occur because of **rupture of the posterior cruciate** (in red).

The **test in lateral rotation-valgus-flexion (Fig. 236)** is carried out in the same way, but the *starting position is in full extension*. The jerk felt at 30° flexion **(Fig. 235)** is caused by anterior subluxation (ASL) of the lateral condyle as it jumps abruptly over the apex of the convex lateral tibial surface (A) from its normal position (arrow 2) on the posterior sloping aspect of the tibial surface to an abnormal position (arrow 1) on the anterior sloping aspect of the tibial surface. This can occur because of rupture of the posterior cruciate.

Three further tests allow the diagnosis of a **tear in the posterolateral corner of the knee and of the lateral collateral ligament** in the absence of a ruptured posterior cruciate.

The **posterolateral drawer test of Hughston:** the patient's feet are placed flat on the board with the hips flexed at 45° and the knees at 90°. By sitting on the patient's foot (see **Fig. 202**, p. 129), the examiner is able to keep the knee locked successively in the neutral position, in 15° lateral rotation and then in 15° medial rotation. Holding the upper end of the tibia tightly in both hands, he *tries to elicit a posterior drawer movement in these three positions*. The test is positive when there is posterolateral subluxation of the lateral part of the tibial plateau while the medial part stays put. When the foot is laterally rotated, this produces a **true rotational drawer movement**, which fades as the foot is moved into the position of null rotation and disappears when the foot is medially rotated because of the tension developed in the intact posterior cruciate.

The **lateral hypermobility test of Bousquet** is performed with the knee flexed at 60°. When pressure is applied to the upper end of the tibia in an attempt to displace it below and behind the condyles, a posterior jerk is felt while the foot is being laterally rotated. This is another example of a *genuine lateral rotational drawer movement*.

The **recurvatum-lateral rotation test**, which requires good relaxation of the quadriceps, can be carried out in two ways:

- **In extension:** the two lower limbs, held by the feet, are lifted into extension and the injured limb displays a genu recurvatum and a lateral rotation indicated by lateral displacement of the anterior tibial tuberosity.
- **In flexion:** while one hand supports the foot and gradually extends the knee, the other hand holding the knee can feel the posterolateral subluxation of the tibia manifested by the combination of genu recurvatum, genu varum and lateral displacement of the tibial tuberosity.

All these tests can be difficult to perform on a tense patient when awake but will produce clear-cut results when the patient is under general anaesthesia.

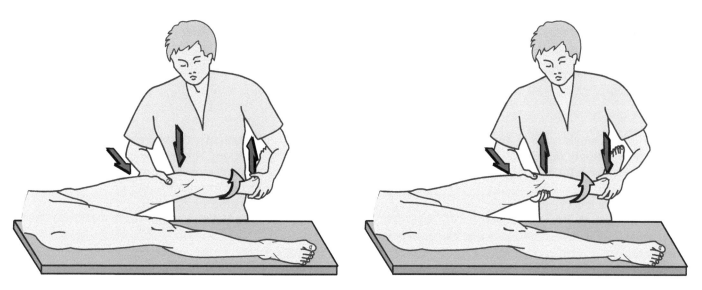

Fig. 233

Fig. 236

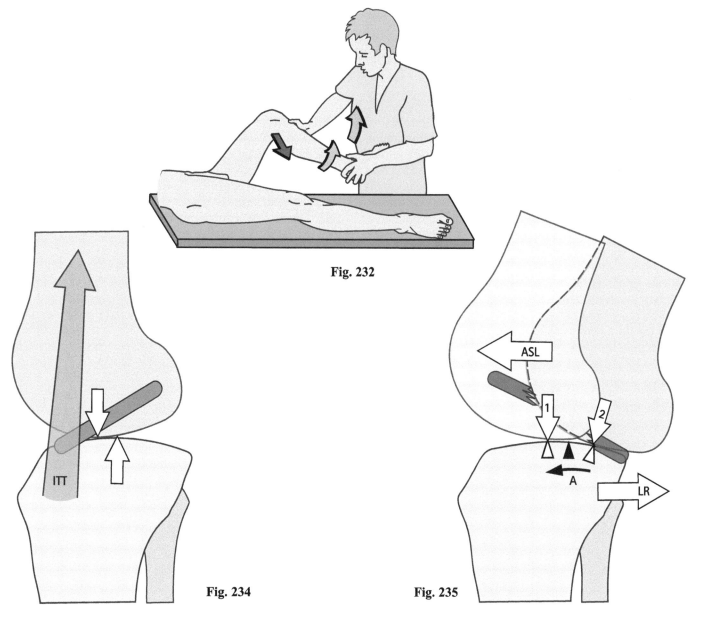

Fig. 232

Fig. 234

Fig. 235

The extensor muscles of the knee

The **quadriceps femoris** is the **extensor muscle of the knee**, and in fact it is the **only muscle** able to extend the knee. It is the **second most powerful** muscle in the body after the gluteus maximus. Its active cross-sectional area is 148 cm², and **with an 8-cm excursion** it develops a force equivalent to 42 kg. It is *three times stronger than the flexors*, since it has to counteract the effect of gravity all the time. We have already seen, however, that when the knee is hyperextended the quadriceps are not required to maintain the erect posture (see p. 114), but, *as soon as any flexion is initiated*, the quadriceps become indispensable and are strongly thrown into action to prevent a fall resulting from knee flexion.

The quadriceps **(Fig. 237)**, as indicated by its name, consist of **four muscles** inserted by a common extensor tendon into the tibial tuberosity (TT):

- three mono-articular muscles: the vastus intermedius (1), the vastus lateralis (2) and the vastus medialis (3);
- one bi-articular muscle, the rectus femoris (4), whose very special physiology will be presented on the next page.

The three mono-articular muscles are *exclusively knee extensors*, but they also have a lateral component of force. More importantly, the vastus medialis is stronger and *descends further than the lateralis*, and its relative predominance is intended to *check any tendency of the patella to dislocate laterally*. The normally balanced contraction of the vasti produces a resultant upward force along the long axis of the thigh, but, if there is an imbalance, e.g. if the lateralis is stronger than a deficient medialis, the patella 'escapes' laterally. This is one of the mechanisms underlying *recurrent dislocation of the patella*, which *always occurs laterally*. Conversely, it is possible to prevent this lateral dislocation by **selectively strengthening the vastus medialis.** The patella is a **sesamoid bone** embedded in the **extensor apparatus of the knee** between the *quadriceps tendon above* and the *patellar ligament below*.

It is an **essential structure** that increases the efficiency of the quadriceps by anteriorly shifting the direction of its muscular pull. This is readily demonstrated using a **parallelogram of forces** with or without the patella.

The force of the quadriceps (Q) applied to the patella (**Fig. 238**: diagram with the patella in place) can be resolved into two vectors:

- a force Q1 acting towards the flexion-extension axis and pressing the patella against the femoral trochlea
- a force Q2 acting along the prolongation of the patellar ligament. In turn Q2, as it acts on the tibial tuberosity, can also be resolved into two orthogonal vectors, i.e. a force Q3, which acts towards the flexion-extension axis and keeps the tibia pressed against the femur, and a tangential force Q4, which is the **only effective extensor component** by *making the tibia slide anteriorly under the femur.*

Let us assume that the patella has been removed (**Fig. 239**: diagram **without** the patella) as in a patellectomy operation, and let us proceed as before. The same force Q now acts tangentially to the femoral trochlea and *directly on the tibial tuberosity*. It can be resolved into two vectors: Q5, a force of coaptation keeping the tibia firmly under the femur, and the tangentially acting Q6, the effective extensor component, now distinctly smaller, while the centripetal component of coaptation Q5 has increased.

If we now compare the effective forces in these two situations (**Fig. 240**: combined diagram), it is clear that Q4 is 50% greater than Q6; hence **the patella, by raising the quadriceps tendon as on a trestle, increases its efficiency.** It is also evident that without the patella the force of coaptation is increased, but this favourable effect is offset by the decrease in the range of flexion secondary to shortening of the extensor apparatus and by its increased susceptibility to injury. **The patella is therefore a very useful structure**, accounting for the rarity and **bad reputation of patellectomy.**

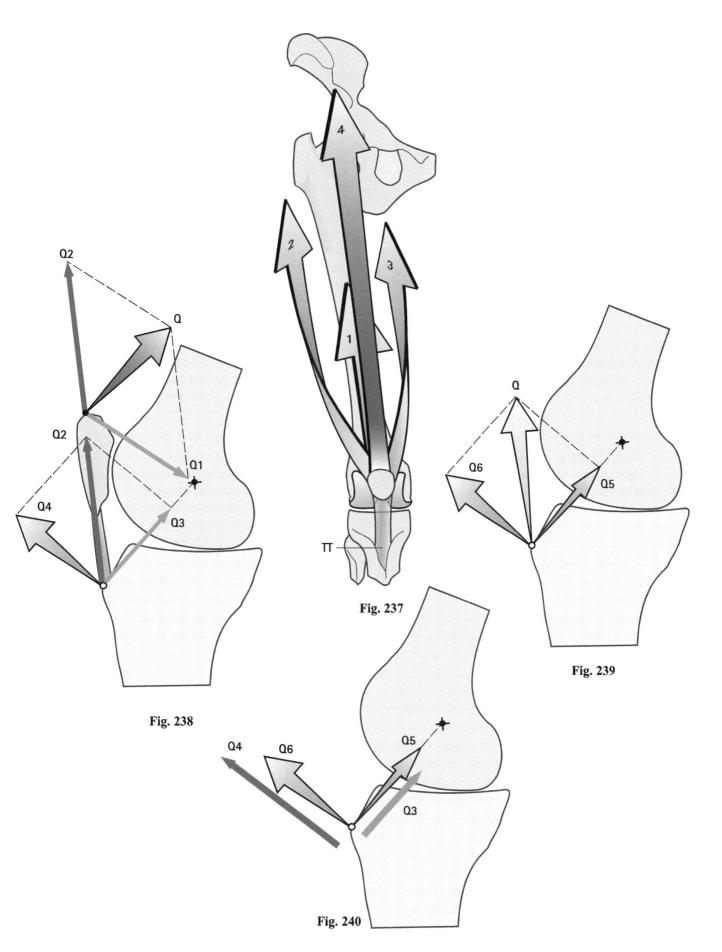

Fig. 238

Fig. 237

Fig. 239

Fig. 240

Physiological actions of the rectus femoris

The **rectus femoris** generates only *one-fifth of the total force of the quadriceps* and cannot by itself produce full extension, but its bi-articular nature gives it *special significance*.

As it runs anterior to the flexion-extension axes of the hip and of the knee, the rectus (red arrow) is at once a hip flexor and a knee extensor (**Fig. 241**: diagram with four positions), but its efficiency as a knee extensor depends on *the position of the hip*, and conversely *its role in hip flexion* depends on *the position of the knee* (**Fig. 242**). This is because the distance between the anterior superior iliac spine (a) and the *superior margin of the femoral trochlea* is shorter (ac) when the hip is in the flexed position II than in the straight position I (ab). This difference in length is due to the *relative* shortening of the muscle when the hip is flexed and the knee flexes passively under the sheer weight of the leg. Under these conditions, *knee extension III is more efficiently produced by the vasti* than by the rectus femoris, which is already relaxed by hip flexion.

On the other hand, if the hip shifts from the straight (I) to the extended (IV) position, the distance between the origin and insertion of the rectus (ad) increases by a length f, and this tenses the muscle. This **relative lengthening** increases its efficiency proportionately. This occurs during running or walking when the *posterior limb provides the propulsive thrust* (**Fig. 245**): the **glutei contract** to *extend* the hip, while the knee and the ankle go into extension. **The power of the quadriceps then reaches its maximum** because of the increased efficiency of the rectus femoris. The **gluteus maximus is therefore an antagonist-synergist of the rectus femoris**, i.e. an antagonist at the hip and a synergist at the knee.

When the swinging limb moves forwards (**Fig. 244**) during the single-limb support phase of walking, the rectus femoris contracts to produce hip flexion and knee extension simultaneously. The bi-articular disposition of this muscle makes it **useful in both phases of walking**, i.e. when the posterior limb provides the propulsive thrust and when the swinging limb moves forwards.

When one gets up from the crouching position, the rectus femoris plays an important role, since it is the only component of the quadriceps *to retain its efficiency* throughout the movement. In fact, as the knee is extended, the hip is also extended by the gluteus maximus, which re-tightens the rectus femoris at its origin, thus maintaining the muscle length constant early in its contraction. This is another example of how the **force** of a powerful muscle located at the root of the limb (the gluteus maximus) can be transferred to a more distal joint via a bi-articular muscle (the rectus femoris).

Conversely, **knee flexion produced by the hamstrings promotes hip flexion through the action of the rectus femoris.** This is useful while jumping with flexed knees (**Fig. 243**) as the recti contribute effectively to flexion of both hips. This is yet another example of antagonism-synergism between the hamstrings (flexors of the knee and extensors of the hip) and the rectus femoris, which flexes the hip and extends the knee.

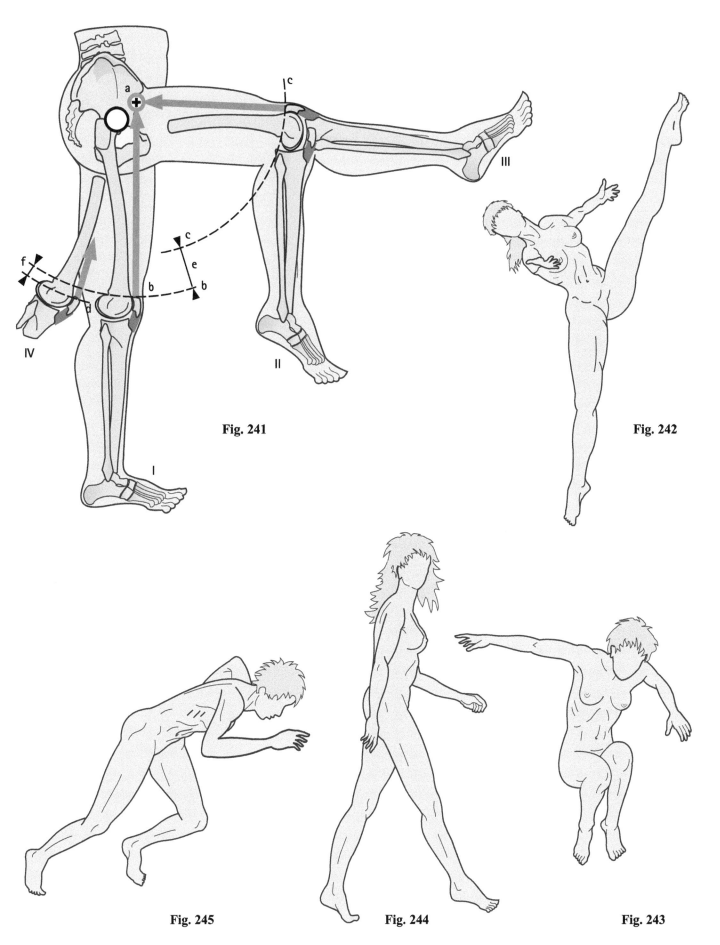

Fig. 241

Fig. 242

Fig. 245

Fig. 244

Fig. 243

The flexor muscles of the knee

The knee flexors are lodged in the *posterior compartment of the thigh* **(Fig. 246)**, and they include the **hamstrings** - the **biceps femoris** (1), the **semitendinosus** (2) and the **semimembranosus** (3); the so-called **anserine muscles** - the **gracilis** (4), the **sartorius** (5) and the **semitendinosus** (which also belongs to the hamstrings); the **popliteus** (see next page); and the **lateral** (6) **and medial heads** (7) **of the gastrocnemius**, which are very weak knee flexors but strong ankle extensors (see p. 212). At the roof of the lower limb can be seen the glutens maximus (8) in the gluteal region.

Nonetheless, the gastrocnemius is an important *knee stabilizer.* Since it takes its origin above the femoral condyles, its contraction during the propulsive phase of the step, i.e. when both the knee and the ankle extend simultaneously, displaces the condyles forwards. It is thus an **antagonist-synergist of the quadriceps.** All these muscles are bi-articular, with two exceptions, i.e. the short head of the biceps femoris and the popliteus, which are both mono-articular (see next page). The bi-articular flexors *extend the hip* simultaneously, and their action on the knee *depends on the position of the hip.*

The **sartorius** (5) is a hip flexor, abductor and lateral rotator and at the same time flexes and medially rotates the knee.

The **gracilis** (4) is a primary adductor and an accessory flexor of the hip, while being also a flexor and a medial rotator of the hip (see p. 148).

The **hamstrings** are both *hip extensors* (see p. 44) and *knee extensors*, and their action depends on the position of the hip **(Fig. 247)**. When the hip is flexed, the distance **ab** between the origins and insertions of these muscles increases regularly, since the centre of the hip joint O, around which the femur rotates, does not coincide with the point of rotation of the hamstrings. Thus as flexion proceeds the hamstrings become relatively longer and *more stretched.* When the hip is flexed at 40° (position II) their relative lengthening can still be offset by passive knee flexion (ab = ab') but, when hip flexion reaches 90° (position III), their relative lengthening is so great that it persists as a significant relative lengthening (f). If hip flexion exceeds 90° (position IV), it becomes very difficult to keep the knee in full extension **(Fig. 248)**, and their relative lengthening (g) is almost totally absorbed by their elasticity, which decreases markedly with lack of exercise. (In position IV knee flexion slackens the hamstrings by bringing back their tibial insertion from position d to position d'.) The tensing up of the hamstrings by hip flexion increases their efficiency as knee flexors when, during *climbing* **(Fig. 249)**, one lower limb swings forwards, and *hip flexion promotes knee flexion.* Conversely, *knee extension promotes hip extension* by the hamstrings: this occurs when one tries to straighten the trunk bent forwards **(Fig. 248)** and also during **climbing** when the previously anterior limb becomes the posterior limb.

If the hip **(Fig. 247)** is fully extended (position V) the hamstrings undergo *relative shortening* (e) with the result that they become weaker knee flexors (see Figure 13, p. 73). These observations stress the usefulness of the monoarticular muscles (popliteus and short head of biceps), which retain the same efficiency regardless of hip position. The aggregate force exerted by the knee flexors is 15 kg, i.e. just over one-third that of the quadriceps.

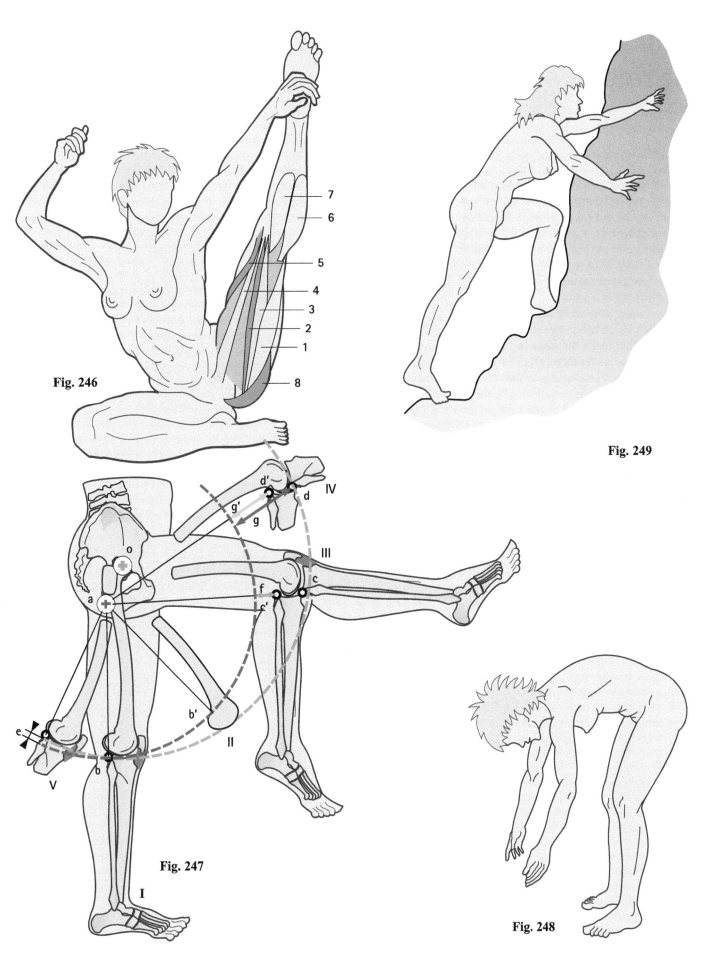

Fig. 246

7
6
5
4
3
2
1
8

Fig. 247

I
II
III
IV
V

a
b
b'
c
c'
d
d'
e
f
g
g'
o

Fig. 249

Fig. 248

147

The rotator muscles of the knee

The knee flexors are also knee rotators and fall into **two groups** depending on their sites of insertion into the bones of the leg (**Fig. 250**: posteromedial view of flexed knee):

- those attached *lateral to the vertical axis* xx' of rotation of the knee, i.e. the **lateral rotators** (**LR**) including (**Fig. 253**) the **biceps femoris** (1) and the **tensor fasciae latae** (2). When these muscles (A) pull posteriorly the lateral part of the tibial plateau (**Fig. 251**: superior view of the tibial plateau), they cause it to rotate in such a way that the tip of the foot *faces more directly laterally*. The **tensor fasciae latae** becomes a flexor-rotator only when the knee is already flexed; with the knee fully extended it *loses its rotator action and becomes an extensor* that **locks the knee in extension**. The **short head (1) of the biceps femoris** (**Fig. 254**: lateral view of the flexed knee) is the *only monoarticular lateral rotator of the knee*, and therefore its action is not affected by the position of the hip.

- those attached *medial to the vertical axis xx'* of rotation of the knee, i.e. **the medial rotators** (MR) represented (**Fig. 253**) by the **sartorius** (3), the **semitendinosus** (4), the **semimembranosus** (5), the **gracilis** (6) and the **popliteus** (7) (**Fig. 254**). When they pull (B) the medial part of the tibial plateau posteriorly (**Fig. 252**: superior view of the tibial plateau), they cause it to rotate so that the tip of the foot looks *medially*. They act as *brakes of lateral rotation when the knee is flexed* and thus protect the joint capsule and its ligaments when they are violently thrown into action during a violent turn to the side opposite the supporting limb. The **popliteus** (7) (**Fig. 256**, posterior view) is the only exception to this general mode of muscle arrangement. Arising by tendon from the lower end of the popliteal groove

on the lateral surface of the lateral femoral condyle, it soon penetrates the knee capsule *(still outside the synovium)* to run between the lateral collateral ligament and the lateral meniscus (**Fig. 254**). It sends a *fibrous expansion to the posterior edge of the lateral meniscus* and then emerges from the capsule under cover of the arcuate popliteal ligament (see also **Fig. 161**, p. 115) before reaching its insertion into the posterior surface of the upper extremity of the tibia. It is the *only monoarticular medial rotator of the knee*. Its action is thus independent of the position of the hip and can be visualized readily on a superior view of the tibial plateau (**Fig. 255**: popliteus as **blue arrow**); it pulls the posterior part of the tibial plateau posteriorly and laterally.

Although it lies behind the knee joint, the popliteus is a *knee extensor*. During flexion, its origin from the femoral condyle shifts superiorly and anteriorly (**Fig. 254**) and stretches the muscle, thus increasing its power as a medial rotator. Conversely, when the knee is flexed and *a fortiori* when it is laterally rotated, its contraction pulls its site of origin *inferiorly and posteriorly*, causing the *lateral femoral condyle to slide into the direction of extension*. The **popliteus** is therefore both an **extensor and a medial rotator of the knee**.

The global force of the medial rotators is only marginally greater (2 kg) than that of the external rotators (1.8 kg).

If one compares the knee with the elbow (its homologue in the upper limb), the knee, unlike the elbow, is the seat not only of flexion but also of axial rotation, thus explaining why none of the motor muscles of the toes have their origins on the femur, and, as a result, do not "cross" the knee joint.

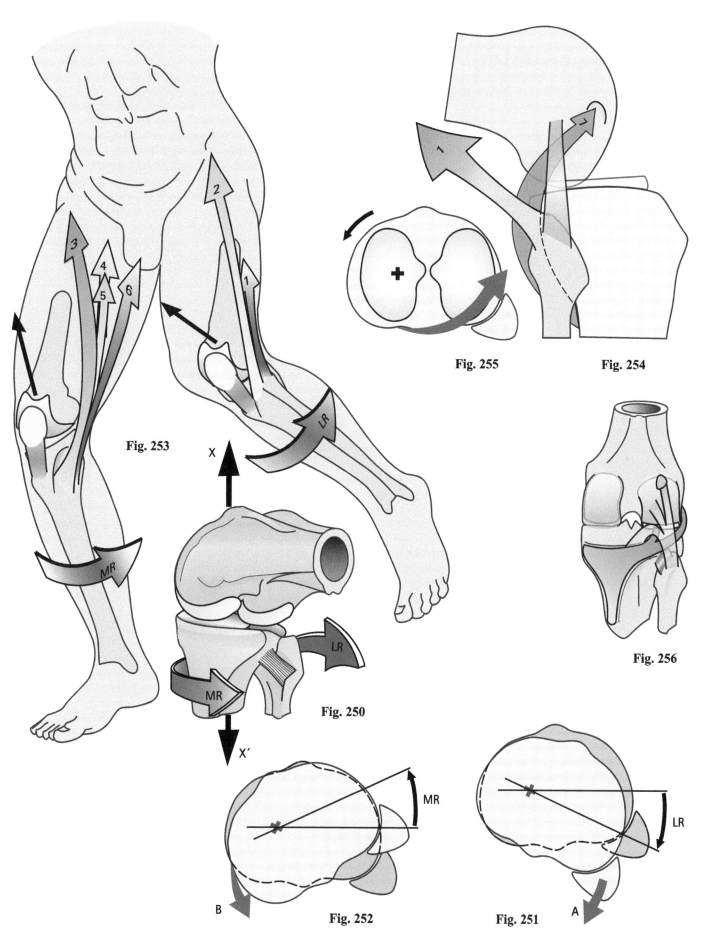

Fig. 253

Fig. 255

Fig. 254

Fig. 256

Fig. 250

Fig. 252

Fig. 251

Automatic rotation of the knee

We have already seen (p. 74) that the final phase of extension is accompanied by a small measure of lateral rotation and that the start of flexion is always combined with some medial rotation of the leg and the foot. These movements of rotation *occur automatically*, i.e. without any conscious desire to rotate the knee. This **automatic rotation** can be displayed on an anatomical preparation based on Roud's *experiment* as follows:

- With the **knee in extension** (**Fig. 257**: superior view of the extended knee), start by driving **two parallel and horizontal pins** in the coronal plane, one into the upper end of the tibia (t) and the other into the lower end of the femur (f).
- If the **femur is flexed at** 90° (**Fig. 258**: superior view of the flexed knee) these two pins are no longer parallel because of the rotation of the femur on the tibia but now form an angle of 30°.
- This becomes evident when the **femoral axis is repositioned in a sagittal plane** (**Fig. 259**): the tibial pin is now oriented mediolaterally and posteroanteriorly, indicating a **medial rotation of the tibia** under the femur, and forms a **20° angle** with the normal to the femoral axis. Therefore knee flexion is coupled with a **20° automatic medial rotation.** This 10° discrepancy occurs because, owing to the physiological valgus, the femoral pin is not perpendicular to the shaft axis but forms an 80° angle (V) with it (see **Fig. 3**, p. 69).
- This experiment can be performed *in reverse*: in the initial position of 90° flexion the pins are divergent (**Fig. 258**), whereas in full extension they are parallel to each other (**Fig. 257**). This shows that **knee extension is automatically coupled with lateral rotation.**

This occurs because the *femoral lateral condyle recedes farther than the medial condyle* during knee flexion (**Fig. 260**: superior view of the tibial plateau) causing the tibia to rotate medially. In the extended knee, the contact points **a** and **b** lie on a transverse axis Ox. During flexion, the medial condyle recedes from a to a' (5-6 mm), while the lateral condyle recedes from b to b' (10-12 mm), and the contact points a' and b' during flexion lie along Oy, which forms a 20° angle xOy with Ox. This differential excursion of the two condyles on the tibial plateau is the cause of the 20° lateral rotation of the tibia during extension.

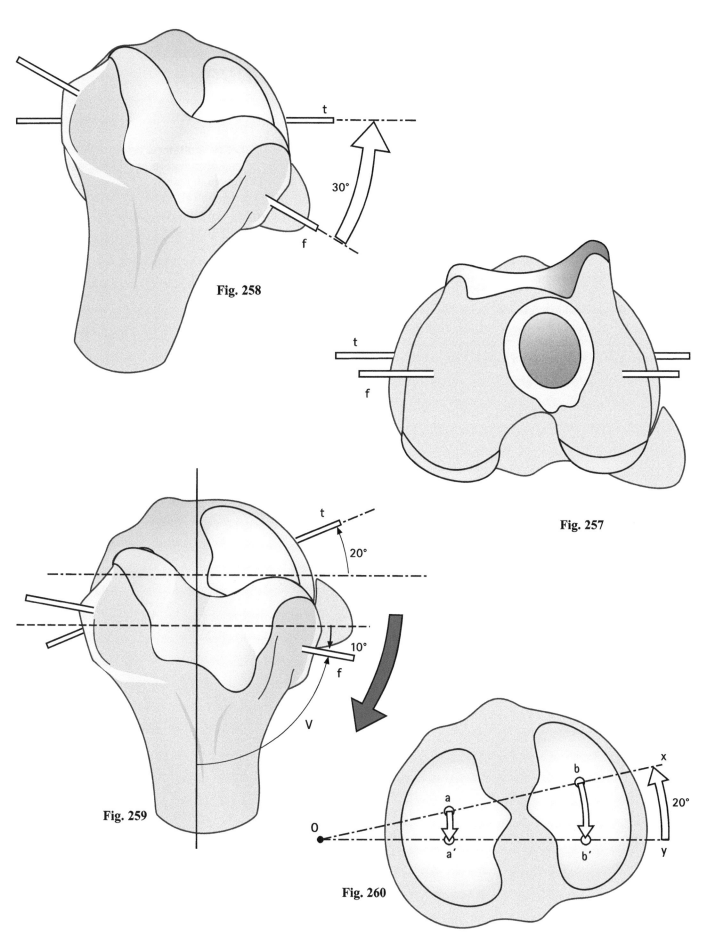

Fig. 258

Fig. 257

Fig. 259

Fig. 260

Automatic rotation of the knee (*continued*)

This differential recession of the condyles is due to **three factors**:

1. The **unequal lengths of the femoral condylar profiles (Figs 261 and 262)**. If the articular surfaces of the medial **(Fig. 261)** and lateral **(Fig. 262)** are rolled out and measured, it is clear that the rolled-out posterior curved surface of the lateral condyle (bd') definitely exceeds that of the medial condyle (assuming that ac' = bc'). This observation partly explains why the *lateral condyle slides over a greater distance than the medial condyle.*

2. The **shape of the tibial articular surfaces**. The medial condyle recedes only a little because it is contained inside a concave surface **(Fig. 263)**, whereas the lateral condyle slides over the posterior border of a concave lateral surface **(Fig. 264)**.

3. The **orientation of the collateral ligaments.**
When the femoral condyles recede on the tibial surfaces, the medial collateral ligament tightens more quickly **(Fig. 263)** than its lateral counterpart, which allows the lateral condyle to recede farther because of its obliquity.

There are also two **rotational force couples** induced by:
- the predominant action of the flexors-internal rotators **(Fig. 265)**, i.e. the anserine muscles (green arrows) and the popliteus (blue arrow)
- the tension in the anterior cruciate (yellow arrow) at the end of extension **(Fig. 266)**: as the ligament comes to lie lateral to the joint axis, this tension produces lateral rotation.

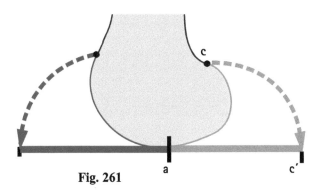

Fig. 261

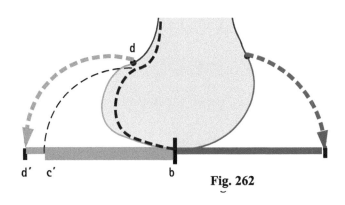

Fig. 262

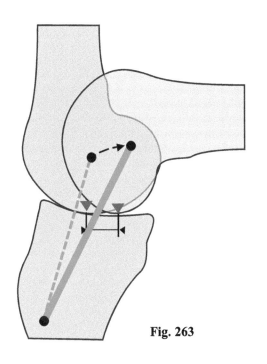

Fig. 263

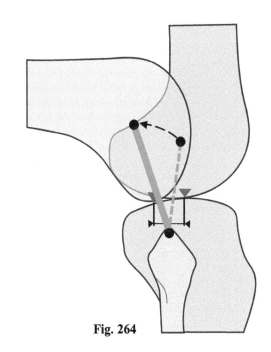

Fig. 264

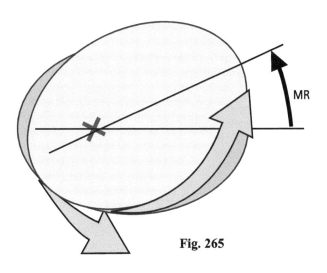

Fig. 265

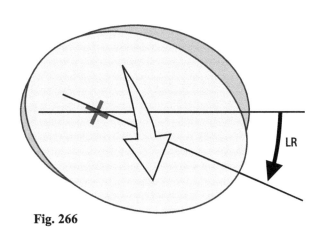

Fig. 266

Dynamic equilibrium of the knee

At the end of this chapter, the stability of this loosely interlocked joint appears to be an **unending miracle.** For this reason, we have tried to provide a **synoptic diagram (Fig. 267)** that correlates the main clinical tests with the underlying anatomical structures: each pointer line corresponds to a possible cause. The choice and the interpretation of these tests, based on recent publications, may be debatable, but *their classification is offered here as purely provisional.*

1. The direct anterior drawer test in null rotation can be weakly positive in normal subjects, and comparison with the presumably normal side is essential. When it is clearly positive (+), it indicates *rupture of the anterior cruciate.* When it is very strongly positive, it indicates *combined rupture of the medial collateral and anterior cruciate ligaments.* Beware, however, of a false positive produced by the *spontaneous reduction of a posterior subluxation* due to rupture of the posterior cruciate…!

2. The anterior drawer test at 15° medial rotation, when positive, is a sure sign of *rupture of the anterior cruciate,* which may be coupled with tearing of the posterolateral corner of the knee.

3. The anterior drawer test at 30° medial rotation, when positive, indicates a *combined rupture of both cruciate ligaments* and, if a *jerk* is also detected, there is also *detachment of the posterior horn of the lateral meniscus.*

4. The lateral Jerk Test in valgus-medial rotation-flexion (the *lateral pivot shift test of MacIntosh)* and the *Jerk Test of Hughston* are diagnostic of *anterior cruciate* rupture.

5. The anterior drawer test in lateral rotation, when moderately positive (+), indicates a tear in the posterolateral corner of the knee and, if associated with a jerk, it indicates *concurrent detachment of the posterior horn of the medial meniscus.*

6. The posterior drawer test in null rotation (the *direct posterior drawer test)* is a sure sign of *rupture of the posterior cruciate.*

7. The lateral Jerk Test in valgus-external rotation-extension (the *pivot shift reverse test)* and the **lateral Jerk Test in valgus-external rotation-flexion** indicate *rupture of the posterior cruciate.*

8. The posterior drawer test in lateral rotation indicates a lesion of the posterolateral corner with or without *rupture of the posterior cruciate.*

9. The posterior drawer test in medial rotation could be a specific sign of *rupture of the posterior cruciate associated with a tear in the posteromedial corner of the knee.*

10. Valgus movement in extension, causing a slight degree of valgus (+), indicates rupture of the *medial collateral ligament.* When the valgus is moderate (++) it indicates a lesion of the *medial condylar plate;* when the valgus is severe (+++), there is also a *rupture of the anterior cruciate.*

11. Valgus movement in slight flexion (10-30°) indicates a *combined rupture of the medial collateral ligament,* of the *medial condylar plate and of the posterolateral corner of the knee* associated with injury to the *posterior horn of the lateral meniscus.*

12. Varus movement in extension, when associated with a moderate degree of varus (+), indicates *rupture of the lateral collateral ligament* with or without *concurrent rupture of the iliotibial tract.* When the varus is severe, there is an *associated rupture of the lateral condylar plate and of the posterolateral corner of the knee.*

13. Varus movement in slight flexion (10-30°) indicates the same lesions as in 12, but without *rupture of the iliotibial* tract.

14. The recurvatum-lateral rotation-valgus test and also *the big toe suspension test* indicate *rupture of the lateral collateral ligament and of the posterolateral corner.*

To understand the mechanics of the knee, one must realize that the active knee is in **dynamic equilibrium** and, above all, one must forgo the idea of *a bifactorial equilibrium* as illustrated by the two plates of a balance. Rather, *windsurfing* **(Fig. 268)** provides a better analogy illustrating a **trifactorial equilibrium:**

- the *sea,* supporting the surfboard, corresponds to the action of the *articular surfaces*
- the *surfer,* steering the board by his *non-stop muscular reactions to the wind and the sea, corresponds to the periarticular muscles*
- the *sail,* the recipient of the force of the wind, corresponds to the *ligamentous complex.*

At all times, the movements of the knee are determined by the **mutual and balanced interactions of these factors,** i.e. articular surfaces, muscles and ligaments an example of a **trifactorial equilibrium.**

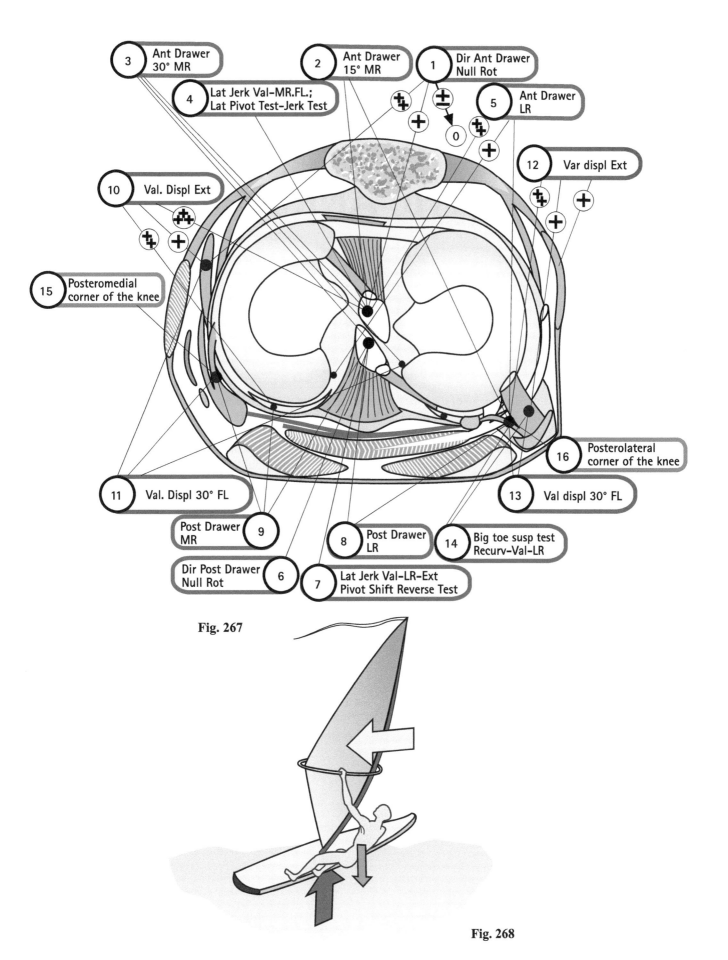

3 Ant Drawer 30° MR

2 Ant Drawer 15° MR

1 Dir Ant Drawer Null Rot

4 Lat Jerk Val-MR.FL.; Lat Pivot Test-Jerk Test

5 Ant Drawer LR

12 Var displ Ext

10 Val. Displ Ext

15 Posteromedial corner of the knee

16 Posterolateral corner of the knee

11 Val. Displ 30° FL

13 Val displ 30° FL

9 Post Drawer MR

8 Post Drawer LR

14 Big toe susp test Recurv-Val-LR

6 Dir Post Drawer Null Rot

7 Lat Jerk Val-LR-Ext Pivot Shift Reverse Test

Fig. 267

Fig. 268

Chapter 3

THE ANKLE

The ankle or talocrural joint is the distal joint of the lower limb. It is a **hinge joint** and has therefore only one degree of freedom. It controls the movements of the leg in the sagittal plane relative to the foot. These movements are essential for walking normally on flat or rough ground.

It is a tightly interlocked joint exposed to extreme mechanical stresses during single-limb support, when it is subjected to the full weight of the body and to the force generated by the dissipation of kinetic energy when the foot rapidly makes contact with the ground during walking, running or jumping. It also supports weights that may be carried by the upper limbs or the trunk (on the shoulders). It is thus easy to imagine the problems involved in the production of total ankle prostheses with guaranteed long-term reliability.

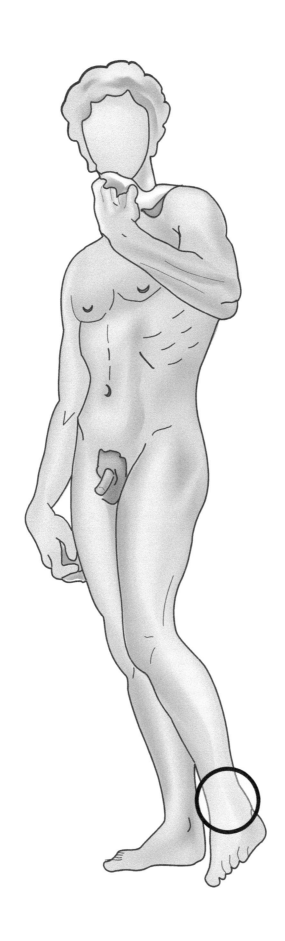

The articular complex of the foot

In fact, the ankle is only the most important or the 'queen' (in Farabeuf's words) of the **entire articular complex of the hindfoot.** This set of joints, assisted by axial rotation of the knee, is equivalent to a single joint with three degrees of freedom and allows the **plantar vault to assume any position in space** in response to any irregularity of the ground. There is a certain similarity with the upper limb, where the articular complex of the wrist, assisted by pronation-supination, allows the hand to assume any position in space, but the *foot enjoys a much more limited range of orientations than the hand.*

The **three main axes** of this joint complex **(Fig. 1)** converge roughly on the hindfoot. When the foot is in the reference position, these three axes are orthogonal. In the diagram, ankle extension changes the direction of the Z axis, while the other two axes remain stationary.

The **transverse axis XX'** passes through the two malleoli and corresponds to the **axis of the ankle joint.** It lies almost entirely in the coronal plane and controls the movements of **flexion and extension** of the foot (see p. 160) that occur in the **sagittal plane.**

The **long axis of the leg Y** is vertical and controls the movements of **adduction and abduction** of the foot occurring in a transverse plane. As shown previously (p. 74) these movements are possible only because of the axial rotation of the flexed knee. To a lesser degree they depend on the joints of the *posterior tarsus*, but they are always combined with movements around the third axis.

The **long axis of the foot Z** is horizontal and *lies in a sagittal plane.* It controls the orientation of the foot and allows it to face directly inferiorly, whether laterally or medially. By analogy with the upper limb, these movements are called **pronation** and **supination**, respectively.

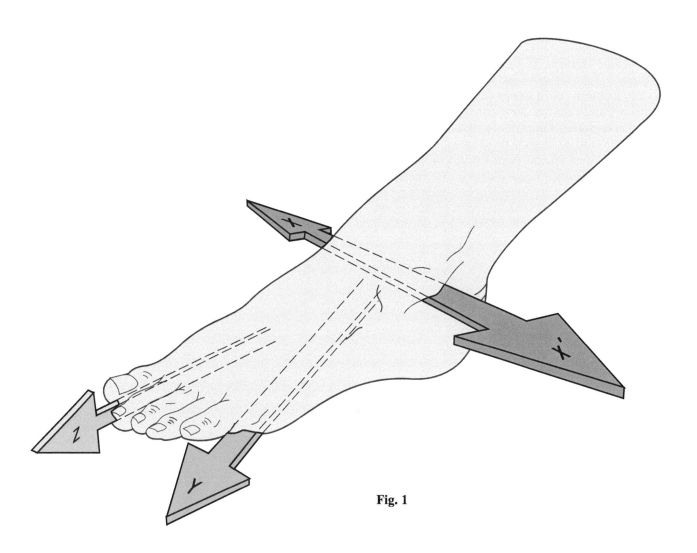

Fig. 1

Flexion-extension

The **reference position (Fig. 2)** is achieved when the sole of the foot is perpendicular to the axis of the leg (A). From this position, **ankle flexion** (B) is defined as the movement that *brings the dorsum of the foot closer to the anterior surface of the leg*. It is also wrongly called dorsal flexion or dorsiflexion, but this is redundant terminology.

Conversely, **ankle extension** (C) moves the foot away from the anterior surface of the leg and tends to bring it into alignment with the leg. It is also called plantar flexion, but **this term is inappropriate**, since flexion corresponds to a distoproximal movement that brings the segments of a limb towards the trunk. Furthermore, it would be illogical for extensor muscles to produce flexion. The term *plantar flexion* deserves to be banned for it is self-contradictory.

In the diagram it is clear that *the range of extension is distinctly greater than that of flexion.* To measure these angles the centre of the ankle joint is not used as the reference point, since it is simpler to measure the **angle between the sole of the foot and the axis of the leg (Fig. 3)**:

- When this *angle is acute* (b), **flexion** is present with a range of 30-50°. The pink zone indicates the margin of individual variations, i.e. 10°.

When the *angle is obtuse* (c), **extension** is present with a range of 30-50°. The margin of individual variations (blue-tinted zone) is larger (20°) than that for flexion.

During extreme movements, the ankle is not the only joint involved: **the tarsal joints contribute their own individual ranges of movement**, which are smaller without being negligible.

- During **extreme flexion (Fig. 4)**, the tarsal joints contribute a few degrees (+) as the plantar vault flattens.
- Conversely, during **extreme extension (Fig. 5)** the additional increase in range (+) results from arching of the vault.

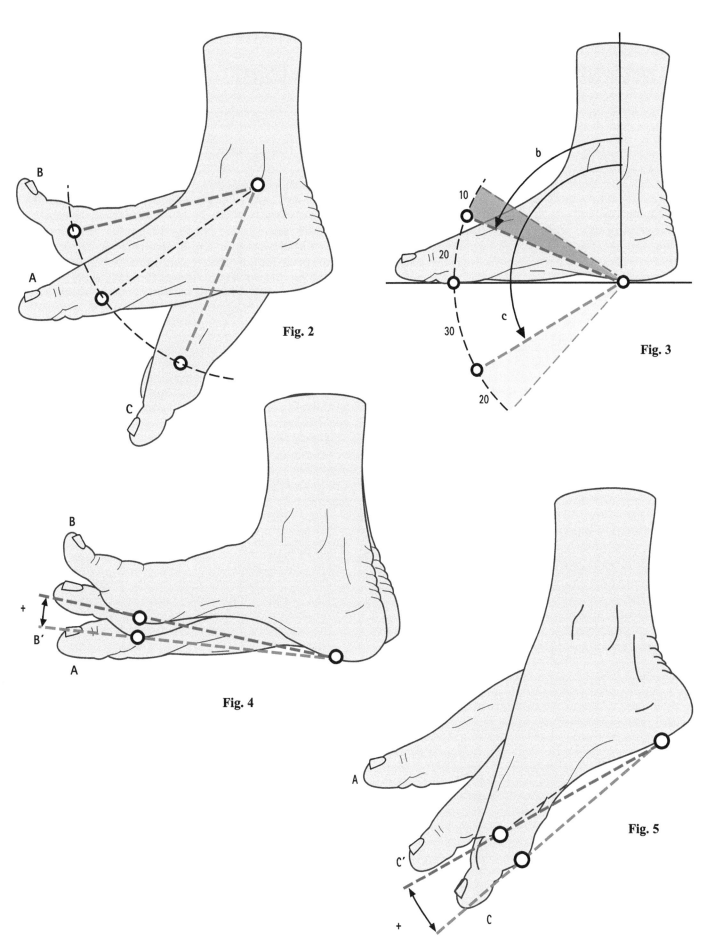

Fig. 2

Fig. 3

Fig. 4

Fig. 5

The articular surfaces of the ankle joint

If the ankle is compared to a **mechanical model (Fig. 6)** it can be described as being composed of the following:

- a *lower piece* (A), the talus, which bears on its superior surface a convex cylindrical structure with a long axis XX running transversely
- an *upper piece* (B), the distal ends of the tibia and of the fibula, forming a single structure (shown here as transparent), whose inferior concave surface contains a segment of a cylinder similar to the one mentioned above.

The *solid cylinder, encased within the segment of the hollow cylinder*, is kept in place laterally by the sides of the upper piece and can perform movements of flexion (blue arrow) and extension (red arrow) around the common axis XX'.

In the actual **skeleton (Fig. 7:** anteromedial view of the 'dismantled' ankle; **Fig. 8:** posterolateral view of the 'dismantled' ankle) the solid cylinder corresponds to the **talar trochlea** with its three surfaces, i.e. a *superior surface* and *two lateral surfaces or cheeks*.

- The **superior surface** or the trochlea proper, convex anteroposteriorly, is depressed centrally by a longitudinal groove (1) with its medial (2) and lateral (3) lips, each edged by one cheek of the trochlea.
- The **medial cheek** (7) is almost flat except anteriorly, where it is inclined medially and is separated from the medial lip of the trochlea (2) by a sharp ridge (11). It articulates with the facet on the lateral surface of the **medial malleolus** (9), which is lined by articular cartilage continuous with that lining the inferior surface of the distal tibia (10).
- The **lateral cheek** (12) is markedly lopsided on its outer aspect **(Fig. 8)** and is concave superoinferiorly **(Fig. 11,** p. 165) and also anteroposteriorly **(Fig. 9,** p. 165). It lies in a slightly oblique plane running anterolaterally. It is in contact with the articular facet (13) on the medial surface **(Fig. 7)**

of the **lateral malleolus** (14). This facet is separated from the tibia by the **interspace of the tibiofibular joint** (15), filled by a synovial fold (16) (see p. 174), which is in contact with the ridge (17) separating the lateral lip from the lateral cheek of the trochlea. This ridge is *bevelled anteriorly* (18) *and posteriorly* (19) (see **Fig. 12**, p. 165). This joint, which is a syndesmosis, is kept in place by the anterior (27) and the posterior (28) tibiofibular ligaments.

The pulley-shaped surface of the talar trochlea corresponds to **an inversely shaped surface on the inferior surface of the distal tibia (Figs 7 and 8)**, which is concave anteroposteriorly **(Fig. 12**, p. 165: sagittal section, lateral view) and contains a blunt sagittal ridge (4) that is bounded posteriorly by the edge of the inferior surface of the distal tibia (10) and sinks into the trochlear groove **(Fig. 11:** coronal section, anterior view), On either side of the ridge, there is a groove, one **medial** (5) and one **lateral** (6), each of which accommodates the corresponding cheek of the trochlea.

This tibial articular surface is bounded posteriorly by the edge of the distal tibia (20), which is also known as *Destot's third malleolus*.

The **lateral ligaments of the ankle joint** are visible in Figure 7 (anteromedial view):

- the anterior talofibular ligament (21)
- the lateral calcaneofibular ligament (22)
- the posterior talofibular ligament (23).

The **medial ligaments of the ankle joint** are visible in Figure 8 (posteromedial view), arranged in a deep and a superficial layer:

- the posterior tibiofibular ligament (24), lying deep
- the anterior tibiofibular ligament (25), lying deep
- the superficial fibres of the deltoid ligament (26), lying superficial.

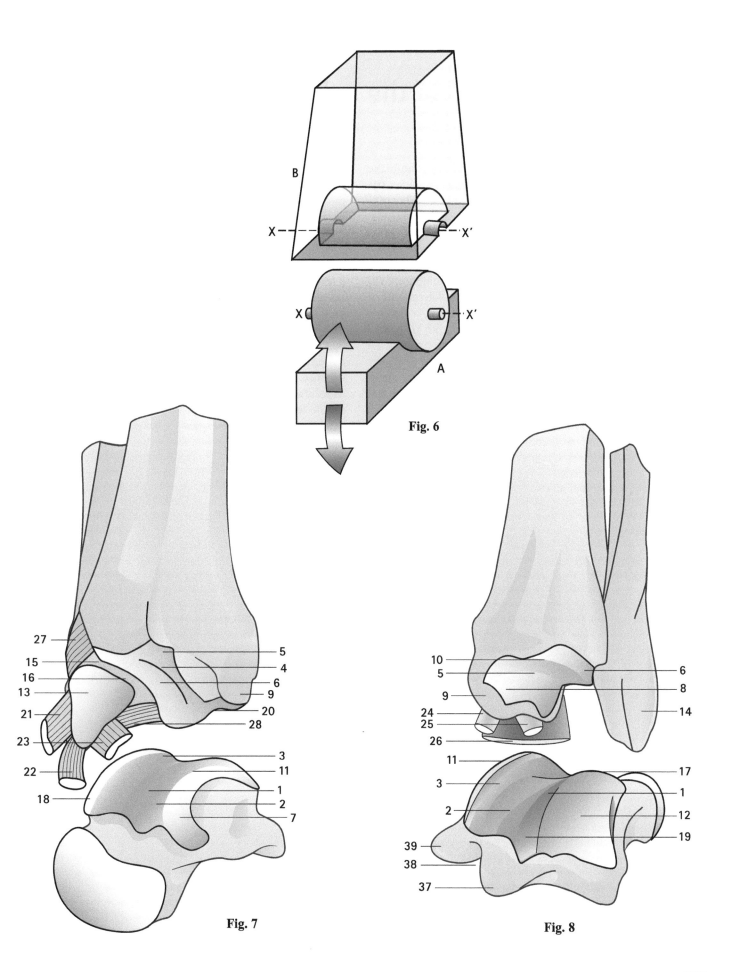

Fig. 6

Fig. 7

Fig. 8

The articular surfaces of the ankle joint (*continued*)

A **superior view** of the ankle joint transected through the malleoli **(Fig. 9)** illustrates perfectly how the talar trochlea **fits snugly** between the two malleoli, i.e. inside the **bimalleolar pincers.** Visible also is the **superior surface of the talar trochlea,** which is wider anteriorly (A) than posteriorly (P). This observation is of great mechanical significance, as will be demonstrated later. This pulley-shaped superior surface has a **medial facet** (2), which forms part of the medial half of the ankle joint (5) and a **lateral facet** (3), which forms part of the lateral half of the ankle joint (6). These two facets are separated by a shallow groove (1), which is not strictly sagittal but is slightly displaced anteriorly and laterally (arrow Z), i.e. in the same direction as the long axis of the foot, whereas the talar neck is directed anteriorly and medially (arrow T). As a result the talus is twisted on itself. The **medial cheek** (7) of the talar trochlea, seen in a medial view of the talus **(Fig. 10),** is sagittal **(Fig. 9)** and practically flat except anteriorly, where it is displaced medially **(Fig. 7).** It articulates **(Fig. 9)** with the articular facet on the lateral aspect of the medial malleolus, which is coated with cartilage continuous with that coating the medial surface of the distal tibia; these two surfaces form a **dihedral angle** (10), which accommodates the **sharp ridge** (11) lying between the medial lip and the medial cheek of the trochlea.

The **lateral** cheek (12), markedly distorted outwards **(Fig. 8),** is concave superiorly **(Fig. 11)** and also anteroposteriorly **(Fig. 9),** and it lies in a plane slightly oblique anteriorly and laterally (broken line). It articulates with the articular facet (13) of the medial surface **(Fig. 7)** of the **lateral malleolus** (14). This facet is separated from the tibial articular facet by the distal tibiofibular **syndesmosis** (15), which is kept in place by the inferior tibiofibular ligaments (40) and is filled by a synovial fold (16) (see also p. 174) in contact with the ridge (17) separating the lateral lip from the lateral cheek of the trochlea. This ridge is bevelled **(Fig. 12)** anteriorly (18) and posteriorly (19), so that only its central part is sharp (see p. 172).

The two cheeks of the talar trochlea are thus tightly kept in place by the malleoli (red arrows). The combination of the tibial distal extremity and the two malleoli is also called the **tibio-fibular mortise.** The characteristics of the malleoli differ symmetrically, as follows:

- the lateral malleolus is *larger* than the medial malleolus;
- it extends *farther distally* m **(Fig. 11)** than the medial malleolus;
- it lies *more posteriorly* **(Fig. 9)** than the medial malleolus **(Fig. 9),** with the result that it lies sightly obliquely (at an angle of 20°) lateral and posterior to the axis XX'.

The term *Destot's third malleolus* **(Fig. 12)** is also applied to the posterior border of the distal tibia (20), which extends farther distally (p) than the anterior border.

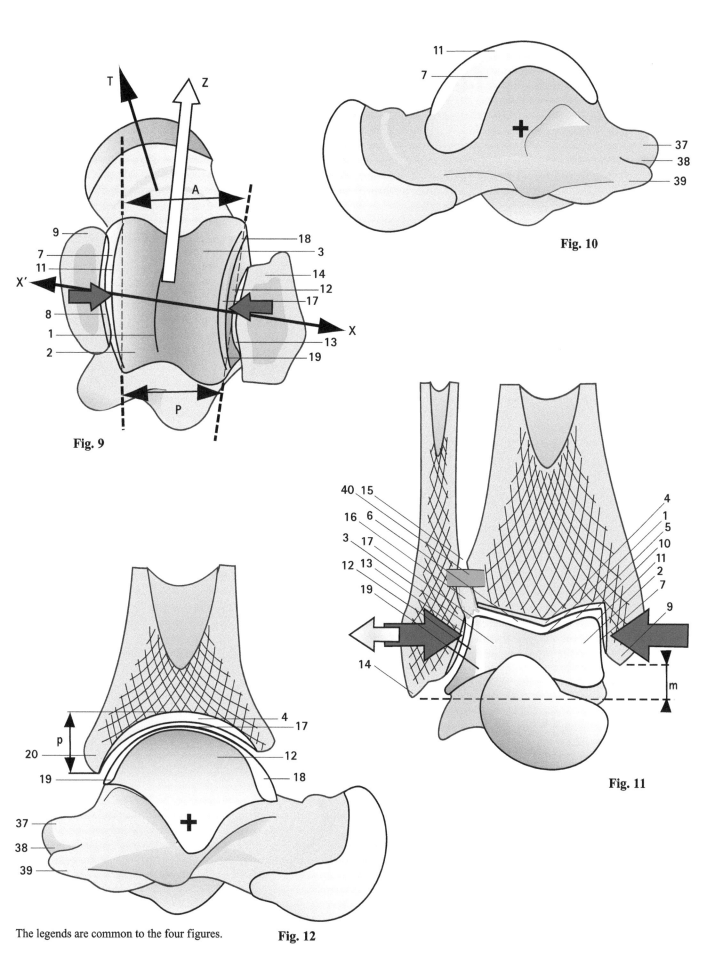

Fig. 9

Fig. 10

Fig. 11

Fig. 12

The legends are common to the four figures.

The ligaments of the ankle joint

The ligaments of the ankle joint consist of two main ligamentous systems, i.e. **the lateral and medial collateral ligaments** and two accessory ligamentous systems, i.e. **the anterior and posterior ligaments.**

The collateral ligaments form on either side of the joint two strong *fan-like fibrous structures*, which are attached above at their apices to the corresponding malleolus near the flexion-extension axis XX′ and which radiate out distally to be inserted into the two bones of the posterior tarsus.

The **lateral collateral ligament (Fig. 13**, lateral view) is made up of **three distinct bands:** two attached to the talus and one attached to the calcaneus.

- The **anterior talofibular ligament** (21), attached to the anterior border of the lateral malleolus (14) runs obliquely inferiorly and anteriorly to be inserted into the talus between the lateral cheek of the trochlear surface and the entrance to the sinus tarsi.

- The **calcaneofibular ligament** (22), arising close to the apex of the lateral malleolus, crosses obliquely inferiorly and posteriorly to its insertion in the lateral surface of the calcaneus. The lateral talocalcanean ligament (32) runs along its inferior border.

- The **posterior talofibular ligament** (23), arising from the medial surface of the lateral malleolus (see **Fig. 7**, p. 163) behind the articular facet, runs horizontally, medially and slightly posteriorly to insert into the lateral tubercle of the talus (37). Because of its location and direction it is more readily seen from behind **(Fig. 14)**. It is continuous with the tiny posterior talocalcanean ligament (31), which classical French authors used to call the 'interosseous hedge' (h).

From the lateral malleolus spring the **two ligaments of the inferior tibiofibular joint (Figs 14 and 15)**: the anterior (27) and the posterior (28), whose role will be discussed later.

The **medial collateral ligament (Fig. 16**, medial view) breaks up into two fibrous sheets, a deep and a superficial.

The **deep fibrous sheet** consists of two talotibial bundles:

The **anterior tibiotalar ligament** (25) runs obliquely inferiorly and anteriorly to be attached to the medial limb of the talar 'yoke'* (seen as transparent in the diagram, **Fig. 16** and also in **Fig. 15**).

The **posterior talotibial ligament** (24) runs obliquely inferiorly and posteriorly to gain insertion into a deep fossa **(Fig. 10)** on the medial cheek of the talar trochlea with its most posterior fibres extending to the medial tubercle (39).

The broad triangular **superficial sheet** makes up the **deltoid ligament** (26). In Figure 15 (anterior view) the deep fibres of the deltoid ligament have been notched and retracted to *reveal its deep anterior bundle* (25), and in Figure 16 (medial view) it is shown as *transparent*. From its tibial origin (36) it fans out *to be inserted along a continuous line* into the navicular bone (33), the medial border of the plantar calcaneonavicular ligament (34) and the sustentaculum tali of the calcaneus (35). Thus this ligament, like the calcaneofibular ligament, is not tethered to the talus.

The **anterior (Fig. 15**, superior view) **and the posterior (Fig. 14**, posterior view) **collateral ligaments** of the ankle are simply localized condensations of the capsule:

- The **anterior ligament** (29) runs obliquely from the anterior margin of the distal tibia to the posterolateral limb of the talar 'yoke' **(Fig. 13)**.

- The **posterior ligament** (30) consists of fibres that start from the tibia and fibula and converge towards their insertion into the medial tubercle of the posterior process of the talus (39), which, along with the *lateral tubercle* of the talus (37), forms the *deep groove for the flexor hallucis longus* (38). This groove is seen to continue distally along the inferior surface of the sustentaculum tali (41).

---

* The talar 'yoke' is a Y-shaped ridge lying transversely on the superior surface of the talar neck; the single limb is medial, and the two bifurcating limbs are posterolateral and anterolateral. It can be seen in Figure 19, p. 189.

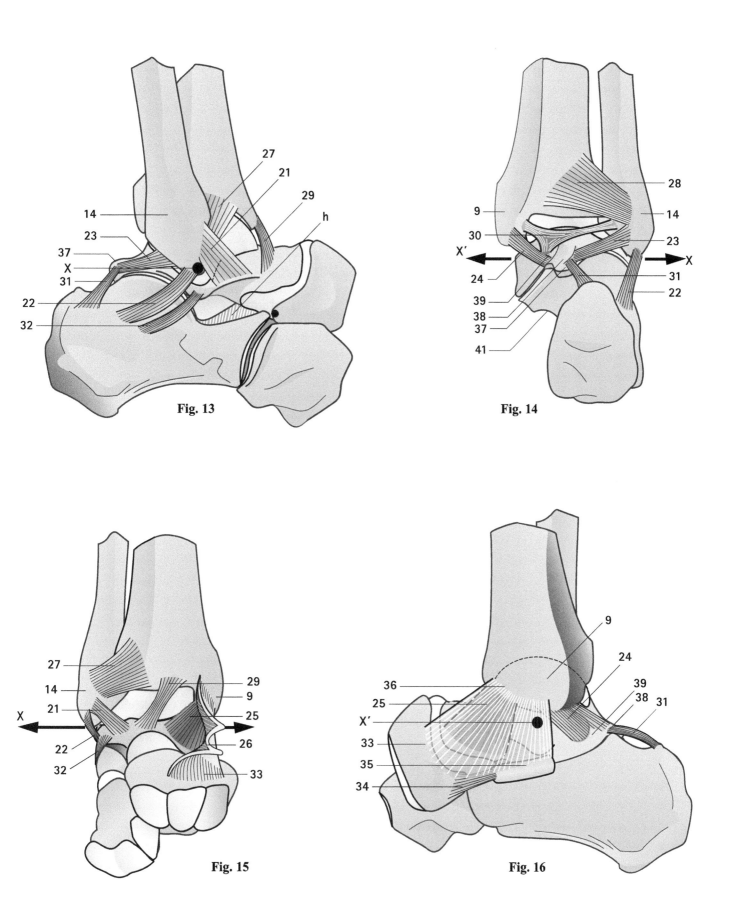

Fig. 13

Fig. 14

Fig. 15

Fig. 16

These four figures are inspired by Rouvière. The legends are common to those on the previous page.

Anteroposterior stability of the ankle and factors limiting flexion-extension

The range of flexion-extension movements is first of all determined by the full arc lengths of the **articular surfaces (Fig. 17**: diagram in profile). The tibial surface is equivalent in length to the arc of a circle subtending an angle of 70° at the centre, and the trochlear surface of the talus is equivalent to the arc of a circle subtending an angle of 140-150° at the centre; therefore by simple subtraction the **total range of flexion-extension** can be deduced to be 70-80°. Since the arc length of the trochlea is greater posteriorly than anteriorly, it follows that *extension has a greater range than flexion.*

Flexion is checked (Fig. 18) by the following factors:

- **bony factors:** During extreme flexion, the superior surface of the talar neck hits (1) the anterior margin of the tibial surface. If flexion continues, the talar neck can break. The anterior part of the capsule is prevented from being nipped between the two bones by being pulled up (2) by contraction of the flexor muscles (arrow), since it has some fibrous attachments to their synovial sheaths
- **capsulo-ligamentous factors:** The posterior part of the capsule is stretched (3) along with the posterior fibres of the collateral ligaments (4)
- **muscular factor:** The *resistance exerted tonically* by the triceps surae (5) is the first to check extension. *Contracture of the muscle* checks flexion prematurely, and the ankle may even be fixed in the position of '**pes equinus.**'* This deformity can be treated by *lengthening the calcaneal tendon.*

Extension (Fig. 19) is limited by identical factors:

- **bony factors:** The talar tubercles (especially the lateral one) come into contact (1) with the posterior margin of the distal tibia. More rarely, fractures of the talar lateral tubercle are caused by ankle hyperextension, but more often the lateral tubercle is anatomically separate from the talus to form the **os trigonum.** *The capsule escapes being nipped* (2) by the same mechanism as operates in flexion
- **capsulo-ligamentous factors:** The anterior part of the capsule is stretched (3) along with the anterior fibres of the collateral ligaments (4)

- **muscular factor:** The tonic resistance of the flexors (5) is the first to check extension. Hypertonicity of the flexors leads to permanent ankle flexion in the position called '**pes talus**' because this foot walks on its heel.

The anteroposterior stability of the ankle and the coaptation of its articular surfaces (Fig. 20) are secured by the *force of gravity* (1, red arrow), which keeps the talus pressed against the distal tibial surface, whose *anterior* (2) and *posterior* margins form bony stops, preventing the talar trochlea from escaping anteriorly or, more often, posteriorly when the foot makes violent contact with the ground. The collateral ligaments (4) are passively responsible for articular coaptation and are assisted by the muscles (not shown here), which all **actively promote coaptation** when the joint is intact.

When flexion-extension movements exceed the range set by mechanical factors, one of the joint components must give way. Thus **hyperextension** can cause either **posterior dislocation (Fig. 21)** with more or less total capsulo-ligamentous rupture or a **fracture of the posterior margin of the tibia (Fig. 22)** followed by posterior subluxation. This lesion tends to recur even after proper surgical reduction – hence the term *irreducible* – if the arc length of the marginal fragment exceeds one-third of that of the tibial surface; fixation with the help of a screw is then necessary.

Similarly, **hyperflexion** can cause either an **anterior dislocation (Fig. 23)** or a **fracture of the anterior margin (Fig. 24).**

When the lateral collateral ligament is sprained, the anterior band **(Fig. 25)** is the first to be affected: at first it is simply 'pulled' in a minor sprain and is torn in a **severe sprain.** It is then possible to demonstrate an **anterior drawer movement** either clinically or – better – radiologically: the talus escapes anteriorly, and the two arcs of a circle constituted by the talar trochlea and the roof of the tibial mortise are no longer concentric. When the centres of curvature are staggered by more than 4-5 mm, **rupture of the anterior band of the lateral collateral ligament has occurred.**

---

* The term *equinus* comes from *equus* = *horse* in Latin: the pes equinus walks on its toes like the horse.

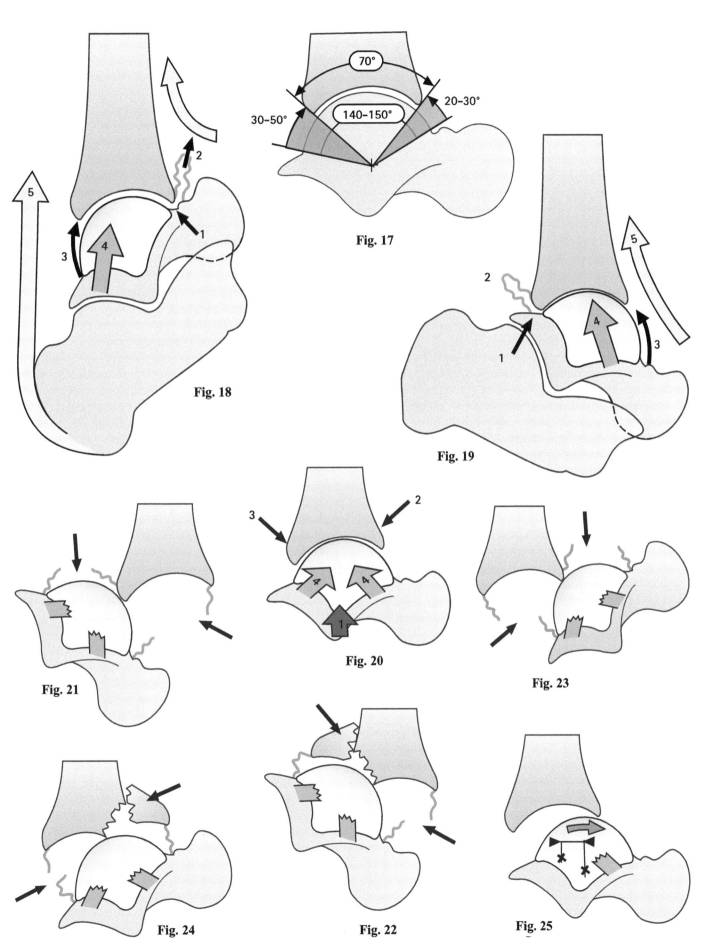

Fig. 17

Fig. 18

Fig. 19

Fig. 20

Fig. 21

Fig. 22

Fig. 23

Fig. 24

Fig. 25

Transverse stability of the ankle joint

As a **joint with only one degree of freedom**, the ankle joint, by virtue of its very make-up, is forbidden any movement around the other two axes in space. It owes **this stability to the very tight interlocking of its articular surfaces** in the manner of a mortise and tenon joint: the talar tenon is tightly held inside the tibiofibular mortise **(Fig. 26)**. The two arms of the **bimalleolar pincers** steady and immobilise the talus on both sides, provided that the distance between the lateral malleolus (A) and the medial malleolus (B) remains unchanged. This condition is fulfilled only when the malleoli and the ligaments of the inferior tibiofibular joint (1) are intact. Furthermore, strong lateral (2) and medial (3) collateral ligaments preclude any rolling movements of the talus around its long axis.

When the foot is violently abducted, the lateral cheek of the talus presses on the lateral malleolus, with the following possible consequences:

- The **bimalleolar pincers are disrupted (Fig. 27)** by the rupture of the ligaments of the inferior tibiofibular joint (1), leading to *diastasis of the tibiofibular joint*. The talus is no longer held in place and can *move from side to side*, i.e. the so-called 'talar rattling'; it can also **(Fig. 28)** *rotate on its long axis* ('talar tilting'), a movement facilitated by a *sprain of the medial collateral ligament* (3). (In the diagram, the ligament is shown as only slightly stretched, i.e. a *mild sprain*.) Finally, the talus can rotate **(Fig. 33)** *around its own vertical axis* (arrow Abd), causing the posterior part of its trochlear surface to break off the posterior margin of the distal tibia (arrow 2).
- If foot abduction continues **(Fig. 32)**, the medial collateral ligament is torn (3), giving rise to a *severe sprain* that may be associated with *diastasis of the tibiofibular joint* (1).
- Or else the **(Fig. 30)** *medial malleolus (B) is fractured at the same time as the lateral malleolus* (A) above the ligaments of the inferior tibiofibular joint (1): this is the 'high' type of **Pott's or Dupuytren's fracture.** At times the fibular fracture occurs much higher at neck level: this is the **Maisonneuve fracture** (not shown here).

- Very often the ligaments of the inferior tibiofibular joint resist injury **(Fig. 29)**, especially the anterior ligament. *Fracture of the medial malleolus* (B) is then combined with fracture of the lateral malleolus just above or through the inferior tibiofibular joint; this is **the 'low' type of Pott's fracture**, one of the variants of this condition **(Fig. 31)** includes the rupture of the medial collateral ligament (3) instead of fracture of the medial malleolus. In these 'low' Pott's fractures there is often an **associated fracture of the distal posterior margin of the tibia**, which is detached as a third fragment continuous with the medial malleolar fragment.

In addition to these abduction-related bimalleolar dislocations there are also **bimalleolar adduction fractures (Fig. 34)**: as the foot is *adducted*, the talus **(Fig. 33)** rotates around its vertical axis (**arrow Add**), and the medial cheek of its trochlear surface fractures the medial malleolus (B) **(Fig. 34)**, while tilting of the talus *fractures the lateral malleolus* (A) at its attachment to the distal tibia.

- Most of the time, however, adduction or inversion of the foot causes not a fracture but a **sprain of the lateral collateral ligament.** In most cases, fortunately, this sprain is mild, with only *stretching rather than tearing of the ligament*, and can be cured without surgery. On the other hand, **in severe sprains** the *lateral collateral ligament is torn*, leading to instability of the ankle joint. An anteroposterior radiograph of the ankle, *taken in forced inversion* (under local anaesthesia if needed), will show **(Fig. 35)** a **tilted talus**: the two lines passing through the articular surfaces of the ankle joint are no longer parallel but *form a 10-12° angle open laterally*. Some ankles are in fact abnormally lax, and it is advisable to have a radiograph of the presumably normal ankle for comparison. A severe sprain often requires surgical intervention.

It goes without saying that **all these lesions of the bimalleolar pincers require meticulous surgical correction** if the stability and functional integrity of the ankle joint are to be restored.

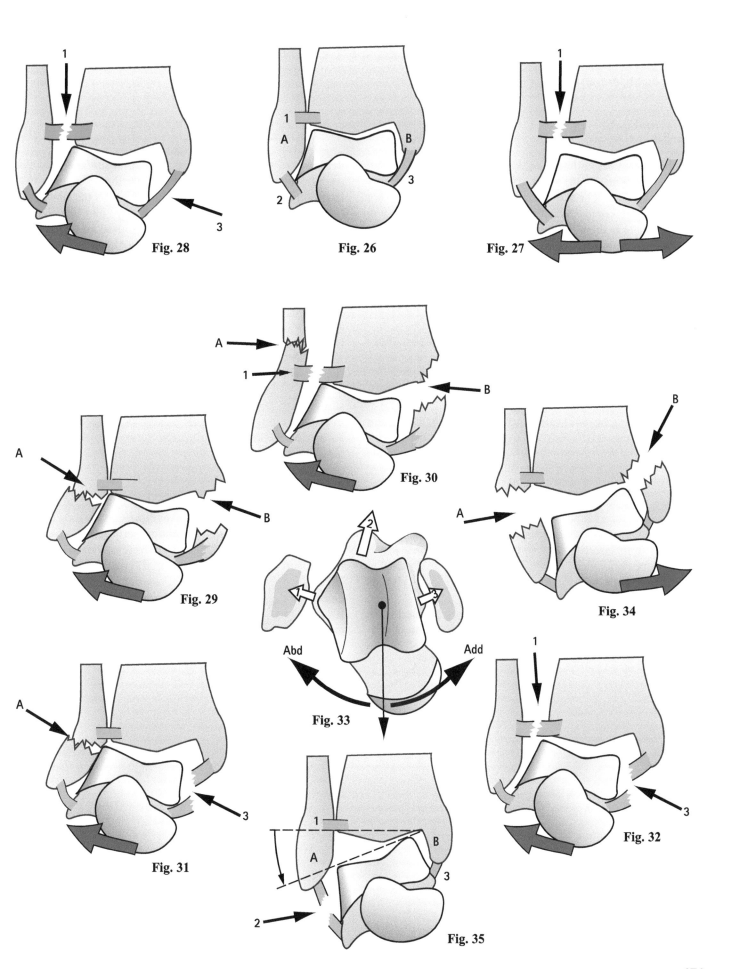

Fig. 28

Fig. 26

Fig. 27

Fig. 30

Fig. 29

Fig. 34

Fig. 31

Fig. 33

Abd

Add

Fig. 32

Fig. 35

The tibiofibular joints

The tibia articulates with the fibula at its two extremities, i.e. at the **superior (Figs 36-38) and the inferior tibiofibular joints (Figs 39-41)**. As will be shown on the next page, these joints are *mechanically linked to each other and to the ankle joint*, making it logical to study them in relation to the ankle.

The **superior tibiofibular joint** is clearly exposed **(Fig. 36**, lateral view) when the fibula is rotated after resecting the anterior tibiofibular ligament (1) and the anterior expansion (2) of the biceps tendon (3). The joint then opens around the hinge formed by the posterior tibiofibular ligament (4). It is a **plane joint** with oval and flat or slightly convex articular surfaces:

- The **tibial articular facet** (5) lies on the posterolateral border of the tibial plateau and *faces obliquely posteriorly, inferiorly and laterally* (white arrow).
- The **fibular articular facet** (6) lies on the superior surface of the fibular head, and its orientation is the *inverse of that of the tibial surface* (white arrow). It is overhung by the fibular styloid process (7), which gives insertion to the biceps femoris tendon (3). The lateral collateral ligament of the ankle joint (8) is attached between the biceps and the fibular facet.

Figure 37 (lateral view of the unopened tibiofibular joint) illustrates clearly how far posteriorly the fibular head is located; it also shows the short quadrilateral anterior tibiofibular ligament (1) and the thick tendinous expansion of the biceps femoris (2) on its way to its insertion into the lateral tibial condyle.

Figure 38 (posterior view) demonstrates the intimate relationship of the popliteus (9) with the superior tibiofibular joint as it runs superficial to the posterior ligament (4).

The **inferior tibiofibular joint (Fig. 39**: joint opened as in **Fig. 36**) contains no articular cartilage and is therefore a **syn-**desmosis (a non-synovial joint). The **tibial surface** is the fairly rough **concave surface** (1) bounded by the bifurcation of the lateral border of the bone and articulates with the fibular facet (2), which is convex, flat or even concave and lies above the fibular articular facet (3) of the ankle joint alongside the insertion of the posterior band of the lateral collateral ligament (4).

The **anterior ligament of the inferior tibiofibular joint** (5), thick and pearly white, runs obliquely inferiorly and laterally **(Fig. 40**, anterior view); its inferior border encroaches on the lateral angle of the ankle mortise, and so during ankle flexion it *bevels* (white arrowheads) the anterior part of the lateral ridge of the talar trochlear surface, which is accordingly flattened.

The thick and broader **posterior ligament** (6) (Fig, 41, posterior view) runs a long way onto the medial malleolus; likewise it bevels the posterior part of the lateral ridge of the trochlear surface during ankle extension.

In addition to the tibiofibular ligaments, the two bones of the leg are joined **(Fig. 39)** by the **interosseous ligament** stretching between the lateral tibial border and the medial fibular surface (green dotted line). It can also be seen in the diagrams showing the leg compartments (p. 210).

In the inferior tibiofibular joint the two bones are not in direct contact but are separated **by fibroadipose tissue**, and this interspace can be shown by radiographs properly centred on the ankle **(Fig. 42)**. Normally the fibular shadow (c) overlaps the anterior tibial tubercle (a) by a distance (8 mm) greater than the distance (2 mm) that separates it from the posterior tubercle (b). If the distance **cb** exceeds **ac**, there is **diastasis of the tibiofibular joint**. It is obvious on a frontal radiograph that the lateral malleolus extends farther *distally* than the medial malleolus.

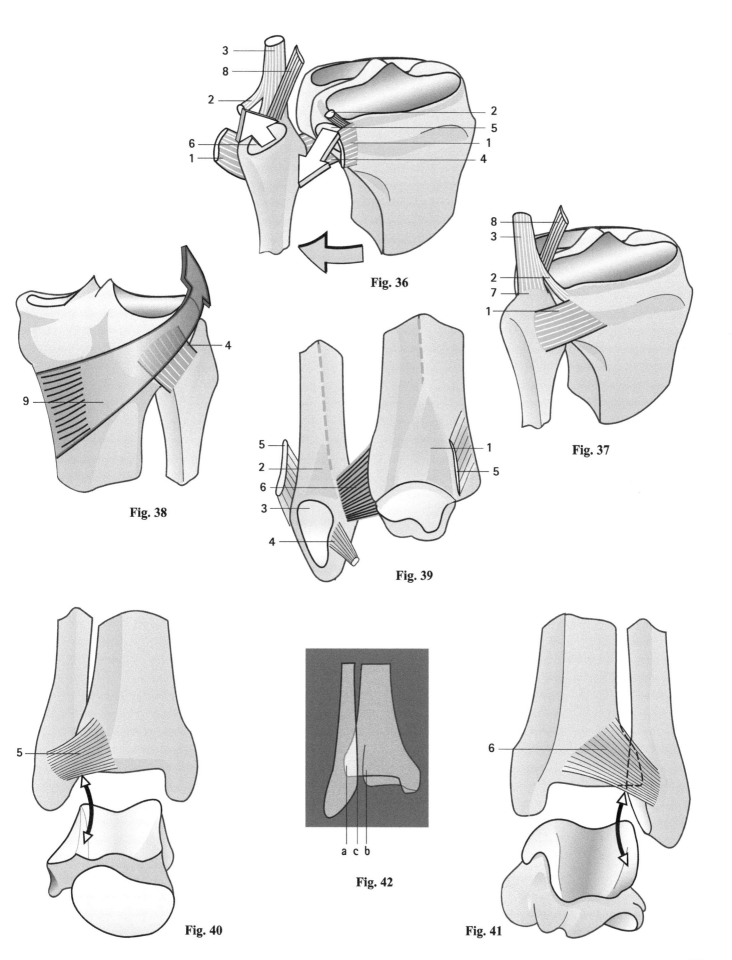

Fig. 36

Fig. 37

Fig. 38

Fig. 39

Fig. 40

Fig. 41

Fig. 42

173

Functional anatomy of the tibiofibular joints

Flexion and extension of the ankle joint *automatically call into action the two mechanically linked tibiofibular joints.*

The **inferior tibiofibular joint is the first to be recruited.** Its mode of action has been well worked out by Pol Le Coeur (1938) and depends above all on the **shape of the talar trochlea** (**Fig. 43**, superior view) with its **medial cheek for the tibia (T)** lying in a sagittal plane and **its lateral cheek for the fibula (F)** lying in a *plane that runs obliquely anteriorly and laterally.* As a result, the width of the trochlear surface is smaller posteriorly (aa') than anteriorly (bb') by 5 mm (e). Therefore, in order to grip tightly both cheeks of the trochlea, the **intermalleolar distance must vary** within certain limits (e): from a *minimum during extension* (**Fig. 44**, inferior view) to a *maximum during flexion* (**Fig. 45**). On anatomical model the ankle can be extended simply by compressing the malleoli firmly from the sides.

It is also obvious *on the skeleton* (**Figs 44 and 45**) that this movement of separation and approximation of the malleoli (e) is followed by *axial rotation of the lateral malleolus* with the *posterior tibiofibular ligament (2) acting as a hinge.* This rotation is easily demonstrated with the use of a pin driven horizontally through the lateral malleolus: between its position (nn') during flexion (**Fig. 44**) and its position (mm') during extension (**Fig. 45**) there is a difference equal to an angle of 30° in the direction of medial rotation. At the same time the anterior tibiofibular ligament (1) is stretched, owing to a change in its obliquity (**Fig. 50**). Note that this medial rotation of the lateral malleolus is less marked in the living subject, but it is nevertheless present. Moreover the **synovial fold** (f), lying within the joint, is displaced as follows: *distally* (1) when the malleoli are approximated during extension (**Fig. 46**) and *proximally* (2) during flexion (**Fig. 47**).

Finally the **fibula moves vertically** (**Figs 48 and 49**: the fibula is represented by a quadrangular ruler). Being attached to the tibia by the *fibres of the interosseous membrane, which run obliquely distally and laterally* (for the sake of clarity only one fibre is included), the fibula is pulled *a little superiorly* as it moves away from the tibia (**Fig. 49**) and is pulled inferiorly as it moves closer to the tibia (**Fig. 48**).

These fibular movements can be summarized as follows:
- **During flexion of the ankle** (**Fig. 50 F**, frontal view):
  - The lateral malleolus *moves away from the medial malleolus (arrow 1).*

- At the same time it is *pulled a little superiorly* (arrow 3), while the fibres of the tibiofibular ligaments and of the interosseous membrane tend to become more *horizontal* (XX').
  - Finally it is **laterally rotated on itself** (arrow 2).
- **During extension of the ankle** (**Fig. 51 E**, frontal view) the converse takes place:
  - The malleoli are (arrow 1) *actively brought closer together*, as demonstrated by Pol Le Coeur: contraction of the fibres of the tibialis posterior inserted into the tibia and fibula tightens the bimalleolar pincers (**Fig. 52**: section of distal fragment of right lower leg with the arrows representing contraction of the tibialis posterior). Thus the talar trochlea is *firmly held in place whatever the degree of ankle flexion or extension.*
  - The lateral malleolus (arrow 2) is *pulled inferiorly* as the ligaments *become vertical* yy'.
  - The lateral malleolus is slightly *rotated medially* (arrow 3).
- The **superior tibiofibular joint** is recruited as a result of these movements of the lateral malleolus:
  - During *ankle flexion* (**Fig. 49**) the fibular facet slides superiorly (h) and the joint space *gaps inferiorly* because of malleolar separation (red arrow) and *posteriorly* because of lateral rotation of the fibula (pink arrow).
  - During *ankle extension* (**Fig. 48**) the converse takes place, i.e. inferior displacement of the fibular facet, narrowing of the joint space and medial rotation of the fibula.

These displacements are small, but not negligible, and the best proof of their occurrence lies in the fact that during the course of evolution the *tibiofibular joint has not yet become fused*, as should have eventually happened in the absence of any functional activity.

Thus, with the help of the tibiofibular joints, the ligaments and the tibialis posterior, the *bimalleolar pincers can constantly adapt* to changes in the width and curvature of the talar trochlea and thus **ensure the transverse stability of the ankle joint.** It is mainly to avoid jeopardizing this adaptability that screws are no longer used in the management of diastasis of the tibiofibular joint.

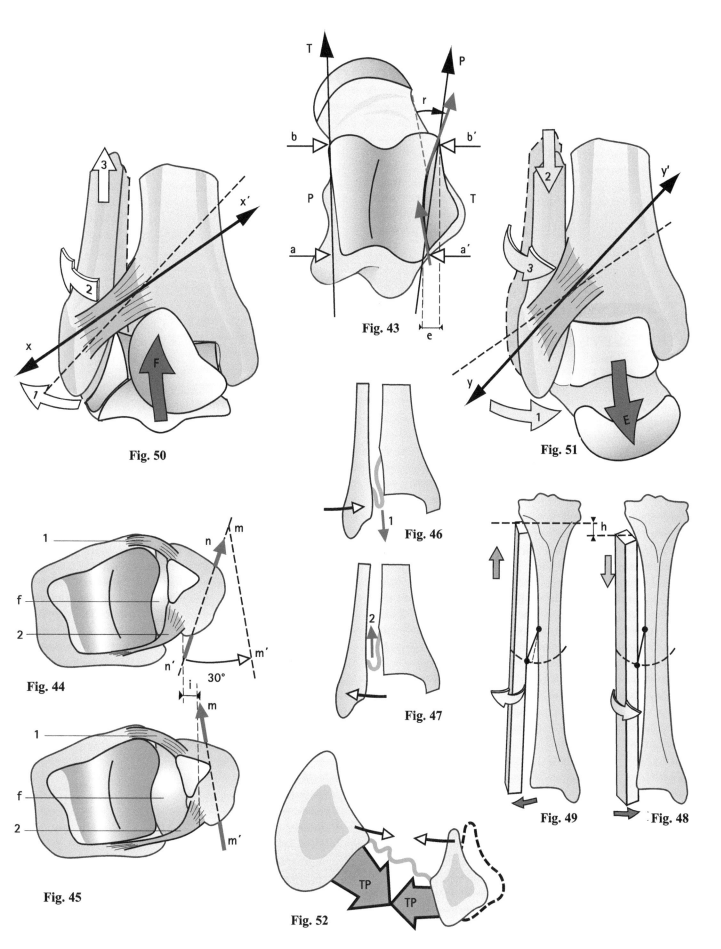

Fig. 50

Fig. 43

Fig. 51

Fig. 44

Fig. 45

Fig. 46

Fig. 47

Fig. 52

Fig. 49

Fig. 48

Why does the leg have two bones?

In Volume 1 we asked the question: 'Why does the forearm have two bones?' and attempted to provide an answer in order to explain pronation-supination (see Volume 1, p. 136). We ask the same question for the leg, but the answer is different, since axial rotation of the leg takes place at the knee joint, provided it is already flexed. **What is the significance of the presence of two bones in the leg?**

An explanation can be found, tentatively, in **Pol Le Coeur's work** (published in his **1938** thesis), where he describes the exceptional functional anatomy of the ankle joint, which is in fact a joint with a 'variable geometry'.

We have already seen the consequences of the unusual shape of the **talar trochlea** (**Fig. 53**: superior view of the talus): wider anteriorly than posteriorly with the curved and oblique profile of its lateral cheek. From extension to full flexion the inferior articular surface of the distal tibia contacts the superior surface of the trochlea in two distinctly different areas (**Fig. 54**).

- **During extension (E)** (blue outline) it is the narrow posterior part of the trochlea that comes into contact with the tibia. The extent of contact is minimal.
- **During flexion (F)** (red outline) the tibia contacts the widest part of the trochlea, where the area of contact is maximal.

If these *two surfaces* (**Fig. 55**) are drawn separately, it is clear that the anterior contact surface is distinctly larger than the posterior one. This is even more obvious if one surface is placed on top of the other (**Fig. 56**); the anterior surface extends beyond the posterior surface on all sides.

As a result of this arrangement, the stresses on the talus during walking are **maximal during the flexion phase**, when the supporting leg swings forward to hit the ground and contact between the two bones is maximal. On the other hand, **during extension the load is reduced**, and there is a lesser need for stability; this is the position of minimal contact between the bones.

As the width of the talar trochlea keeps changing, **the intermalleolar distance needs to change accordingly**, and this is achieved by a split in the tibiofibular mortise, which requires the presence of *two constituent bones*. This explains why there are two bones!

There is still a critical problem to be resolved, i.e. **the constant adjustment of the intermalleolar distance**, which increases during flexion F and decreases during extension E, as shown in the mechanical model (**Fig. 57**) representing the talar trochlea and the two extreme positions of the bimalleolar pincers. This fine-tuning mechanism (a stroke of *genius*!) is entrusted (**Fig. 58**: posterior view of the leg bones) to the tibialis posterior (1), which extends the ankle and arises from both tibia and fibula. Therefore, during ankle extension this muscle produces **simultaneously** ankle extension and approximation of the malleoli, thus accommodating the smaller width of the talar trochlea; it is assisted in this action, but to a lesser degree, by the flexor hallucis longus (2). Hence the adaptation of the bimalleolar pincers during extension is active and of muscular origin. On the other hand, their adaptation during flexion is passive: the intermalleolar distance is forcibly increased by the progressive widening of the talar trochlea, which is slowed down by the ligaments and also by the above-mentioned muscles, which oppose ankle flexion.

It is also clear that the curved profile of the lateral cheek of the talus ensures that the pressure exerted on the fibular articular facet is always perpendicular to its surface, giving rise to the **automatic rotation of the fibula** on its long axis.

The appearance of these **two bones in the intermediate segment of each of the four limbs** goes back 400 million years (**Fig. 59**: transformation of the fin (a) into a leg (b and c)), when during the middle Devonian period, our remote ancestor, an obscure crossopterygian fish (the Eusthenopteron, **Fig. 60**) left the sea *after its fins had evolved into legs* and became a *tetrapod*, similar to a modern-day lizard or crocodile. The progressive reorganization of its fins led to the retention of a single ray h in the proximal segment (**Fig. 59**), the development of two rays side by side in the intermediate segment (the future radius r and ulna u or tibia and fibula in the leg) and the subsequent formation of the carpal and tarsal bones and of the five rays of the hands and toes, thus providing the prototype for all vertebrates.

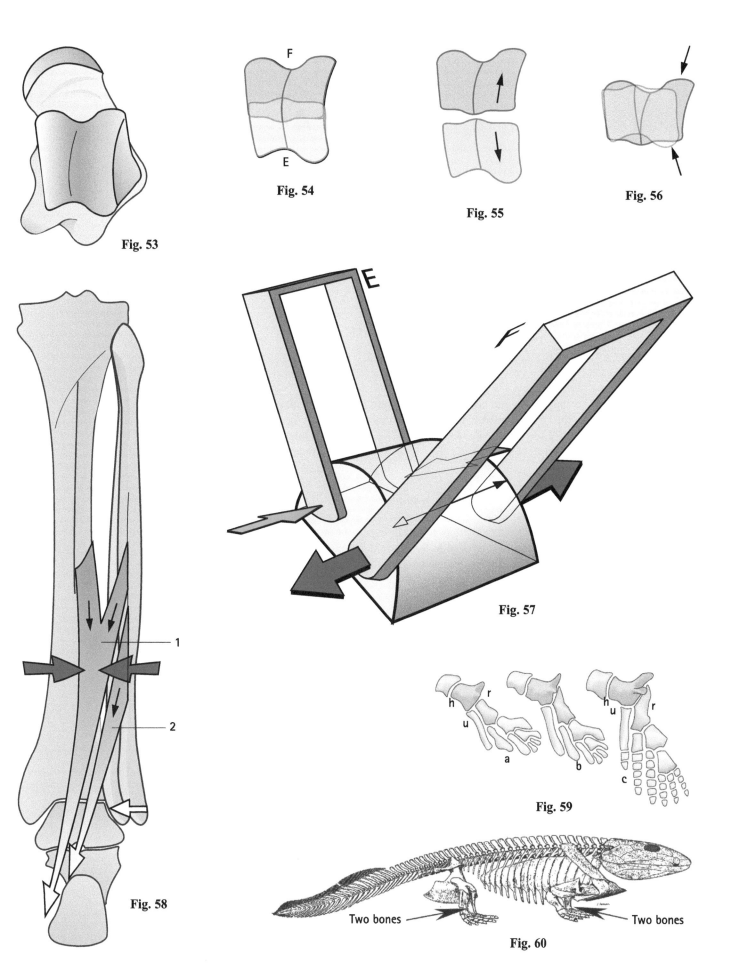

Fig. 53

Fig. 54

Fig. 55

Fig. 56

Fig. 57

Fig. 58

1

2

Fig. 59

Fig. 60

Two bones

Two bones

Chapter 4

THE FOOT

The joints of the foot are numerous and complex and fall into two groups: those among the tarsal bones and those between the tarsal and metatarsal bones. They include the following:

- the subtalar joint
- the transverse tarsal joint
- the tarsometatarsal joint
- the cuboidonavicular joint and the cuneonavicular joints.

These joints have a double function:

1. Since the ankle joint is responsible for orientation of the foot in the sagittal plane, they **orient the foot** relative to the sagittal plane, so as to ensure that the sole of the foot faces the ground appropriately, whatever the position of the leg and the slope of the ground.

2. They **alter the shape and curvature of the plantar vault** to allow the foot to adapt to any unevenness of the terrain and also to interpose a *shock-absorber* between the ground and the weightbearing limb, thereby imparting elasticity and suppleness to the step.

These joints therefore play a vital role. On the other hand, the joints involving the toes, i.e. the metatarsophalangeal and interphalangeal joints, are *far less important than their counterparts in the hand*. One of these joints, however, is crucial during the loading response of the gait cycle*, i.e. the metatarsophalangeal joint of the big toe.

---

* In all vertebrates, this intermediate segment or zeugopod always contains two bones, which are modified and adapted during evolution.

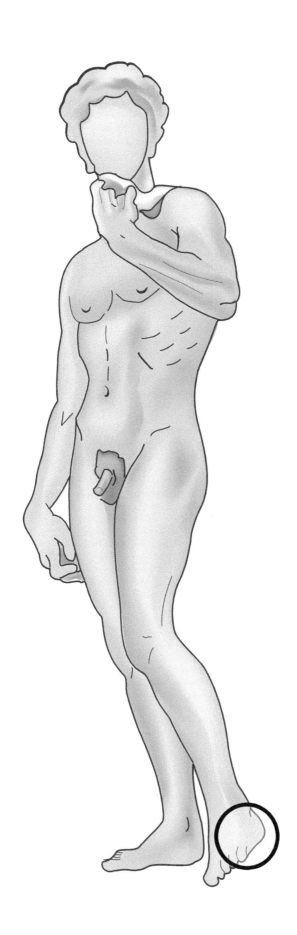

Axial rotation and side-to-side movements of the foot

In addition to movements of flexion and extension that occur at the ankle, the foot can move around the **vertical axis of the leg** (axis Y, p. 159) and its **own horizontal and longitudinal axis** (axis Z).

Around the **vertical axis** Y **(Fig. 1)** occur movements of adduction-abduction:

- **adduction (Fig. 2)**, when the tip of the foot moves medially towards the plane of symmetry of the body
- **abduction (Fig. 3)**, when the tip of the foot moves laterally away from the plane of symmetry of the body.

The **total range of adduction-abduction movements**, when they occur exclusively in the foot, is from 35-40° (Roud). These movements of the tip of the foot in the horizontal plane, however, can also be produced by lateral-medial rotation of the leg with the knee flexed or rotation of the whole lower limb with the knee extended. They then have a greater range, attaining a maximum of 90° each way, as in ballerinas.

Around the **longitudinal axis Z** the foot turns so that the sole faces:

- medially **(Fig. 4)**: by analogy with the upper limb this movement is defined as **supination**
- laterally **(Fig. 5)**: this movement is called **pronation.**

The range of **supination** is 52° (Biesalski and Mayer) and exceeds that of **pronation**, which is only 25-30°.

These movements of abduction-adduction and pronation-supination, as just defined, do not actually occur in the pure state in the joints of the foot. In fact, it will be shown later that these joints are so built that any movement in one of the planes must be associated with movement in the other two planes of space. Thus *adduction is necessarily accompanied by* **(Figs 2 and 4)** *supination and slight extension.* This triad of movements is typical of the so-called **position of inversion.** If the extension component is cancelled by an equivalent flexion at the ankle, the foot is in the **varus position.** Finally, when lateral rotation at the knee offsets the adduction, then the movement obtained is an *apparently pure form of supination.*

Conversely **(Figs 3 and 5)**, *abduction is necessarily associated with pronation and flexion* leading to the **so-called position of eversion.** If the flexion is cancelled by an equivalent extension at the ankle (in the diagrams extension is overcompensated), the foot is in the **valgus position.** If, in addition, medial rotation of the knee cancels the abduction, then the movement obtained is an *apparently pure form of pronation.*

Thus, barring any compensating movements taking place at joints outside the foot, adduction can never be associated with pronation, and, vice versa, abduction can never be combined with supination. **There are, therefore, combinations of movements that are forbidden by the very architecture of the joints of the foot.**

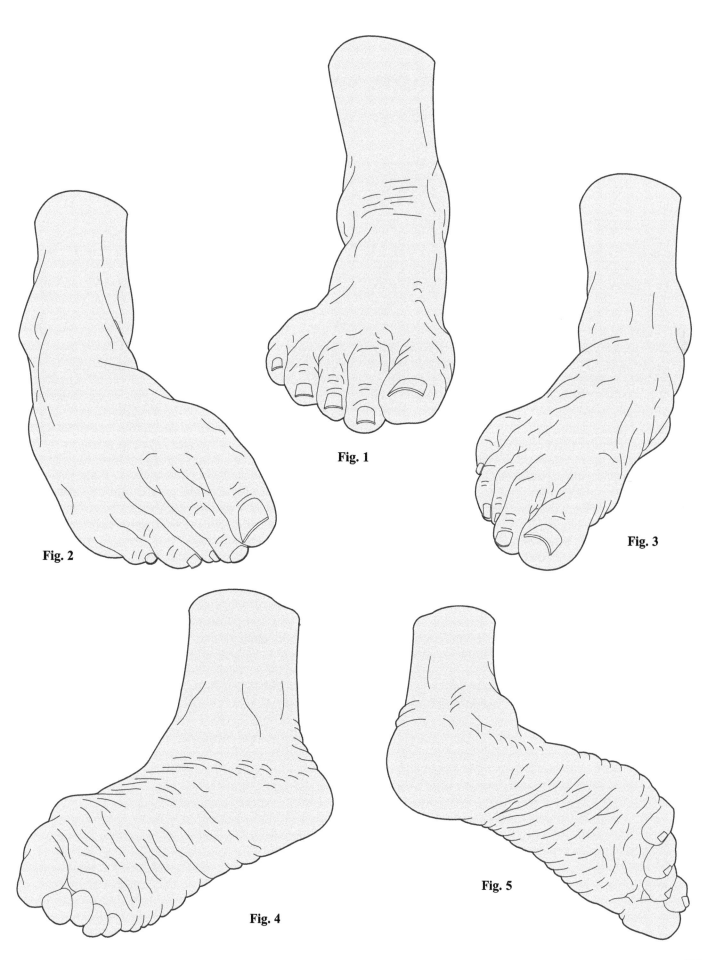

Fig. 1

Fig. 2

Fig. 3

Fig. 4

Fig. 5

The articular surfaces of the subtalar joint

(The legends are common to all the diagrams.)

The inferior surface of the talus A (**Fig. 6**: the talus has been separated from the calcaneus and rotated on its hinge axis xx') articulates with the superior surface of the calcaneus B. These two bones are in contact at two articular facets that make up the subtalar joint:

- **The posterior facet of the talus a** is in contact with the **large posterior calcaneal facet a'** for the talus (also known as the thalamus of Destot). These two surfaces are united by ligaments and a capsule in such a way that the joint is anatomically independent.
- The **small facet b** on the inferior surface of the neck and head of the talus comes to rest on the **anterior calcaneal articular facet for the talus b'**, which is obliquely set and is supported by the anterior process of the calcaneus and the sustentaculum tali. These two, the talar and calcaneal facets, belong to a much larger joint that also includes the **posterior surface of the navicular** (d') and forms with the talar head (d) the **medial part of the transverse tarsal joint.**

Before examining the function of these joints, one must understand the **shapes of their articular facets**. These joints are of the **plane variety:**

- The **large posterior calcaneal facet** for the talus (a') is roughly oval, with its great axis running obliquely anteriorly and laterally; it is *convex* along its great axis (**Fig. 7**, lateral view and **Fig. 8**, medial view) and *straight* or slightly concave along the other orthogonal axis. It can therefore be likened to a segment of a cylinder (f), whose axis would run *obliquely, posteroanteriorly, lateromedially and slightly superoinferiorly.*
- The **corresponding talar articular facet** (a) also has this cylindrical shape with a similar radius and a similar axis, except that the talar cylinder corresponds to a **segment of a concave cylinder (Fig. 7)**, whereas the calcaneal cylinder corresponds to **a segment of a convex cylinder.**

- On the whole, **the talar head is spheroidal**, and the bevelled surfaces on its circumference can be viewed as *facets chiselled out on the surface of a sphere* (broken red line) with centre g (**Fig. 6B**). Hence the **anterior surface of the calcaneus b'** is *biconcave*, while the opposite talar surface is reciprocally biconvex. Quite often the calcaneal surface b' is waisted in its middle part and resembles the sole of a shoe (**Fig. 6**); occasionally it is even *subdivided into two facets* (**Figs 7 and 8**): the one (e') resting on the sustentaculum tali, and the other (b') on the anterior calcaneal process. The stability of the calcaneus has been found to be proportional to the surface area of the latter facet. The talus may also have two separate articular facets **b** and **e**. The anterior surface of the calcaneus contains the articular surface (h) for the cuboid.

The **calcaneal surface b' + e'** is itself part of a much larger concave spherical surface that also includes the **posterior surface of the navicular d'** and the dorsal surface of the plantar **calcaneonavicular ligament c'** Along with the **deltoid ligament** 5 and the capsule, these surfaces form a *spherical socket* for the talar head. On the talar head (**Fig. 6A**), corresponding articular facets are present: the bulk of its articular surface d lodges inside the navicular, and between this surface d and the calcaneal facet b lies the *triangular area* c, with its base located medially and corresponding to the plantar **calcaneonavicular ligament c'**.

This combination of *two different types of articular surfaces* (**Fig. 6C**), i.e. spherical and cylindrical, within the same joint, reveals the very special nature of the biomechanics of this joint, which can only have a *single position of articular surface congruence*, i.e. the weight-bearing position, where the *forces are transmitted in their entirety*. In other positions, there is a **significant degree of obligatory mechanical play**, which is secondary to the non-congruence of the articular surfaces and is of little importance mechanically, *since the stresses are not then transmitted*. This is an example of what could be called **fuzzy mechanics** as compared to industrial mechanics, which is precise and well regulated.

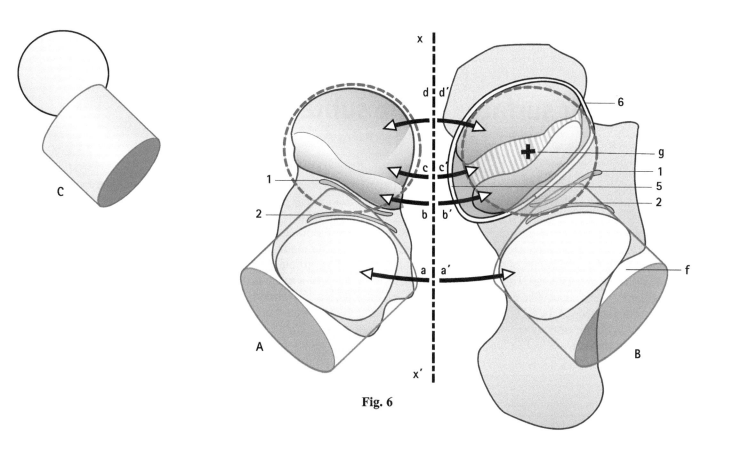

Fig. 6

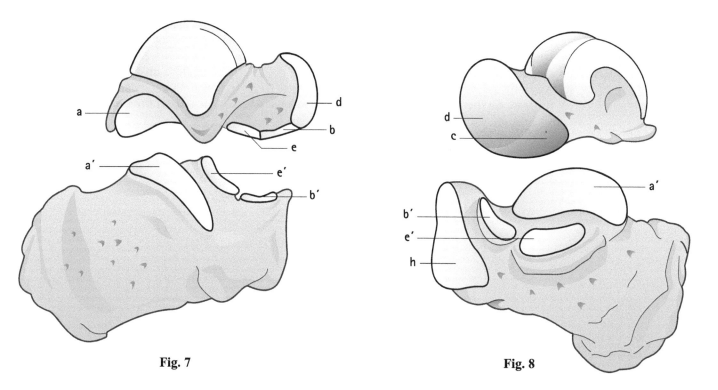

Fig. 7   Fig. 8

Congruence and incongruence of the articular surfaces of the subtalar joint

(The legends are common to all the diagrams on the next page but do not correspond to those on the previous page.)

The description of the joint given on the previous page allows one to understand the arrangement and conformity of the articular surfaces but not to grasp their peculiar *modus operandi*. For this purpose, the articular surfaces of the anterior subtalar joint must be described in greater detail. The joint is opened around its axis of rotation XX' and shown like the pages of an open book in Figure 9 (inferior surface of the talus flipped over alongside the calcaneus) and in Figure 10 (superior surface of the calcaneus). **On the inferior surface of the talar neck (Fig. 9)** the **facet b** corresponds to the **facet b'** on the **superior surface of the calcaneus (Fig. 10)** near the sustentaculum tali. The **talar head** also contains **(Fig. 9)** the articular facets for the navicular bone (e) and for the subtalar joint (d).

On the other hand, the cartilage-coated surface beyond the subtalar joint is subdivided into **three facets** (labelled mediolaterally as c_1, c_2 and c_3) corresponding to the anterior process of the calcaneus, which is itself subdivided into two facets (c'_1 and c'_2 mediolaterally). Posteriorly are visible the two articular surfaces of the posterior subtalar joint, i.e. the **posterior talar facet on the calcaneus** (a') and the **inferior facet on the body of the talus** (a).

There is only a **single position of articular congruence for the subtalar joint:** the **intermediate position**, where the foot lies straight under the talus without any inversion or eversion; it is the position adopted by a normal foot (neither flat nor arched) when one stands erect and still on a horizontal surface with symmetrical bilateral limb support. The articular surfaces of the posterior part of the subtalar joint are *perfectly congruent*: the facet of the talar neck (b) rests on the facet (b') on the

sustentaculum tali, and the middle talar articular facet c_2 rests on the horizontal facet c_1 of the anterior process of the calcaneus. This orthostatic position, where the articular facets are coapted by the force of gravity and not by the ligaments, is **stable** and can be maintained for a long time because of the congruence of the articular surfaces. **All other positions are unstable and lead to a more or less severe degree of incongruence.**

During eversion, the anterior tip of the calcaneus (**Fig. 11:** superior view of the right side with the blue talus assumed transparent) is shifted laterally and tends to 'lie down' (**Fig. 12,** anterior view). During this movement, the **two facets b and b'** stay coapted and form a **pivot**, while the subtalar articular surface a slides inferiorly and anteriorly on the posterior talar facet a' before hitting the floor of the sinus tarsi, and the posterosuperior surface of the posterior talar facet becomes 'uncovered' a' (**Fig. 11**). Anteriorly, the **small talar facet c_3** slides on the surface (**Fig. 12**) of the oblique facet c'_2 of the calcaneus. For this reason, the two facets c_1 and c'_2 deserve the name of '**facets of eversion**'.

During inversion the calcaneus is displaced in the opposite direction, with its anterior tip moving medially (**Fig. 13**) and its lateral surface tending to '*lie flat*' (**Fig. 14**). These **two pivot-like facets stay in contact;** meanwhile the large talar articular surface of the subtalar joint 'climbs' on to the posterior calcanean facet for the talus a', uncovering its anteroinferior part (**Fig. 13**), and anteriorly the talar facet of inversion c_1 comes to rest on the horizontal facet c'_1 on the anterior process of the calcaneus (**Fig. 14**).

These two positions are therefore **unstable with incongruent articular surfaces** *and require full ligamentous support.* **They can be maintained only for a short time** and are not supported.

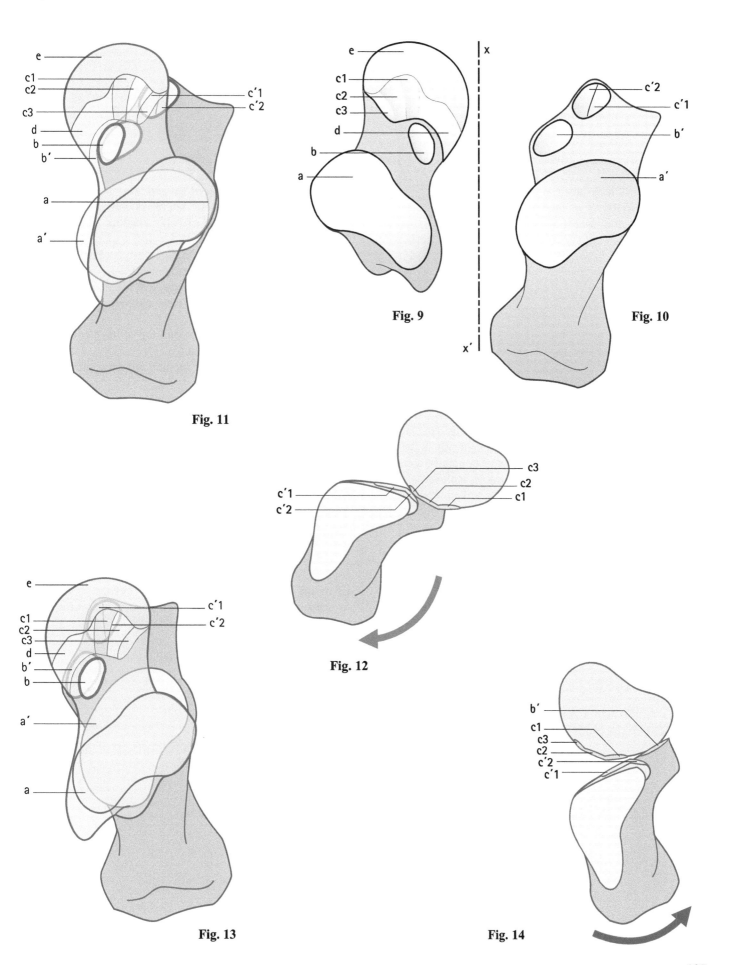

Fig. 9

Fig. 10

Fig. 11

Fig. 12

Fig. 13

Fig. 14

The talus: the unusual bone

The posterior tarsus contains the talus, which is an unusual bone in three ways:

First, because of its location at the apex of the posterior tarsus, it acts as a **distributor** of the weight of the body and of other loads *over the entire foot* **(Fig. 15)**.

Its **superior articular surface**, i.e. the trochlea, receives the weight of the body (arrow 1) and the loads transmitted by the bimalleolar pincers and transmits these stresses in three directions:

- **posteriorly**, towards the heel (**arrow 2**), i.e. the posterior calcaneal tuberosity, via the posterior part of the subtalar joint and the posterior talar facet for the calcaneus
- **anteriorly and medially (arrow 3)**, towards the medial arch of the plantar vault via the talonavicular joint
- **anteriorly and laterally (arrow 4)** towards the lateral arch of the plantar vault via the anterior part of the subtalar joint.

It is **subjected to compressive forces** and plays a *considerable mechanical role*.

Second, it has **no muscular attachments (Fig. 16)**, but it is hemmed in on all sides by leg muscles on their way to the foot; hence the nickname of '**encaged bone**', i.e. held in a cage of muscle tendons. The muscles, 13 in number, include:

- the four tendons of the extensor digitorum communis (1)
- the fibularis tertius (often absent) (2)
- the fibularis brevis (3)
- the fibularis longus (4)
- the calcaneal tendon i.e. the tendon of insertion of the triceps surae (5)
- the tibialis posterior (6)
- the flexor hallucis longus (7)
- the flexor digitorum longus (8)
- the extensor hallucis longus (9)
- the tibialis anterior (10).

Third, it is **entirely covered by articular surfaces and ligamentous insertions (Fig. 17**, lateral view; and **Fig. 18**, medial view), justifying its name of **relay station.** These ligaments include the following:

- the interosseous or inferior talocalcanean ligament (1)
- the lateral talocalcaneal ligament (2)
- the posterior talocalcaneal ligament (3)
- the anterior band of the lateral collateral ligament of the ankle joint (4)
- the deep fibres of the anterior band of the medial collateral ligament of the ankle joint (5)
- the posterior band of the medial collateral ligament of the ankle joint (6)
- the posterior band of the lateral collateral ligament of the ankle joint (7)
- the anterior capsule of the ankle joint reinforced by the anterior collateral ligament (8)
- the posterior collateral ligament of the ankle joint (9) reinforcing the capsule
- the talonavicular ligament (10).

Since it bears no muscular attachments, the talus is nourished only by blood vessels coming from the ligament insertion sites and by a few direct blood vessels; this arterial supply is *just adequate under normal conditions*. After fractures of the talar neck, especially when combined with subluxation of the talar body, its blood supply may be compromised beyond repair, leading to **pseudarthrosis of the talar neck** or, even worse, **aseptic necrosis of the body of the talus.**

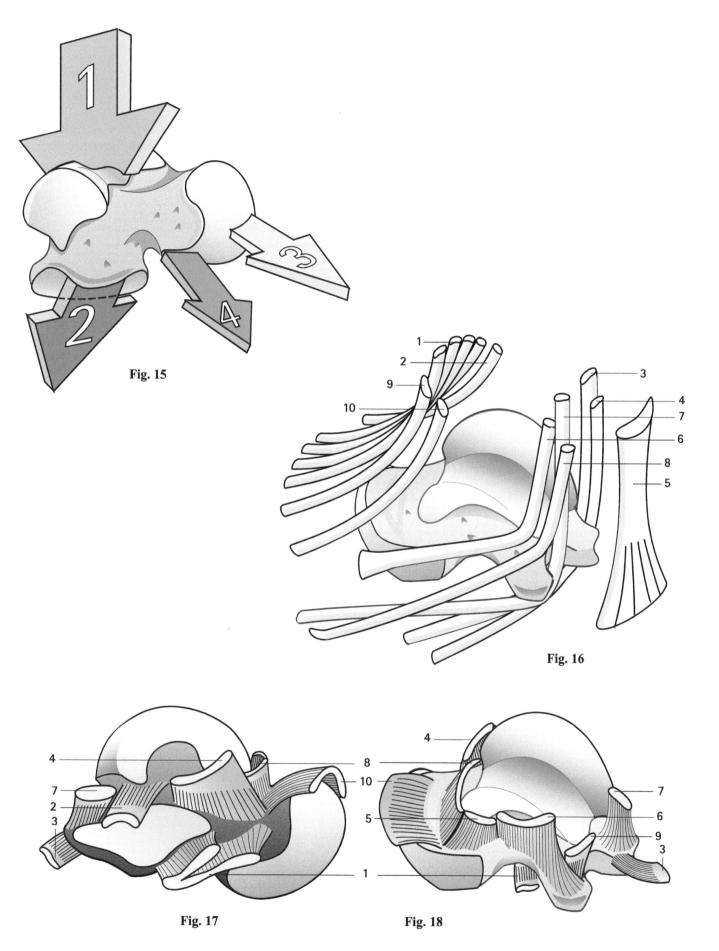

Fig. 15

Fig. 16

Fig. 17

Fig. 18

The ligaments of the subtalar joint

The talus and the calcaneus are united by *short and powerful ligaments*, since they are subjected to **sizeable stresses** *during walking, running and jumping*.

The main ligament is the **interosseous talocalcaneal ligament** (**Fig. 19**, anterolateral view), made up of **two thick quadrilateral fibrous bands** filling the *sinus tarsi*, which is a fairly large interosseous groove located between the inferolateral aspect of the talar neck and the superior surface of the anterior half of the calcaneus.

- The **anterior band** (1) is attached to the *sinus calcanei* (the floor of the sinus tarsi just superior to the anterior process of the calcaneus). Its dense and pearly-white fibres run *obliquely superiorly, anteriorly and laterally* to insert into the *sinus tali* on the inferior surface of the talar neck (the roof of the sinus tarsi; see **Fig. 6A**, p. 183) just posterior to the edge of the cartilage-coated articular facet of the talar head.
- The **posterior band** (2) is inserted posterior to the anterior band into the floor of the sinus tarsi, i.e. just anterior to the posterior talar facet. Its thick fibres run *obliquely superiorly, posteriorly and laterally* to gain insertion into the roof of the sinus tarsi (see **Fig. 6A**, p. 183) just anterior to the posterior talar surface.

The arrangement of these two bands becomes obvious when the talus is separated from the calcaneus, *assuming that the ligaments are elastic* (**Fig. 20**: anterolateral view, with the ligaments shown as extensible).

The talus is also bound to the calcaneus by two other less important ligaments (**Figs 19 and 20**):
- The **lateral talocalcaneal ligament** (3), which springs from the lateral tubercle of the talus and runs obliquely inferiorly and posteriorly parallel to the intermediate band of the lateral collateral ligament of the ankle joint, to be inserted into the lateral calcaneal surface;
- the **posterior talocalcaneal ligament** (4), a thin fibrous slip running from the lateral talar tubercle to the superior calcaneal surface.

The interosseous talocalcaneal ligament is of **paramount importance in the statics and dynamics** of the subtalar joint. In fact, it holds a central position as shown by the diagram (**Fig. 21**: superior view of the four tarsal bones), where a transparent talar trochlea has been placed on top of the calcaneal articular facets. It is clear that the weight of the body, transmitted by the leg bones to the talar trochlea, is spread over the posterior talar facet of the calcaneus and the anterior calcaneal facets of the talus, i.e. the anteromedial b'1 and the anterolateral b'2 facets. It is also clear that the interosseous talocalcaneal ligament (visible through the transparent talar trochlea as two green lines) lies exactly along the prolongation of the axis of the leg (cross in circle) so that it is equally **active during torsion and elongation of the foot** (see p. 198).

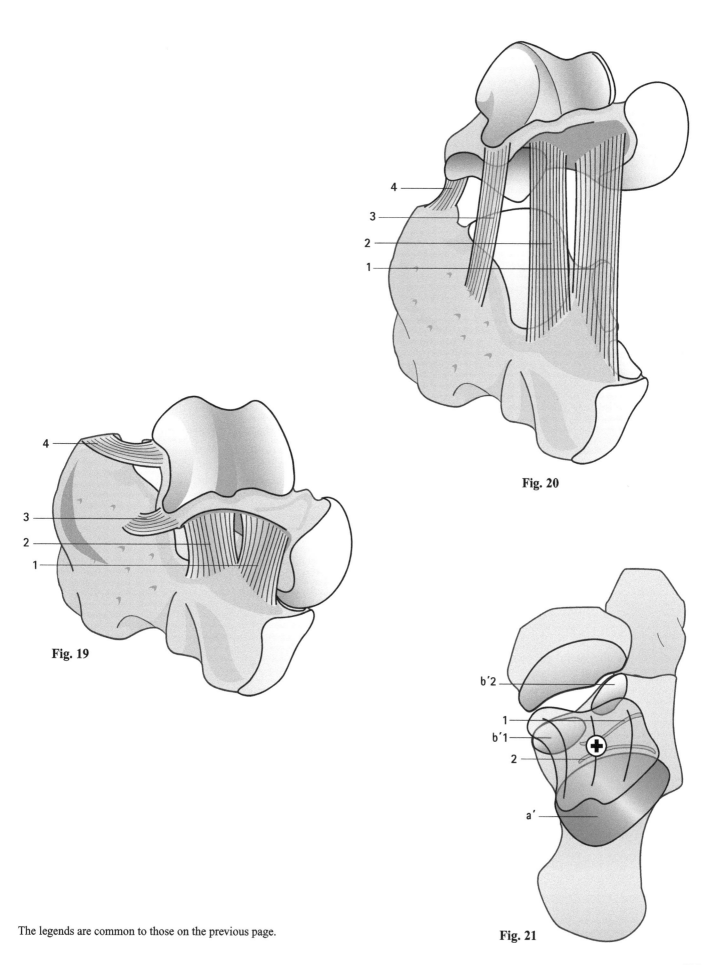

Fig. 20

Fig. 19

Fig. 21

The legends are common to those on the previous page.

The transverse tarsal joint and its ligaments

When the joint is opened anteriorly and the navicular and cuboid bones are displaced distally (**Fig. 22**, inspired by Rouvière), it is seen to consist of the posteriorly concave **talonavicular joint** medially (**Fig. 6B**, p. 183) and of the slightly anteriorly concave **calcaneocuboid joint** laterally, in such a way that the joint space resembles an elongated italicized S in the transverse plane when viewed from above.

The **anterior calcaneal surface** (e) has a complex shape: *transversely it is concave in its superior part and convex in its inferior part*; thus supero-inferiorly it is at first concave and then convex. The corresponding **posterior articular surface of the cuboid** (e') is reciprocally shaped, but often (**Fig. 27**: posterior view of the navicular-cuboid pair) it is extended by a facet (e'2) on the navicular, whose lateral extremity rests on the cuboid. The two bones articulate via **two plane facets h and h'** and are solidly united by **three ligaments**, i.e. a lateral dorsal ligament (5), a medial plantar ligament (6) and a short thick interosseous ligament (7). (Here the two bones have been artificially separated.) The ligaments of the transverse tarsal joint are five in number:

* The **plantar calcaneonavicular ligament** c' or the spring ligament unites the calcaneus and the navicular (**Fig. 23**) and also provides an articular surface (see p. 183); its medial border gives insertion to the **base of** the deltoid ligament (**Fig. 16**, p. 167)
* The **dorsal talonavicular ligament** (9) running from the dorsal surface of the talar neck to the dorsal surface of the navicular (**Figs 22 and 26**)
* The **bifurcated ligament (Figs 23 and 26)**, which lies in the midline and forms the keystone of the transverse tarsal joint, comprises **two bands** arising together (10) from the anterior calcaneal process near its anterior edge. The **medial band** (11) or the lateral calcaneonavicular ligament lies in a vertical plane and is inserted into the lateral surface of the navicular, while its inferior border occasionally blends with the plantar calcaneonavicular ligament to split the joint into two distinct synovial cavities. The **lateral band** (12) or the medial calcaneocuboid ligament, less thick than the previous

ligament, runs horizontally to be inserted into the dorsal aspect of the cuboid. These two bands therefore form a solid right angle open superiorly and laterally (**Fig. 25**: anterior view, diagrammatic).

* The **dorsal calcaneocuboid ligament** (13) is a thin slip (**Figs 23 and 26**) stretched over the superolateral surface of the calcaneocuboid joint;
* The **plantar calcaneocuboid ligament**, dense and pearly white, carpets the plantar aspect of the tarsal bones and consists of two distinct layers:
  - A **deep layer** (14), which unites (**Fig. 24**: dorsal view after the superficial layer has been cut and pulled back) the anterior calcaneal tubercle and the plantar surface of the cuboid just posterior to the groove for the fibularis longus tendon (FL). (Note also the insertion of the tibialis posterior TP into the navicular tuberosity, **Figs 22-24 and 27**).
  - A **superficial layer** (15), attached posteriorly to the plantar surface of the calcaneus between its posterior tubercles and its anterior tubercle and anteriorly to the plantar surface of the cuboid anterior to the groove for the fibularis longus. It sends **expansions** (16) for insertion into the bases of the four metatarsals. Thus the groove on the cuboid is transformed into a fibro-osseous canal (17), which the fibularis longus FL traverses lateromedially (**Figs 24 and 26**); on its medial side runs the flexor hallucis longus tendon (FHL) under the sustentaculum tali and under the plantar calcaneonavicular ligament. If two paramedian sections are taken through the posterior tarsus (**Fig. 28**: directions of the two planes of section), a medial view (**Fig. 29**: lateral part of the section) shows the fibularis longus FL tendon leaving the cuboid and the anterior (1) and posterior (2) bands of the talocalcaneal ligament. The large plantar calcaneocuboid ligament with its deep (14) and superficial (15) fibrous bands is one of the essential structures for sustaining the plantar vault (see **Fig. 100**, p. 219).

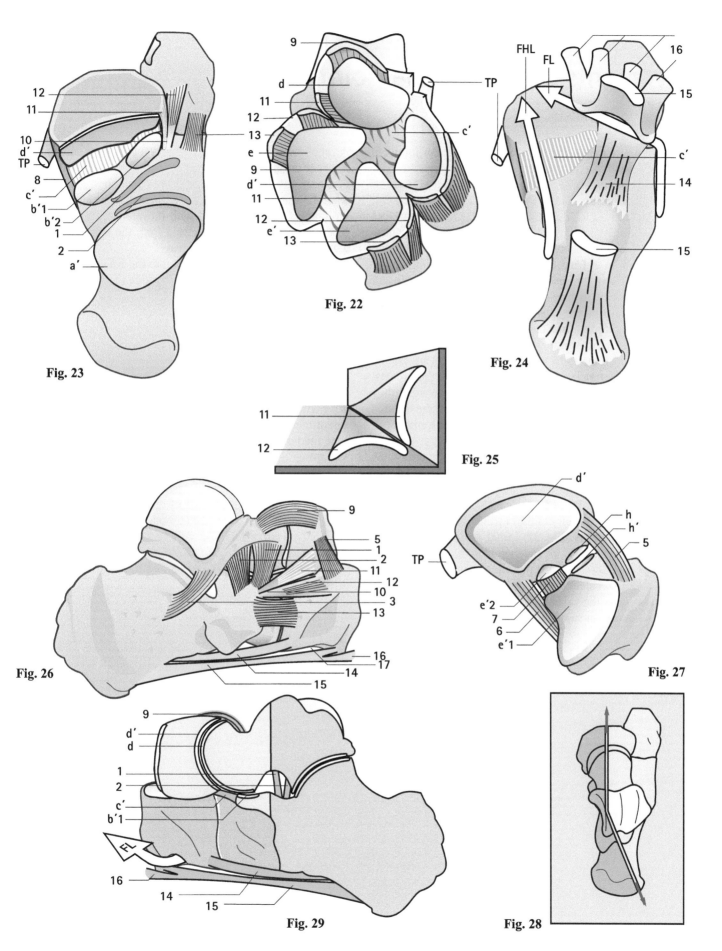

Fig. 22

Fig. 23

Fig. 24

Fig. 25

Fig. 26

Fig. 27

Fig. 28

Fig. 29

Movements at the subtalar joint

Taken separately, each of the surfaces of the subtalar joint can be roughly likened to a geometrical surface. The posterior talar facet is a *segment of a cylinder*; the talar head is a *segment of a sphere*. This joint, however, must be viewed as a plane joint, since it is geometrically impossible for two spherical surfaces and two cylindrical surfaces contained within the same mechanical unit to slide simultaneously on one another without a gap appearing between at least one of the two interacting sets of surfaces, i.e. without a more or less extensive **loss of contact** between the opposing surfaces. Thus the joint has some measure of play by virtue of its very structure and stands in sharp contrast to a very tight joint, like the hip joint, where the articular surfaces are geometrical and congruent with minimal play.

On the other hand, if the surfaces of the subtalar joint are exactly congruent in the intermediate position, i.e. where the greatest degree of contact is needed to transmit the body weight, they become frankly incongruent in extreme positions where the area of contact is reduced, but then the stresses are much smaller or almost nil.

Starting from the **intermediate position (Fig. 30**: anterior view of the transparent calcaneus-talus couple), movements of the calcaneus on the talus (assumed to be fixed) occur simultaneously **in the three planes of space.** During foot inversion **(Fig. 2, p. 181)** the anterior extremity of the calcaneus undergoes **three elementary movements (Fig. 31**: initial position shown by a blue broken line):

- a slight depression (t) leading to a slight extension of the foot
- a medial displacement (v) with adduction of the foot
- a rotation (r) as the calcaneus tends to lie down flat on its lateral surface with supination of the foot.

A set of exactly converse elementary movements can be shown to occur during foot eversion.

Farabeuf gave the perfect account of this complex movement when he said that 'the calcaneus pitches, turns and rolls under the talus'. This comparison with movements of a boat is perfectly justified **(Fig. 34)**. Starting from the stable position (a), when the boat is exposed to a wave:

- it **pitches** as its stem plunges into the wave (b)
- it **turns** as its stem moves to one side (c)
- it **rolls** to one side (d).

These elementary movements around the axes of pitching, turning and rolling are automatically combined as the ship 'dips' obliquely relative to the wave (e).

It can be shown geometrically that a movement whose elementary movements about three axes are known *can be reduced to a single movement occurring about a single axis oblique to these three axes*. For the calcaneus, shown here diagrammatically as a parallelepiped **(Fig. 32)** this axis **mn** is oblique superoinferiorly, mediolaterally and anteroposteriorly. Rotation about this axis **mn (Fig. 33)** results precisely in the movements described above. This axis, demonstrated by Henke, enters the superomedial surface of the talar neck, runs through the sinus tarsi and emerges at the lateral process of the calcaneal tuberosity (see p. 199 and also the mechanical model of the foot at the end of this book). **Henke's axis**, as will be shown later, is not only the axis of the subtalar joint but also the axis of the transverse tarsal joint, and it **controls all the movements of the posterior tarsus under the ankle.**

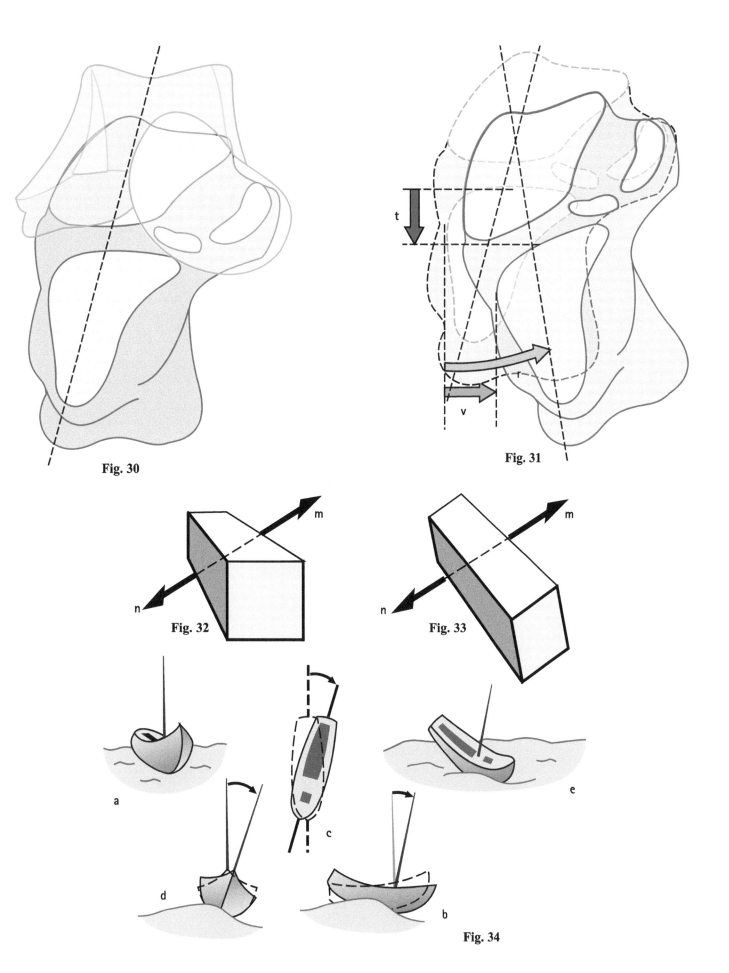

Fig. 30

Fig. 31

Fig. 32

Fig. 33

Fig. 34

Movements at the subtalar and transverse tarsal joints

The **relative movements of the posterior tarsal bones** are easily analysed with the use of an anatomical specimen X-rayed in the positions of inversion and eversion. If each bone is transfixed with a metal pin and labelled as **a** for the talus (blue), **b** for the calcaneus (red), **c** for the navicular (green) and **d** for the cuboid (orange), then their angular displacements can be measured.

On superior **radiographs taken vertically**, with the talus staying put, the change from eversion (Fig. 35) to inversion (Fig. 36) is associated with the following angular displacements:

- The **navicular** (c) (Fig. 36) slides medially on the talar head and turns through a 5° angle
- The **cuboid** (d) follows the navicular, turning also through a 5° angle, and slides medially relative to the calcaneus and the navicular
- The **calcaneus** (b) moves anteriorly slightly and rotates on the talus, also through a 5° angle.

These three elementary rotations occur in the same direction, i.e. in the direction of **adduction**.

Anteroposterior radiographs, with the talus still considered to be stationary, show the following displacements **during passage from eversion** (Fig. 37) **to inversion** (Fig. 38):

- The **navicular** (c) rotates through an angle of 25° and slightly overshoots the talus medially.

- The **cuboid** (d) disappears medially completely behind the shadow of the calcaneus and rotates through an 18° angle.
- The **calcaneus** (b) slides medially under the talus and rotates through a 20° angle.

These three elementary rotations take place in the same direction, i.e. in the direction of **supination** with the navicular rotating more than the calcaneus, and especially more than the cuboid. Finally, **lateral radiographs taken** during the **passage from eversion** (Fig. 39) **to inversion** (Fig. 40) show the following displacements:

- The **navicular** (c) *literally slides under the talar head* and turns on itself through a 45° angle so that its anterior surface tends to face inferiorly.
- The **cuboid** (d) also slides inferiorly in relation to both the calcaneus and the talus. This descent of the cuboid with respect to the talus is distinctly greater than that of the navicular on the talus. At the same time the cuboid rotates through a 12° angle.
- The **calcaneus** (b) moves anteriorly relative to the talus, whose posterior border clearly overhangs the calcaneus behind its posterior talar facet. At the same time it turns through a 10° angle in the direction of extension, like the navicular.

These three elementary movements occur in the same direction, i.e. in the direction of **extension**.

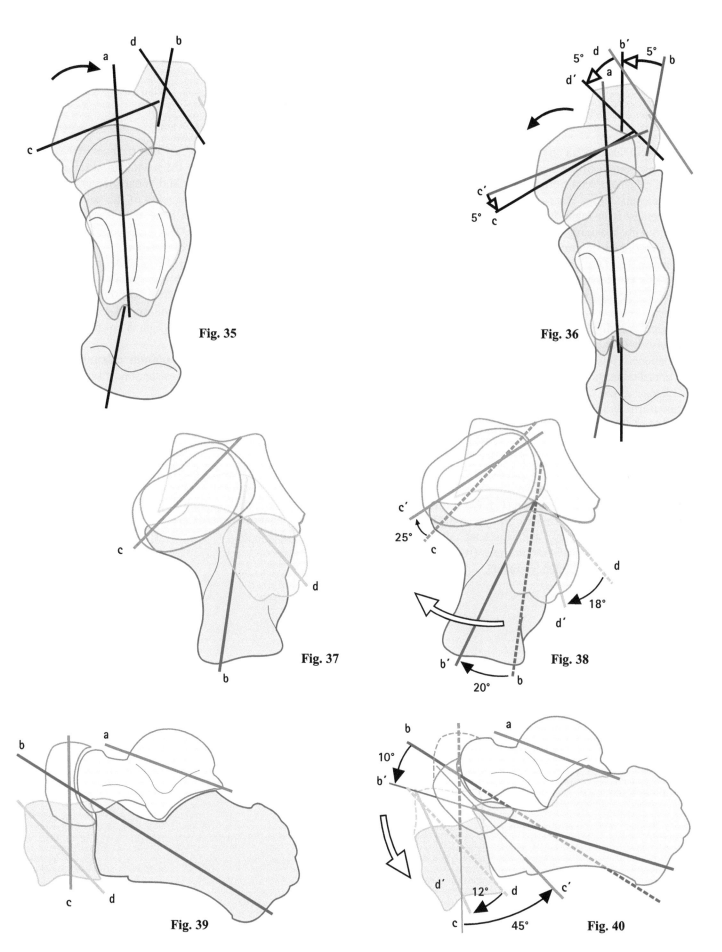

Fig. 35

Fig. 36

Fig. 37

Fig. 38

Fig. 39

Fig. 40

Movements at the transverse tarsal joint

These movements depend on the shape of the articular surfaces and the disposition of the ligaments. On the whole (**Fig. 41**: talus and calcaneus seen from the front), the articular surfaces are set along an axis xx' that runs obliquely superoinferiorly and mediolaterally at an angle of 45° with the horizontal plane and serves, roughly speaking, as a **hinge** for inferior and medial as well as superior and lateral **movements** of the navicular-cuboid pair (arrows S and C). The surface of the ovoid talar head with its long axis yy' at a 45° angle with the horizontal (the angle of 'rotation' of the talar head) is elongated in the direction of this movement.

The **navicular is displaced on the talar head** medially **(Fig. 42)** and inferiorly **(Fig. 43)** by the pull of the tibialis posterior (TP), whose tendon is inserted into the navicular tubercle. The tension in the dorsal talonavicular ligament (a) checks these movements. This change in the orientation of the navicular produces, via the cuneiform and the first three metatarsals, **adduction and hollowing of the medial arch of the foot** (see p. 230).

At the same time, the navicular moves **into eversion** relative to the calcaneus (**Fig. 44**: superior view after removal of the talus) and the spring ligament (b), the inferior border of the deltoid ligament (c) and the medial band of the bifurcated ligament (d) become taut. During **foot inversion (Fig. 45)** contraction of the tibialis posterior (TP, not shown) brings the navicular closer to the calcaneus (blue arrow) and causes the talus to ride over the posterior talar facet of the calcaneus (red arrow), thereby relaxing the above-mentioned ligaments.

This explains why the anterior articular surfaces of the calcaneus do not extend right down to the navicular, since an articular surface supported by a bony and consequently rigid bracket would not permit these movements of the navicular relative to the calcaneus. On the other hand, the pliable surface of the spring ligament (b) is essential (see p. 230) for the elasticity and hollowing of the medial arch of the foot.

Movements of the cuboid on the calcaneus are very limited superiorly (**Fig. 46**, medial view) as a result of two factors:

- the **beak-like projection of the anterior process** of the calcaneus (black arrow), which impedes movement on the superior aspect of the joint, which is covered by the **calcaneocuboid ligament** (e).
- the **tension in the powerful plantar calcaneocuboid ligament** (f), which rapidly stops the joint from gapping inferiorly (a).

On the other hand (**Fig. 47**), the cuboid descends easily on the convex surface of the calcaneal articular facet; this movement is checked by the **tension of the lateral band (1) of the bifurcated ligament.**

In the transverse plane (Fig. 48: horizontal section at level AB of **Fig. 41**) the cuboid *slides more easily medially*, being checked only by the tension of the **dorsal calcaneocuboid ligament** (g). On the whole, movement of the cuboid takes place *preferentially inferiorly and medially.*

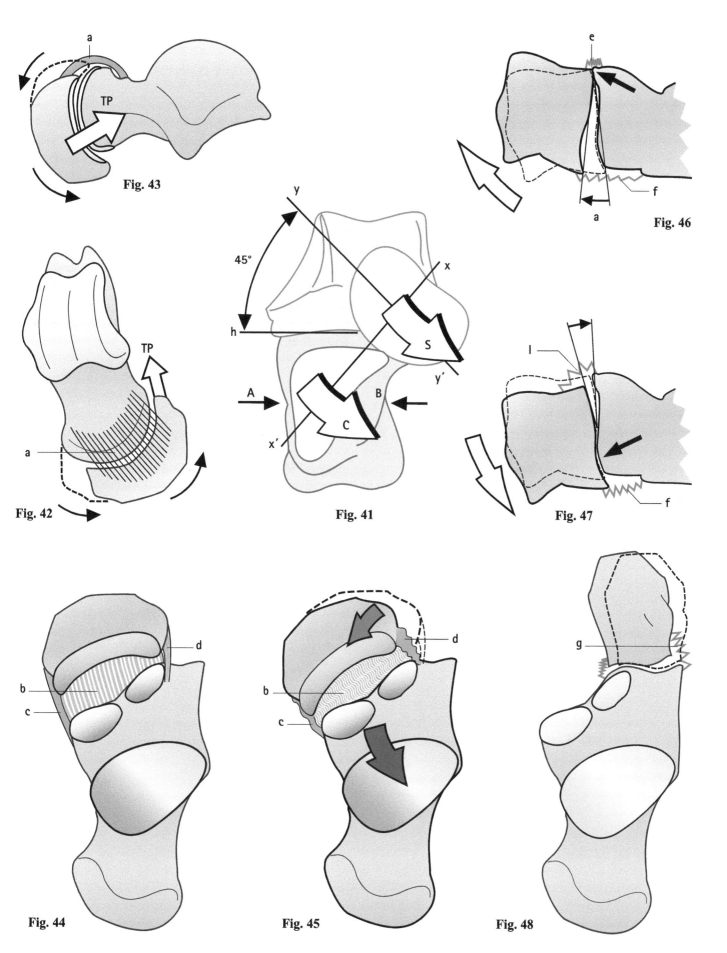

Fig. 43

Fig. 42

Fig. 41

Fig. 46

Fig. 47

Fig. 44

Fig. 45

Fig. 48

The overall functioning of the posterior tarsal joints

It is clear from examining and manipulating an anatomical specimen of the posterior tarsus that all these joints constitute an inseparable functional unit: the **articular complex of the hindfoot**, entrusted with adapting the orientation and shape of the entire plantar vault.

The subtalar and the transverse tarsal joints are mechanically linked and together form the **equivalent of a single joint with one degree of freedom** around **Henke's axis mn** (see also the model of the foot at the end of this book).

The diagrams on the next page show the four bones of the posterior tarsus from two different viewpoints: **anterolateral** views **(Figs 49 and 51)** and **anterior** views **(Figs 50 and 52)**. In each of these diagrams, the positions corresponding to **inversion I (Figs 49 and 50)** and to **eversion** E **(Figs 51 and 52)** in the vertical plane have been juxtaposed. As a result it is possible to appreciate the *changes in direction of the navicular-cuboid pair* relative to the talus, which stays put by definition.

Movement of inversion (Figs 49 and 50)

- The tibialis posterior pulls on the navicular **Nav** exposing the superolateral part of the talar head **d.**
- The navicular drags along the cuboid **Cub** with the help of the naviculocuboid ligaments.
- The cuboid in turn pulls the calcaneus **Calc**, which dives anteriorly under the talus **Tal** (d).
- The sinus tarsi gaps maximally **(Fig. 49)**, while the two bands of the interosseous ligament (1 and 2) become taut.
- The posterior talar facet of the calcaneus a' is laid bare anteroinferiorly, while the talocalcaneal joint gaps superiorly and posteriorly.

To sum up

- The navicular-cuboid pair **(Fig. 50)** is drawn medially (red arrow **Add**) causing the forefoot to move anteriorly and medially (red arrow, **Fig. 49**).

- At the same time, the navicular-cuboid pair rotates around an anteroposterior axis running through the bifurcated ligament, which actively resists elongation-torsion stresses. This rotation is due to the combined lowering and rotation of the navicular and depression of the cuboid and produces supination of the foot (red arrow): the sole of the foot moves to face medially **as the lateral plantar arch is depressed;** the cuboid articular facet for the fifth metatarsal Vm faces inferiorly and anteriorly; **elevation of the medial plantar arch** causes the navicular anterior facet for the first cuneiform Ic to face directly anteriorly.

Movement of eversion (Figs 51 and 52)

- The fibularis brevis, inserted into the tuberosity of the bone of the fifth metatarsal, pulls the cuboid laterally and posteriorly.
- The cuboid drags along the navicular, exposing the superomedial part of the talar head, while the calcaneus dips posteriorly below the talus (d).
- The sinus tarsi closes down **(Fig. 51)**, and the movement is checked by the impact of the talus on the floor of the sinus tarsi.
- The posterosuperior part of the posterior talar facet of the calcaneus **a'** is laid bare.

To sum up

- The navicular-cuboid pair **(Fig. 52)** is pulled laterally (blue arrow Abd) so that the forefoot comes to face anteriorly and laterally (blue arrow, **Fig. 51**).
- At the same time the navicular-cuboid pair rotates on itself in the direction of **pronation** Pron (blue arrow) as a result of depression of the navicular and abduction of the cuboid, whose articular facet Vm now looks anteriorly and laterally.

The author uses first (C1), second (C2) and third (C3) for medial, intermediate and lateral cuneiforms.

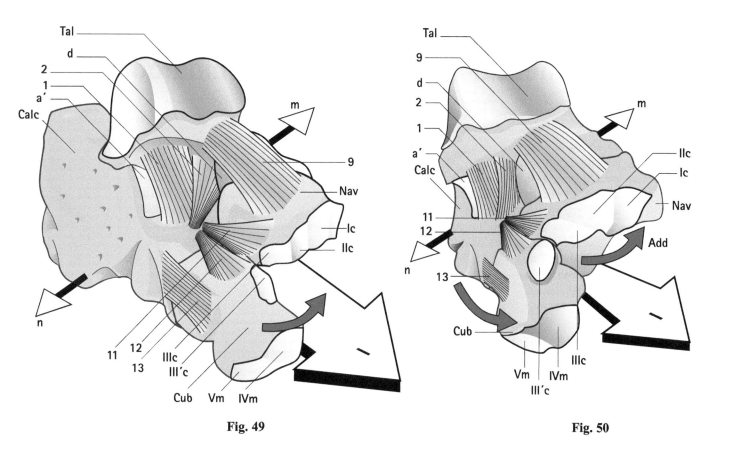

Fig. 49

Fig. 50

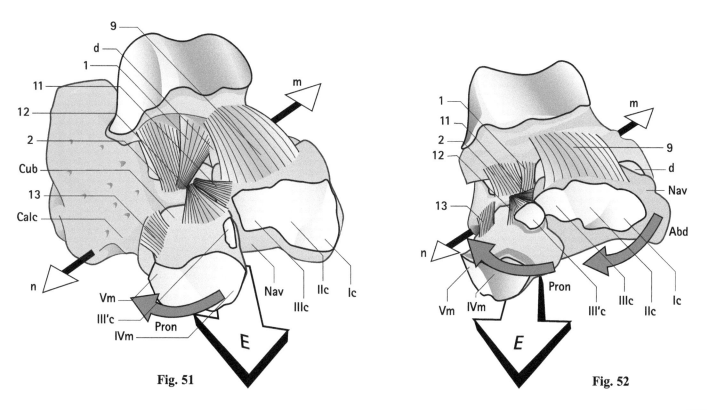

Fig. 51

Fig. 52

The heterokinetic universal joint of the hindfoot

Henke's axis, which we have just defined, is not fixed and unchanging, as one might think. In reality, it is a **mobile axis**, i.e. shifting in space during movements. This conclusion can be drawn from a study of successive radiographs of the posterior tarsus taken during movements of inversion-eversion. When instantaneous centres of rotation are superimposed on corresponding pairs of radiographs, they do not coincide. This observation justifies the hypothesis that a mobile Henke's axis **(Fig. 53)** shifts from an **initial position** (1) to a **final position** (2) along a crooked path that maps all its intermediate locations. The mathematical demonstration of this hypothesis needs to be done on a computer.

In the hindfoot, there are **two successive nonparallel axes**, i.e, **the axis of the ankle joint** and **Henke's axis** which, as we have just seen, represents the global axis of the subtalar and transverse tarsal joints. It is thus possible to use the universal joint* as the mechanical model for the articular complex of the hindfoot.

In **industrial mechanics** the universal joint **(Fig. 54)** is defined as a joint with two orthogonal axes and two rotating shafts. Such a joint transmits the rotational movement from one shaft to the other, whatever the angle between them within certain limits, e.g., 45°. In cars with front-wheel drive it is inserted between the drive shaft and the axle shaft linking the two driving wheels. It is also called a *homokinetic joint*, since the driving couple of force remains the same regardless of the positions of the shafts.

In **biomechanics** there are **three joints of this type:**
- the sternoclavicular joint - a saddle joint
- the wrist joint - an articular complex of condyloid type
- the trapeziometacarpal joint, another saddle joint, described in detail in Volume 1.

In the hindfoot, the critical difference lies in the fact that the universal joint is of the heterokinetic type, i.e. *the joint is not regular.* Instead of being orthogonal, i.e. perpendicular to one another in space, **its axes are oblique with respect to one another.** For the purpose of demonstration, a mechanical model of this heterokinetic joint **(Fig. 55)** has been superimposed on a diagram of the ankle containing the following:
- the leg skeleton A and the forefoot skeleton B
- the transverse axis of the ankle joint XX' running slightly obliquely anteriorly and medially
- Henke's axis YY' running obliquely in a posteroanterior, inferosuperior and lateromedial direction
- an intervening piece C, which *has no bony equivalent* but represents a distorted tetrahedron whose opposite corners contain the two shafts of the joint.

The **non-orthogonal nature of these axes gives rise to a differential bias** in the movements of the articular complex of the hindfoot. The muscles, organized in relation to these two axes (see p. 220), can produce only two types of movements, with other types being mechanically prohibited:
- **inversion (Fig. 56)**, which extends the foot and turns its plantar surface to face medially
- **eversion (Fig. 57)**, which flexes the foot on the leg and turns its plantar surface to face laterally.

Understanding the mechanism of this heterokinetic universal joint is basic to our understanding of the actions of the muscles of the foot, and of the orientation of the sole of the foot as well as of its static and dynamic characteristics.

---

* The joint called "cardan" in French and "universal joint" in English was invented by Girolamo Cardano (1501-1576); hence its name in French. It allowed compasses to be installed on ships despite their rolling and pitching and greatly assisted in maritime exploration. In English it is called the universal joint, which is wrong because the adjective would better suit a ball-and socket joint.

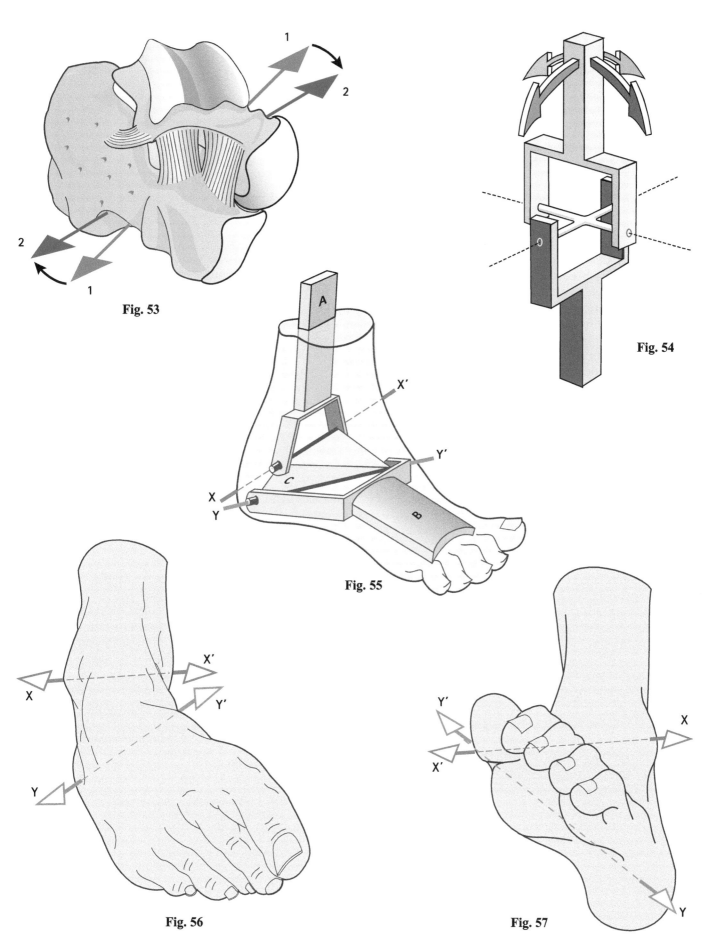

Fig. 53

Fig. 54

Fig. 55

Fig. 56

Fig. 57

The ligamentous chains during inversion and eversion

Movements of inversion and eversion of the foot are limited by two types of resisting factors:
- bony impacts
- the ligamentous systems of the hindfoot.

Factors restricting the movement of inversion

As shown previously, during inversion the calcaneus dips inferiorly and medially, causing the talus to climb towards the superior part of the calcaneal posterior talar facet, where it meets no bony resistance. Meanwhile, the anteroinferior part of the posterior talar facet is laid bare, as is the talar head when the navicular slides inferiorly and medially without encountering any bony obstacle.

Therefore, inversion is not restricted by any bony cheeks except for the medial malleolus, which keeps the talar trochlea in place.

Hence inversion is limited only by a **chain of ligaments**, which are tightened and generate two lines of tension **(Fig. 58)**.

1. **The main line of tension:**
- starts from the lateral malleolus
- then runs along the anterior band of the lateral collateral ligament (1) of the ankle joint
- bifurcates to reach the calcaneus and the cuboid via:
  - the interosseous ligament (2 and 3)
  - the **lateral** calcaneocuboid branch of the bifurcated ligament (7)
  - the superolateral or dorsal calcaneocuboid ligament (6)
  - the **plantar calcaneocuboid ligament** (not shown here)
  - the navicular branch of the bifurcated ligament (8)
- and finally spreads from the talus to the navicular via the dorsal talonavicular ligament (5).

2. **The accessory line of tension** starts from the medial malleolus and follows the posterior band of the medial collateral ligament of the ankle joint (not shown here) and then the posterior talocalcaneal ligament (not shown here).

Therefore, during inversion, the talus acts as a relay station for the ligaments with **two coming towards it and three leaving it.**

Factors restricting the movement of eversion

During eversion **(Fig. 59)**, the main posterior facet of the inferior surface of the talus slides down along the slope of the posterior talar facet of the calcaneus before hitting the superior surface of the calcaneus at the level of the floor of the sinus tarsi. The lateral cheek of the talus is pulled laterally and hits the lateral malleolus with the risk of fracture if the movement is not checked. **Thus bone-to-bone contacts play a predominant role in limiting eversion.**

The **ligamentous chain limiting eversion** also gives rise to *two lines of tension*:

1. **The main line of tension**
- starts from the medial malleolus and proceeds via the two planes of the anterior band of the medial collateral ligament of the ankle joint:
  - the superficial plane (the deltoid ligament 9), linking the malleolus directly to the navicular and the calcaneus, which are themselves united by the spring ligament (11)
  - the deep plane (10), linking the malleolus to the talus via the anterior tibiofibular ligament (not shown here) and then to the calcaneus via the interosseous ligament (12).
- spreads to the calcaneus, which is bound to the cuboid and the navicular by the bifurcated ligament, which forks into two branches, one for the cuboid (7) and the other for the navicular (8). It is clear that this ligament keeps these three bones tightly bound during both inversion and eversion
- spreads along the sole of the foot via the plantar calcaneonavicular ligament (not shown).

2. **The accessory line of tension**
- starts from the lateral malleolus
- spreads to the talus via the posterior band of the lateral collateral ligament of the ankle joint (not shown) and thence to the calcaneus via the lateral talocalcanean ligament (13)
- spreads also directly to the calcaneus via the middle band of the lateral collateral ligament of the ankle joint (4).

In sum, the talar relay station **receives two ligaments and gives origin to two ligaments.**

One can draw the overall conclusion that **inversion tears the ligaments**, particularly the anterior band of the lateral collateral ligament of the ankle joint, causing severe sprains, whereas **eversion leads to fractures of the malleoli, starting with the lateral malleolus.**

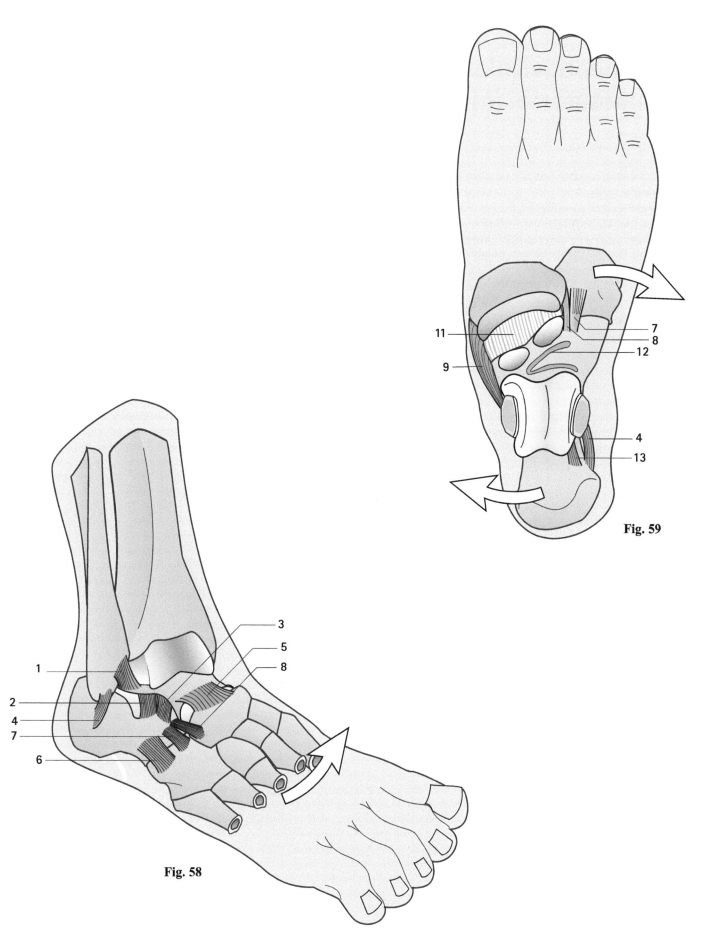

Fig. 59

Fig. 58

The cuneonavicular, intercuneiform and tarsometatarsal joints

All these joints are **plane joints** with small-range gliding and gapping movements.

The navicular-cuboid pair (**Fig. 60**, frontal view) has **three navicular facets: Ic, IIc and IIIc** articulating with the **medial (C1), intermediate (C2) and lateral (C3) cuneiforms** respectively and **three cuboid facets** articulating with the **fifth metatarsal (Vm), fourth metatarsal (IVm)** and the **lateral cuneiform (III'c)**, respectively. The cuboid also supports the lateral extremity of the navicular at the cubonavicular joint (arrows).

A **blown-up anterolateral view (Fig. 61)** illustrates how the artificially raised block of the **three cuneiforms** articulates with the navicular-cuboid pair: the double arrow shows how the lateral cuneiform rests on the cuboid, i.e. on a facet (III'c) lying just anterior to the articular facet for the navicular and belonging to the cuneocuboid joint.

The **intercuneiform joints (Fig. 62**: superior view of the cuneonavicular and intercuneiform joints and partially of the tarsometatarsal joints) have articular facets and interosseous ligaments: the one between the C1 and C2 has been cut (19), and the other between the C2 and C3 cuneiforms (20) is left in place.

The **tarsometatarsal joint** consists proximally (**Fig. 64**, superior view) of the three cuneiforms medially, of the cuboid (Cub) laterally, and distally of the bases of the **five metatarsals M1, M2, M3, M4 and M5**; it is made up of a *succession of tightly interlocked plane joints*. A dorsal view of the opened joint (**Fig. 63**, inspired by Rouvière) shows the various articular facets of the tarsal bones and the corresponding facets of the metatarsals.

The base of the **second metatarsal M2** with its three facets fits snugly into the cuneiform mortise formed by the medial facet IImC3 of the lateral cuneiform C3, the anterior facet IImC2 of the intermediate cuneiform C2 and the lateral facet IImC1 of the medial cuneiform C1. The tarsometatarsal joints are also held together by **powerful ligaments** that become visible **(Fig. 62)** when the joints are opened from above, the first metatarsal is rotated on its axis (arrow 1) and the third metatarsal is pulled laterally (arrow 2). The ligaments are these:

- medially, the **strong bifurcated ligament** (18), running from the lateral aspect of C1 to the medial aspect of the base of the second metatarsal; *it is the critical ligament in midfoot disarticulations*
- laterally, a **ligamentous system** comprising straight fibres (21) between (C2) and the second metatarsal (M2) and between C3 and M3 as well as crossed fibres (23) between C3 and M2 and between C2 and M3 (24).

The **robustness of the tarsometatarsal joint** also depends on numerous ligaments (**Fig. 64**, dorsal view and **Fig. 65**, plantar view) stretching from the base of each metatarsal to the corresponding tarsal bone and to the bases of the neighbouring metatarsals. Particularly on the dorsal aspect **(Fig. 64)**, ligaments radiate from the base of the second metatarsal to all the neighbouring bones; on the plantar aspect **(Fig. 65)** there are ligaments running from the medial cuneiform to the first three metatarsals. Into the plantar aspect of the base of the first metatarsal is inserted the fibularis longus (FL) after emerging from its plantar groove (white arrow). The fibularis brevis (FB) is inserted into the tuberosity on the base of the fifth metatarsal.

The **joint space of the tarsometatarsal joint** is shown in these two diagrams as a red broken line.

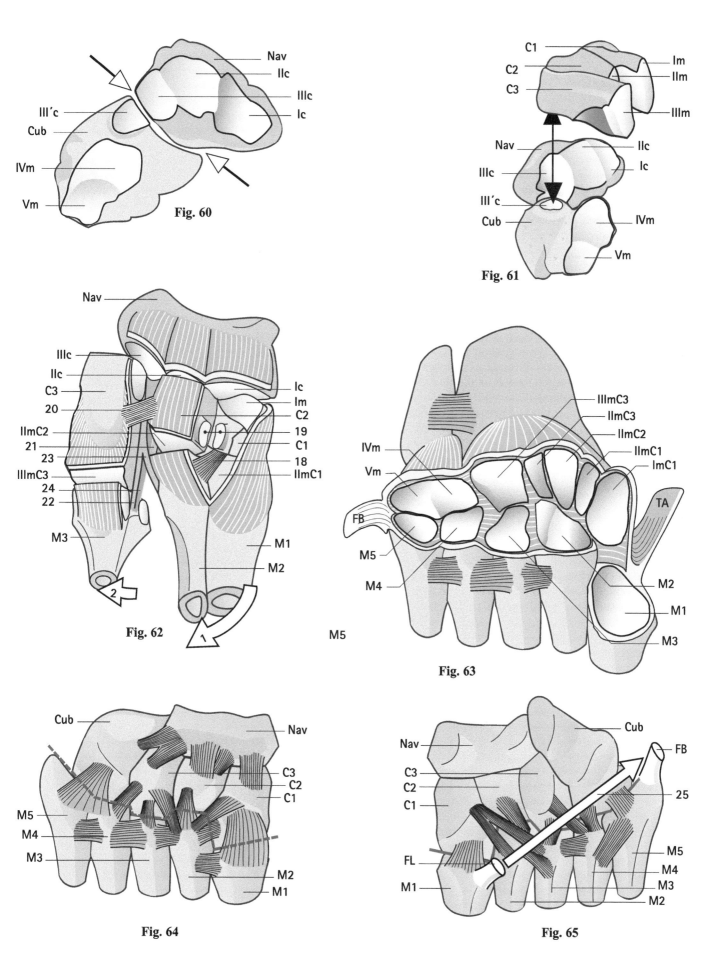

Fig. 60

Fig. 61

Fig. 62

Fig. 63

Fig. 64

Fig. 65

Movements at the anterior tarsal and tarsometatarsal joints

The **intercuneiform joints (Fig. 66**: coronal section) allow small vertical movements to occur and alter the transverse curvature of the plantar vault (see p. 241). The lateral cuneiform (C1) rests on the cuboid (Cub), whose medial third (dark) supports the cuneiform arch. **Along the long axis of the foot (Fig. 67**: sagittal section) small displacements of the cuneiforms relative to the navicular contribute to the changes of curvature of the medial arch (see p. 236).

The movements in the tarsometatarsal joints (Fig. 68, superior view) can be deduced from the shape of the joint interspaces and the orientation of their articular surfaces (very well described in anatomy textbooks):

- **Overall**, the combined interspace of the tarsometatarsal joints is oblique mediolaterally, superoinferiorly and anteroposteriorly, with its medial end lying 2 cm anterior to its lateral end. The **general obliquity** of this axis of flexion-extension of the metatarsals, like Henke's axis, contributes to the **movements of eversion-inversion** (see mechanical model of the foot at the end of this volume).
- The degree of overshooting of the cuneiforms follows a geometric progression: the lateral cuneiform (C1) overshoots the cuboid (Cub) by 2 mm; the lateral cuneiform overshoots the intermediate cuneiform (Ci) by 4 mm; and the medial cuneiform (Cm) overshoots the intermediate by 8 mm.

Thus is constituted the **cuneiform mortise** for the base of the second metatarsal, which is therefore the **least mobile** of all the metatarsals and serves as the **ridge-tile of the plantar vault** (see p. 240).

- The two outermost segments of the joint space have an **inverse obliquity:** the space between M1 and Cm is oblique anteriorly and laterally and, when produced, it runs through *the middle of M5*; the space between M5 and Cub is oblique anteriorly and medially and, when produced, ends up near the head of M1.

The flexion-extension axis of the two outermost metatarsals (which are the most mobile) is thus not perpendicular but **oblique** to their long axes. As a result, these **outermost metatarsals do not move in the sagittal plane** but along a conical surface; during flexion they both move simultaneously towards the axis of the foot (**Fig. 70**: diagrammatic superolateral view of the tarsometatarsal joint space with the outermost metatarsals).

- The movement *aa' of the head* of M1 has a flexion component F and an abduction component Abd of 15° range (inspired by Fick).
- In symmetrical fashion, the movement **bb'** of the head of M5 consists of a flexion component F associated with an adduction component **Add.**

Therefore the heads of these metatarsals move simultaneously interiorly and towards the axis of the foot, and this increases **(Fig. 70)** the curvature of the anterior arch with **hollowing of the anterior part of the plantar vault** along the curved line a'b' (red broken line). Conversely, extension of the metatarsals is followed by flattening of the anterior arch (see mechanical model of the foot at the end of this volume).

This movement of bringing closer together the two outermost metatarsals is also assisted (**Fig. 69**: anterior view of the anterior surfaces of the cuboid and cuneiforms) by the obliquity of the transverse axes xx' and yy' of their articular facets; it is represented by the thick double-headed arrows. These movements of hollowing and flattening of the anterior arch are shown diagrammatically in Figure 71.

Therefore, the changes in the curvature of the anterior arch result directly from the movements taking place at the tarsometatarsal joints.

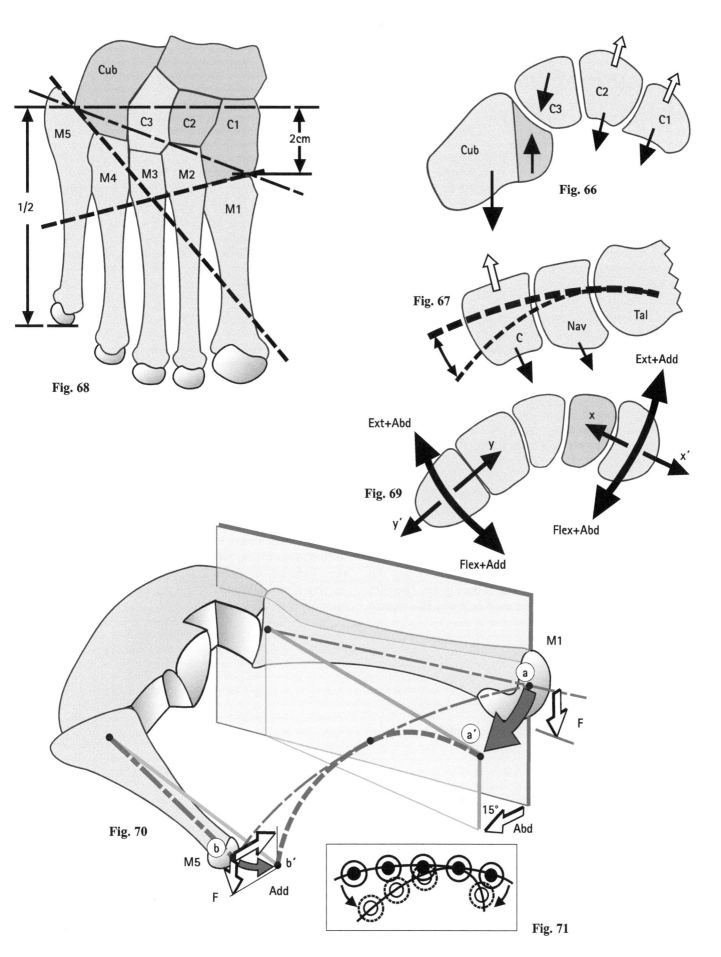

Cub

C3

C2

C1

M5

M4

M3

M2

M1

2cm

1/2

Fig. 68

Cub

C3

C2

C1

Fig. 66

Fig. 67

C

Nav

Tal

Ext+Add

Ext+Abd

y

x

x′

Fig. 69

y′

Flex+Abd

Flex+Add

M1

a

a′

F

15°

Abd

Fig. 70

b

M5

b′

F

Add

Fig. 71

207

Extension of the toes

The metatarsophalangeal and the interphalangeal joints of the toes will not be described, since they are identical to those of the fingers (see Volume 1) except for **some functional differences** regarding the metatarsophalangeal joints. Whereas flexion at the metacarpophalangeal joints has a greater range than extension, extension has the greater range at the metatarsophalangeal joints:

- **Active extension** has a range of 50-60°, and active flexion only 30-40°.
- **Passive extension (Fig. 72)**, which is essential in the last phase of the step, reaches or exceeds 90°, compared to a 45-50° range for active flexion.

Side-to-side movements of the toes at the metatarsophalangeal joints have a much smaller range than those of the fingers. In particular, the human big toe, unlike that of the monkey, has lost its potential for opposition as a result of the adaptation of the human foot for bipedal walking on the ground.

Active extension of the toes is produced by three muscles: two extrinsic muscles - the extensor hallucis longus and the extensor digitorum longus; and one intrinsic muscle - the extensor digitorum brevis.

The **extensor digitorum brevis (Fig. 73)** lies entirely in the dorsum of the foot. Its four fleshy bellies arise from the *sulcus calcanei* in the floor of the sinus tarsi and from the stem of the inferior extensor retinaculum. Their thin tendons blend with the tendons of the extensor digitorum longus for the four medial toes, except that its first tendon is inserted directly into the dorsal surface of the proximal phalanx of the big toe. The fifth toe thus receives no tendon from the short extensor. This muscle therefore extends the metatarsophalangeal joints of the first four toes **(Fig. 74)**.

The extensor digitorum longus and the extensor hallucis longus are lodged in the anterior compartment of the leg, and their tendons are inserted into the phalanges in a manner that will be studied later (see p. 214).

The **tendon of the extensor digitorum longus (Fig. 75)** descends along the anterior surface of the instep inside the lateral loop of the stem of the inferior extensor retinaculum before dividing into **four tendons** destined for the four lateral toes (see **Fig. 98**). The fifth toe therefore is extended only by the long extensor, which is not only a toe extensor as indicated by its name but **also and above all an ankle flexor** (see p. 220). Hence its pure extensor action on the toes is only apparent when combined with **contraction of the synergistic-antagonistic** ankle extensors, mainly the triceps surae (shown as a white arrow).

The **tendon of the extensor hallucis longus (Fig. 76)** passes inside the medial loop of the superior limb of the inferior extensor retinaculum and then deep to its inferior limb (see also **Fig. 98**, p. 219) to be inserted into the two phalanges of the big toe, i.e. into the medial and lateral margins of the proximal phalanx and into the dorsal surface of the base of the distal phalanx. It is therefore **an extensor of the big toe but also and above all an ankle flexor.** Just like the **extensor digitorum longus**, it needs contraction of the synergistic-antagonistic extensors of the ankle in order to produce isolated extension of the big toe.

For Duchenne de Boulogne, the true extensor of the toes is the extensor digitorum brevis; we shall offer support for this opinion later.

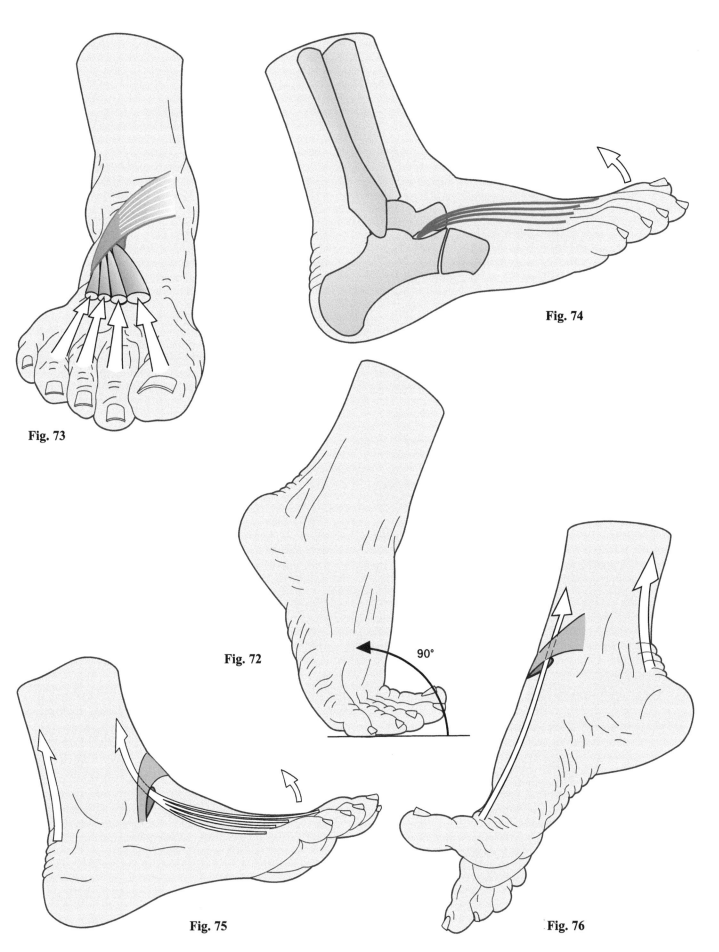

Fig. 73

Fig. 74

Fig. 72

90°

Fig. 75

Fig. 76

The compartments of the leg

Just as the forearm contains the extrinsic muscles of the hand and fingers, the leg contains the extrinsic muscles of the foot and toes. Figures 77 and 79 (distal surfaces of cross-sections taken respectively from the upper third and from lower down in the right leg) show clearly how the muscles surround the two leg bones, i.e. the tibia (T) and the fibula (F). Between these two bones lies the **interosseous membrane** (1) like a median partition, while the leg is wrapped inside a continuous and inextensible **superficial fascia** (2). Medially, the superficial fascia covers directly the medial surface of the tibia, which is thus immediately subcutaneous; laterally, on the other hand, the fibula lies deep and is connected to the superficial fascia by **two fibrous septa**, i.e. the **lateral intermuscular septum** (3) and the **anterolateral intermuscular septum** (4).

As a result the leg has **three spaces** and **four fascial compartments** (**Fig. 78**, posterolateral view in perspective: the tibia has been transected at a higher level than the fibula):

- On the anterior surface of the leg, **the anterior compartment** (arrow 1) is enclosed by the interosseous membrane and the anterolateral intermuscular septum and holds the ankle flexors and the toe extensors.
- On the anterolateral aspect of the fibula lies the **anterolateral compartment** (arrow 2) bounded by the two intermuscular septa and filled with the fibularis muscles.
- On the posterior surface of the leg lies the **posterior compartment**, which is in turn subdivided into two parts by the deep fascia (5) stretching between the medial border of the tibia and the posterolateral border of the fibula: the **deep posterior compartment** (arrow 3), lying between the tibia and the interosseous membrane, contains the toe flexors and some ankle extensors; the **superficial posterior compartment** (arrow 4), lying between the deep fascia and the superficial fascia, contains the powerful ankle extensor, i.e. the triceps surae.

The **anterior compartment** (**Fig. 80**: anterior view of the leg) contains four muscles mediolaterally:

- The **tibialis anterior** (6) arises from the tibia, the medial half of the interosseous membrane (1) and the upper one-fourth of the deep surface of the superficial fascia (7). Its fleshy belly, occupying the inner half of the compartment, gives rise to a strong distal tendon TA, which is held against the front of the ankle by the **superior (8) and inferior (9) limbs of the inferior extensor retinaculum.**
- The **extensor hallucis longus** (10) lies slightly more distal than the tibialis anterior and arises from the medial surface of

the fibula and the interosseous membrane; its tendon of insertion (EHL) runs parallel to that of the tibialis anterior and deep to the two limbs of the inferior extensor retinaculum.

- The **extensor digitorum longus** (11) arises proximally and laterally to the extensor hallucis from the fibula, the interosseous membrane and the upper one-fourth of the deep surface of the deep fascia (12), and its distal tendon (EDL) runs lateral to the two preceding muscles deep to the lateral part of the extensor retinaculum.
- The **fibularis tertius** (13) (often absent) arises from the lower half of the lateral surface of the fibula, and its rather thin tendon (FT) runs deep to the most lateral part of the extensor retinaculum.
- The **anterior tibial artery** (14 in the diagrams opposite) with its *accompanying veins* traverses the oval aperture formed by the two bones and the superior border of the interosseous membrane and runs deep inside the anterior compartment, flanked by the anterior tibial nerve (15) (shown in these cross-sections).

The **anterolateral compartment** (**Fig. 81**: lateral view of the leg) lodges the two fibular muscles:

- The **fibularis longus** (16) arises from the lateral surface of the fibula (17), the lateral intermuscular septum (3), the anterolateral intermuscular septum (4) and the deep surface of the upper one-fourth of the deep fascia. Its **tendon** (18) descends towards the posterior border of the lateral malleolus.
- The **fibularis brevis** (19) arises distal to the fibularis longus from an area (20) encompassing the lateral aspect of the fibula and the two intermuscular septa. Its tendon (21) descends along and anterior to that of the fibularis longus before they both enter the **osteo-fibrous tunnel** that lies on the posterior border of the lateral malleolus and holds them down regardless of the position of the ankle. On emerging from this tunnel they veer towards the lateral border of the cuboid.

The **fibular artery** (22) flanked by the **fibular nerve** (23) (also shown in the cross-sections) crosses the lateral intermuscular septum before entering the upper corner of the lateral compartment. It sends a branch that goes through the anterolateral septum (24) and anastomoses with the anterior tibial artery. It then descends in the anterolateral compartment, and halfway down the leg it penetrates the anterolateral septum (25) before rejoining the anterior tibial artery. Also visible in Figures 77 and 79 are the long saphenous vein (LSV) and the short saphenous vein (SSV) embedded in the subcutaneous fat.

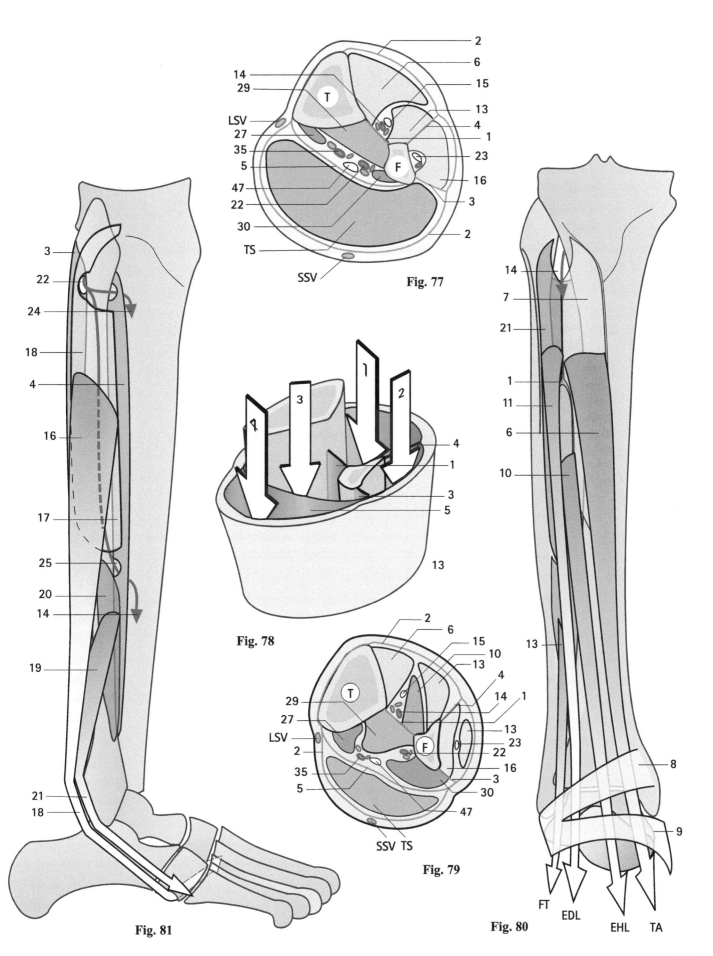

Fig. 77

Fig. 78

Fig. 79

Fig. 80

Fig. 81

FT EDL EHL TA

211

The compartments of the leg (*continued*)

The posterior space contains two compartments:

1. A deep compartment (**Fig. 82**, posterior view with the triceps surae removed) containing four muscles:

- The **popliteus** (26), is really a knee muscle and runs obliquely superolaterally to quickly leave the region.
- The **flexor digitorum longus** (27) is the most medial muscle and arises over a large area on the medial aspect of the posterior tibial surface and also from the fibula across a fibrous arcade (28); on its way down, its tendon (FDL) crosses the posterior margin of the talus before passing below the sustentaculum tali of the calcaneus.
- The **tibialis posterior** (29) arises, as we have already seen (see **Fig. 58**, p. 177), from the interosseous membranes and from both leg bones. Its tendon (TP) runs under the arcade formed by the flexor digitorum longus (white arrow) before skirting the posterior border of the medial malleolus and changing direction as it proceeds to the forefoot.
- The **flexor hallucis longus** (30) arises from the fibula distal to the preceding muscle, and its tendon (FHL) courses in the groove between the medial and lateral tubercles on the posterior surface of the talus before sliding under the sustentaculum tali on its way to the forefoot.

2. A superficial compartment (**Figs 83 and 84**) containing essentially the **triceps surae** with its two deep and superficial planes:

1. The deep plane (**Fig. 83**) lodges two muscles:

- The **soleus** (31) is a very wide muscle arising from a strong aponeurosis (32) that runs along two lines (33), one deep to the gastrocnemius and the other on the head of the fibula. These two sites of origin are bridged by a fibrous band that arches (34) over the tibial artery as it runs alongside the posterior tibial nerve (visible in the cross-sections) as it enters the deep compartment before dividing into the posterior tibial (35) and common fibular (**Fig. 79**, 22) nerves. The muscle belly of the soleus terminates on a wide aponeurosis that contributes to the formation of the calcaneal tendon (36) (see p. 224).

- The **plantaris** (37), a slender muscle arising from the lateral condylar plate and from the sesamoid bone, is unusual in having a thin and very long tendon (38) (almost as long as the leg) that runs along the medial border of the soleus and of the calcaneal tendon to share a common insertion into the calcaneus. This muscle is a weak ankle extensor, but, although it is often absent, it is of great value, since it provides an easily accessible tendon for transplantation.

2. The superficial plane (**Fig. 84**) contains the double-headed **gastrocnemius**, which arises above the knee and is therefore bi-articular. Its two heads arise separately, but they merge in the midline to terminate on the aponeurotic calcaneal tendon (see p. 224).

- The **medial head** (39) arises from the medial condylar plate and from the long tendinous band (40) attached above the medial condyle. The muscle fibres and the tendinous band course lateral to the tendons of the semimembranosus (41) and of the semitendinosus (42) with an intervening bursa (not shown here).
- The **lateral head** (43) has a similar supracondylar origin to that of the medial head. Its muscle fibres and its tendinous band (44) course medially alongside the biceps femoris (45).

It is important to be able to visualize these compartments in order to understand the **compartment syndrome** commonly seen after injuries. Obstruction to venous return caused by the injury can cause **oedema to develop in the muscles** within the compartment, increasing the pressure within the compartment and setting up a vicious circle, which worsens the venous stasis and hence the oedema. The increased pressure within the compartment will stop the arterial supply and thus *endanger the viability of the distal extremity of the limb* and, worse, *cause ischaemia of the nerves included in the compartment* at the risk of prolonged impairment of nerve conduction and eventually of nerve damage.

The compartment syndrome must be diagnosed as soon as possible in order to initiate the only possible form of treatment, i.e. section of the superficial fascia, which will reduce the pressure inside the compartment and break the vicious circle.

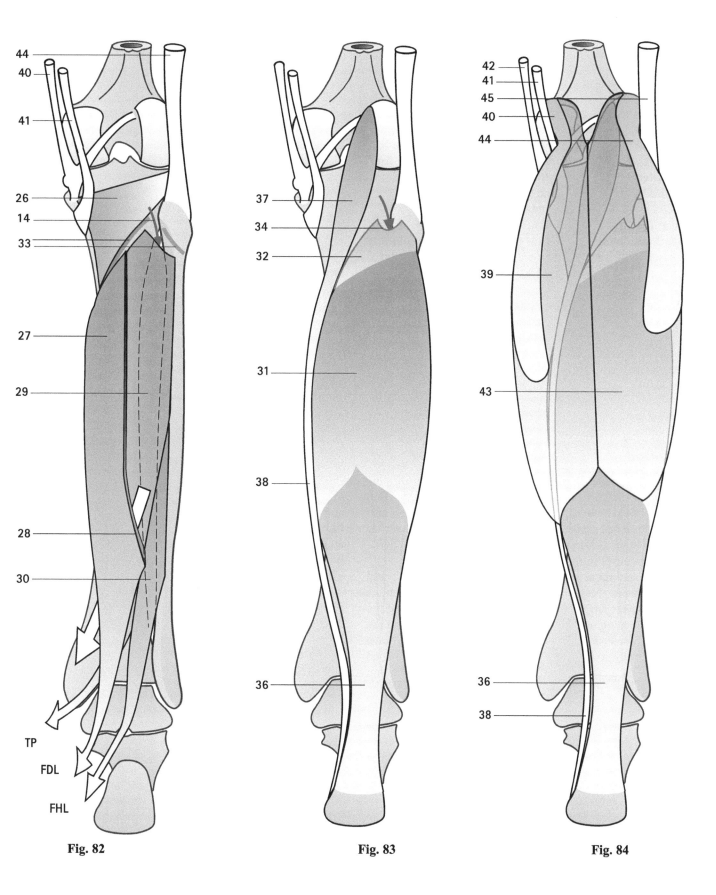

44
40
41
26
14
33
27
29
28
30
TP
FDL
FHL

Fig. 82

37
34
32
31
38
36

Fig. 83

42
41
45
40
44
39
43
36
38

Fig. 84

213

The interosseous and the lumbrical muscles

(The legends are the same for all the diagrams.)
As in the hand, the **interossei** fall into two groups **dorsal** and **plantar**, but their arrangement is slightly different in the foot (**Fig. 85**: frontal section, posterior slice shown). The **four dorsal interossei** (1) are centred on the second metatarsal (not on the third, as in the hand) and are inserted (white arrows) into the second toe (first and second interossei) or into the toe next in order, i.e. the third interosseus is inserted into the third toe and the fourth into the fourth toe (**Fig. 92**). The **three plantar interossei** (2) arise from the medial aspects of the last three metatarsals and are inserted (**Fig. 93**) into the corresponding toes.

The **mode of insertion of the interossei** of the foot (**Fig. 86**: dorsal view of the extensor apparatus; **Fig. 88**: lateral view of the muscles of the toe) is similar to that of the interossei of the hand. Each one is inserted into the **lateral aspect of the base of the proximal phalanx** (3) and sends a **tendinous slip** (4) into the lateral band (5) of the dorsal digital expansion. The tendon of the extensor digitorum longus (EDL) is inserted into the three phalanges, just as the extensor longus is inserted into the fingers, by some fibres into the sides of the proximal phalanges (6) and not into their bases, and by two lateral bands (5) into the base of the distal phalanx. Proximal to the metatarsophalangeal joint (**Fig. 87**, dorsal view), the tendons of the extensor longus for the second, third and fourth toes are joined by the corresponding thin tendon of the extensor digitorum brevis (EDB). Figure 85 also shows on the dorsal aspect of the foot the tendons of the extensor digitorum longus (EDL), of the extensor hallucis longus (EHL) and of the extensor digitorum brevis (EDB).

As in the hand, there are **four lumbricals (Figs 85, 87 and 90)** arising from the tendons of the flexor digitorum longus (19) (the counterpart of the flexor digitorum profundus of the hand), whose margins (see **Fig. 97**) receive the insertion of the quadratus plantae or flexor digitorum accessorius (not shown here, since it lies in the same plane as the flexor longus). Each lumbrical runs medially (**Fig. 97**, p. 217) to insert by tendon (**Figs 87 and 88**) like an interosseus, i.e. into the base of the

proximal phalanx (8) and into the lateral band of the dorsal digital expansion (9).

The tendon of the flexor digitorum longus (19), like the flexor digitorum profundus in the hand (**Figs 88 and 97**), runs along the fibrocartilaginous plate (10) of the metatarsophalangeal joint and then 'perforates' the tendon of the flexor digitorum brevis (24) to insert into the base of the distal phalanx. The quadratus plantae, an intrinsic muscle of the foot, is thus analogous to the flexor digitorum sublimis of the hand: it is superficial and is perforated by the flexor digitorum longus before inserting into the lateral margins of the middle phalanges. The flexor digitorum longus flexes the distal phalanx on the middle phalanx (**Fig. 90**); the quadratus plantae flexes the middle phalanx on the proximal phalanx. The interossei and the lumbricals (**Fig. 89**) (as in the hand) flex the proximal phalanx and extend the middle and distal phalanges. They are crucial for the stabilization of the toes: by flexing the proximal phalanx they provide a solid point of support for the toe extensors in their action as ankle flexors. Thus a deficiency of the interossei and of the lumbricals causes the **claw foot deformity** of the toes (**Fig. 91**), since the proximal phalanx, no longer stabilized by the interossei, is hyper-extended by the pull of the extensor and slides on to the dorsal surface of the metatarsal head. This deformity becomes fixed by the **dorsal luxation of the interossei** above the axis of the metatarsophalangeal joint (+). Furthermore, the middle and distal phalanges are flexed by the relative shortening of the flexors, and the toes become fixed in this deformity by subluxation of the proximal interphalangeal joint (arrow) between the lateral bands of the extensor expansion, so that the action of the extensor is now reversed.

As in the hand, the position of the toes depends therefore on the balance struck among different muscles. Thus it becomes clear, as stated by Duchenne de Boulogne, that the extensor digitorum brevis (EDB) is the true extensor of the toes, since the extensor digitorum longus (EDL), **is in fact an ankle flexor and would have 'benefited' from a direct insertion into the metatarsals** (according to Duchenne).

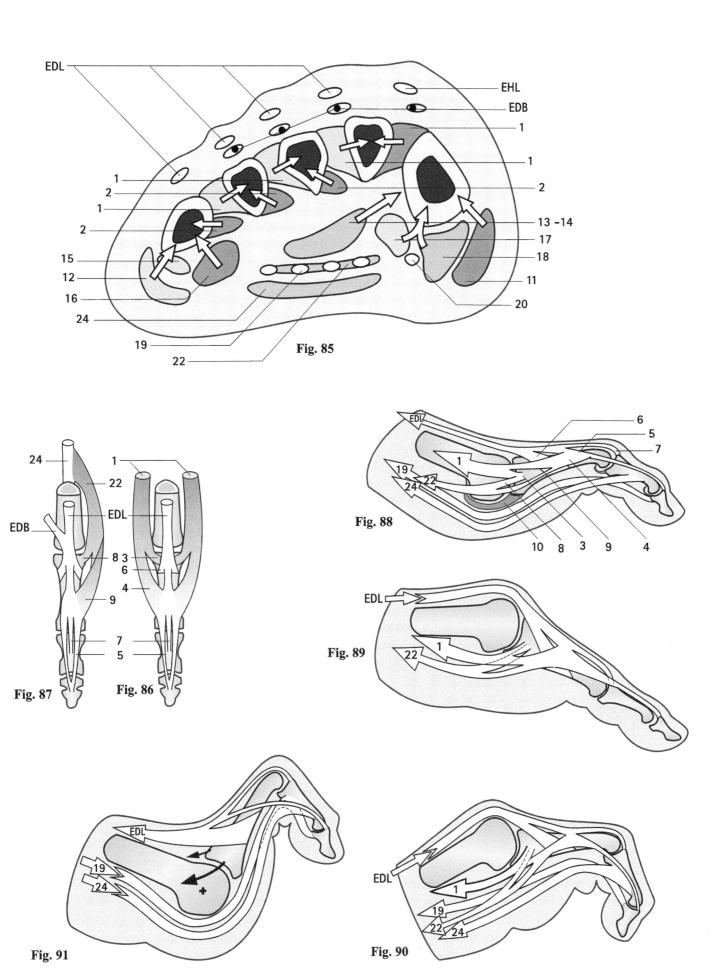

Fig. 85

Fig. 86

Fig. 87

Fig. 88

Fig. 89

Fig. 90

Fig. 91

215

The muscles of the sole of the foot

(The legends are the same as on the previous page.)
The plantar muscles are arranged in **three layers** from deep to superficial:

1. The **deep layer** consists of the **dorsal** (1) and **plantar interossei** (2) and the muscles attached to the fifth toe and to the big toe as follows:

- The **dorsal interossei** (1) (**Fig. 72**, plantar view), in addition to being flexors-extensors of the toes, also pull the toes away from the axis of the foot running through the second metatarsal and the second toe. The big toe is abducted by the **abductor hallucis** (11), which arises from the medial process of the calcaneal tuberosity, and the little toe by the **abductor digiti minimi** (12). These two muscles are equivalent to the dorsal interossei.

- The **plantar interossei** (2) (**Fig. 93**, plantar view) pull the last three toes closer to the second toe. The big toe is brought closer to the axis of the foot by the **adductor hallucis**, which has an **oblique head** (13) arising from the bones of the anterior tarsus and a **transverse head** (14) arising from the plantar metatarsophalangeal ligaments of the third, fourth and fifth toes and from the deep transverse metatarsal ligaments. It pulls the proximal phalanx of the big toe directly laterally and plays a part in supporting the anterior arch (see **Fig. 28**, p. 241).

- The **muscles of the fifth toe** (**Fig. 94**, dorsal view) are three in number and lie within the lateral plantar compartment of the foot.
  - The **opponens digiti minimi** (15) is the deepest of these muscles; it runs from the anterior tarsus to the fifth metatarsal and has a similar action to that of the opponens of the fifth finger but is less efficient. It hollows the plantar vault and the anterior arch.
  - The other two muscles are both inserted into the lateral tuberosity of the base of the proximal phalanx: the **flexor digiti minimi brevis** (16) arises from the anterior tarsus and the **abductor digiti minimi** (12) arises from the lateral process of the calcaneal tuberosity and from the tuberosity of the fifth metatarsal (**Fig. 95**) and helps to support the lateral arch (see **Fig. 18**, p. 239).

- The **muscles of the big toe** (**Fig. 94**) are three in number and lie in the medial plantar compartment of the foot (except for the abductor). They are inserted into the lateral surface of the base of the proximal phalanx and into the two sesamoid bones related to the metatarsophalangeal joint of the big toe; hence their name of sesamoid muscles.

- On the medial side, one sesamoid bone and the proximal phalanx give insertion to the *medial part* of the **flexor hallucis brevis** (17) and to the **abductor hallucis** (11), which arises from the medial process of the calcaneal tuberosity (**Fig. 95**) and helps to support the medial arch (see p. 237, **Fig. 7**).

- On the lateral side, one sesamoid bone and the proximal phalanx receive the insertions of the **two heads of the adductor hallucis** (13 and 14) and the **lateral head of the flexor hallucis brevis** (18), which arises from the anterior tarsal bones.

These sesamoid muscles are **strong flexors of the big toe.** They are crucial for the stabilization of the big toe, and their deficiency causes a claw-toe deformity due to the unbalanced action of the extensor hallucis. They are also very active during the last phase of the step (see **Fig. 50**, p. 247).

2. The **intermediate layer** is made up of the **long flexor muscles** (**Fig. 96**). The **flexor digitorum longus** (19) crosses the deep surface of the **flexor hallucis longus** (20) after the latter emerges from its groove beneath the sustentaculum tali and after they **exchange tendinous interconnections.** The long flexor then divides into four tendons for the last four toes. The **lumbricals** (22) take origin (**Fig. 97**) from two adjacent tendons of the long flexor except for the first lumbrical (22'). The tendons of the flexor digitorum longus perforate those of the flexor digitorum brevis before inserting into the distal phalanges. The oblique pull of these tendons is offset by the action of a flat muscle that runs along the axis of the foot (**Fig. 97**) between the two processes of the calcaneal tuberosity to the lateral border of the flexor digitorum longus tendon for the fifth toe. It is the **quadratus plantae** (23), whose simultaneous contraction reduces the obliquity of these tendons.

The **flexor hallucis longus** (20) (**Figs 94 and 96**) runs between the two sesamoid bones to insert into the distal phalanx of the big toe, which it flexes powerfully.

3. The **superficial layer** (**Fig. 95**) consists of one muscle lying in the middle plantar compartment alongside the flexor longus. It is the **flexor digitorum brevis** (24), which arises from the processes of the posterior calcaneal tuberosity and is inserted into the last four toes. It is analogous to the flexor digitorum sublimis of the hand. Its perforated tendons (**Fig. 97**) are inserted into the middle phalanges, which they flex.

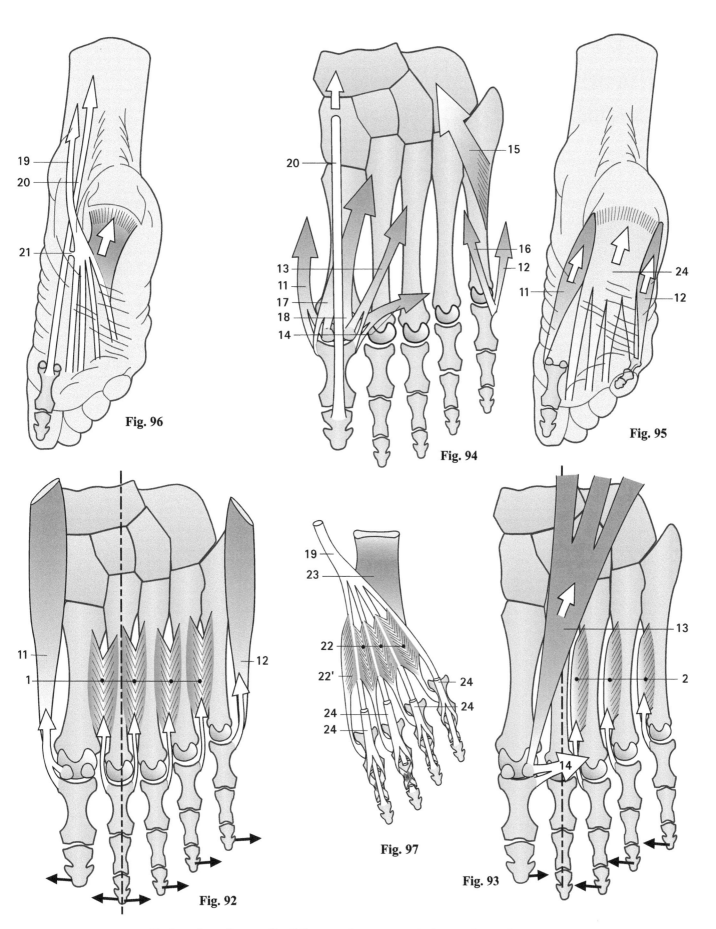

Fig. 96

Fig. 94

Fig. 95

Fig. 92

Fig. 97

Fig. 93

The legends are the same for all figures and are common to those on the previous page.

The fibrous tunnels of the instep and of the sole of the foot

The **inferior extensor retinaculum of the ankle (Fig. 98)** braces the four dorsal tendons of the foot against the tarsal bones in the anterior concavity of the instep and serves as a **reflecting pulley**, whatever the degree of ankle flexion. It starts from the floor of the sinus tarsi on the superior surface of the anterior process of the calcaneus and soon divides into two divergent limbs:

- **a distal limb** (a) fanning out towards the medial margin of the foot
- **a proximal limb** (b) terminating in the tibial crest near the medial malleolus.

Medially their deep and superficial lamellae embrace the **tibialis anterior** (1), which is invested in a synovial sheath starting two fingers' breadths proximal to the superior border of the retinaculum (s).

Laterally, the stem of the retinaculum originating from the sinus tarsi contains **two loops:**

- the **medial loop** containing the **extensor hallucis longus** (2), which is invested in a synovial sheath that barely overshoots the retinaculum proximally
- the **lateral loop** (not shown) for the tendons of the **extensor digitorum longus** (3) and of the **fibularis tertius** (4), which are invested in a common synovial sheath extending farther proximally than that for the extensor.

All the other tendons descend in the **retromalleolar grooves.**

Posterior to the lateral malleolus the lateral retromalleolar groove (**Fig. 99**, lateral view) lodges an osteofibrous tunnel (5), which arises from the stem of the inferior extensor retinaculum and contains the two parallel tendons of the fibularis brevis (6) (in front and above) and of the fibularis longus (7) (behind and below). They bend sharply at the malleolar tip and stay tethered to the lateral surface of the calcaneus inside two osteofibrous tunnels (8 and 9) resting on the fibular tubercle (10). At this point their common synovial sheath divides into two. The fibularis brevis is inserted into the lateral tuberosity of the fifth metatarsal (11) and into the base of the fourth metatarsal. A short segment (12) of this tendon has been resected to reveal the tendon of the fibularis longus as it changes direction and enters the groove on the undersurface of the cuboid (13). It is seen again (14) in the sole of the foot (**Fig. 100**: inferior view of the bones of the foot), where it is wrapped inside a synovial sheath and veers obliquely anteriorly and interiorly in yet another osteofibrous tunnel formed superiorly by the tarsal bones and interiorly by the superficial band of the long plantar ligament

(deep fibres shown, 15), running from the calcaneus (16) to the cuboid and the bases of all the metatarsals and also by the terminal expansions of the tibialis posterior tendon (17). The fibularis longus tendon inserts mainly into the base of the first metatarsal (18) but sends slips to the second metatarsal and to the medial cuneiform. As it enters the plantar tunnel it is almost always associated with a sesamoid bone (32) that allows it to be reflected.

Therefore the plantar surface of the foot is carpeted by **three sets of fibrous sheets (Fig. 100)**:

- the **longitudinal** fibres of the long plantar ligament arranged in two layers (the diagram shows only the deep layer, 15)
- the fibres of the tendon of the fibularis longus (7) **running obliquely anteriorly and medially** (14)
- the expansions of the posterior tibialis tendon (21), which run **obliquely anteriorly and laterally** towards the tarsal and metatarsal bones, except for the two outermost metatarsals.

Posterior to the medial malleolus (Fig. 101, medial view inside the medial retro-malleolar gutter) there are **three tendons** contained within distinct tunnels and sheaths derived from the extensor retinaculum. These tendons are arranged anteroposteriorly and mediolaterally as follows:

- The **tibialis posterior** (19) runs close to the malleolus and bends slightly inside its *tunnel* (20) at the malleolar tip to gain insertion into the navicular tuberosity (21) while sending many plantar expansions.
- The **flexor digitorum longus** (22) runs alongside the tibialis posterior and then along the inner margin of the sustentaculum tali (23) (see also **Fig. 103**) before crossing the deep surface (24) of the extensor hallucis longus tendon.
- The **flexor hallucis longus** (25) runs between the medial and lateral tubercles of the talus (26) (see also 38, **Fig. 14** p. 167), and then underneath the sustentaculum tali (27) (see also **Fig. 103**). It thus changes direction twice.

Two coronal sections of the right foot (anterior aspects) taken at two levels A and B indicated by arrows A and B in Figures 99 and 101, illustrate clearly the arrangement of these tendons and of their synovial sheaths in the retromalleolar grooves: section A (**Fig. 102**) is taken through the malleoli; section B (**Fig. 103**) is more anterior and runs through the sustentaculum tali and the fibular tubercle. They show the adductor hallucis (28), the abductor digiti minimi (31), the quadratus plantae (29) and the flexor digitorum brevis (30).

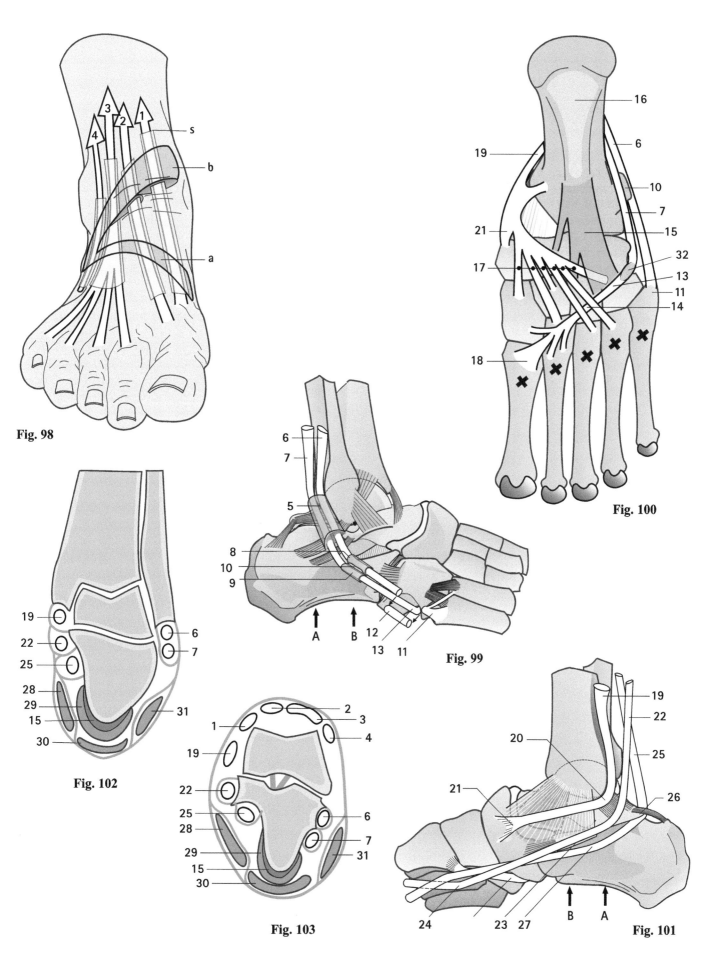

Fig. 98

Fig. 99

Fig. 100

Fig. 101

Fig. 102

Fig. 103

The flexor muscles of the ankle

The foot and the hindfoot are mobilized by the ankle flexors and extensors using **the axes of the articular complex of the posterior tarsus**, as demonstrated previously in relation to the heterokinetic universal joint (**Fig. 55**, p. 201). (We think that it is best to discard Ombredanne's original diagram (**Fig. 105**), where the axes XX' and ZZ' are orthogonal, since it fails to fit with the facts.) By definition, the axes XX' and UU' of the heterokinetic joint are not orthogonal (**Figs 104 and 105**), thus introducing a **directional bias** for the movements, a bias reinforced by the unequal distribution of the muscles. These two axes create **four quadrants** containing **10 muscles and 13 tendons (Fig. 104)**. All the muscles lying anterior to the transverse axis XX' are **ankle flexors**, but they can be further subdivided into **two groups** according to their relationship to *Henke's axis* UU':

- The two muscles lying *medial to this axis*, i.e. the **extensor hallucis longus** (EHL) and the **tibialis anterior** (TA) are at the same time *adductors and supinators* proportionately to their distance from this axis; thus the tibialis anterior is a stronger adductor-supinator than the extensor hallucis longus;
- The two muscles lying *lateral to this axis*, i.e. the **extensor digitorum longus (EDL)** and the **fibularis tertius (FT)** are at the same time *abductors and pronators*. For the same reason as above, the fibularis tertius is a stronger abductor-pronator than the extensor digitorum longus.

To obtain **pure ankle flexion** without an adduction-supination or an abduction-pronation component, these two muscle groups must contract simultaneously and in a balanced fashion as **antagonists-synergists** (these actions can be reproduced in the mechanical model of the foot included at the end of this volume).

Two of the four ankle flexors are inserted directly into the tarsal or metatarsal bones:

- The **tibialis anterior** (TA) **(Fig. 106)** is inserted into the medial cuneiform and the first metatarsal;
- The **fibularis tertius** (FT) **(Fig. 107)**, which is present only in 90% of cases, is inserted into the base of the fifth metatarsal.

Their action on the foot is thus direct and needs no assistance from other muscles.

This is not the case with the other two ankle flexors, i.e. the **extensor digitorum longus** (EDL) and the **extensor hallucis longus** (EHL), which act on the foot via the toes. Thus if the toes are stabilized in the straight position or in flexion **(Fig. 107)** by the interossei (Ix), the extensor digitorum longus flexes the ankle, but if there is insufficiency of the interossei, then ankle flexion occurs at the expense of a *claw deformity of the toes* **(Fig. 111)**. Similarly, **(Fig. 106)** stabilization of the big toe by the sesamoid muscles (S) allows the extensor longus to flex the ankle. If there is insufficiency of the sesamoid muscles, then ankle flexion will be accompanied by a *claw deformity of the big toe* **(Fig. 109)**.

When the muscles of the anterior compartment of the leg are paralysed or weak (a relatively frequent occurrence), the tips of the toes cannot be raised **(Fig. 108)** giving rise to a **pes equinus** (*equus* (Latin) = horse, which walks on tiptoe). Thus, during walking, the patient must lift the whole leg high up for the tips of the toes to clear the ground, i.e. high-steppage gait **(Fig. 109)**. In some cases, the extensor longus retains some of its strength **(Fig. 110)**, and the dropped foot is also deviated laterally: this is the pes valgus equinus.

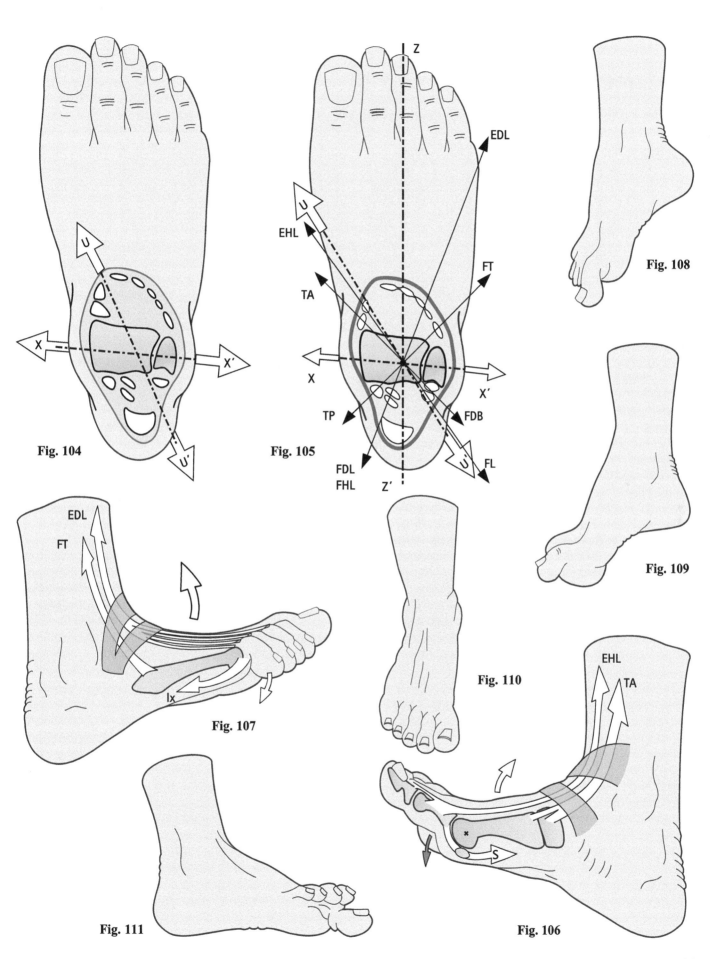

Fig. 104

Fig. 105

Z
EDL
FT
EHL
TA
X
X'
TP
FDB
FDL
FHL
FL
Z'

Fig. 108

Fig. 109

Fig. 107

EDL
FT
Ix

Fig. 110

Fig. 111

Fig. 106

EHL
TA
S

The triceps surae

All ankle extensors descend posterior to the flexion-extension axis XX' (**Fig. 105**, p. 221). Theoretically, there are **six extensors of the ankle joint** (discounting the functionally negligible plantaris). In practice, however, *only the triceps surae is effective*: it is after all one of the most powerful muscles in the body after the gluteus maximus and the quadriceps. Besides, its more or less axial position makes it primarily an *extensor*.

As its name indicates, the **triceps surae** consists of *three muscle bellies* (**Fig. 112**, posterior view) converging into a common tendon - the **calcaneal tendon or the Achilles tendon** (1) - for insertion into the posterior surface of the calcaneus (see next page).

Of these three muscles *only one is monoarticular*, i.e. the **soleus** (2), arising from the tibia, the fibula and the *soleal arch* (3), which is a fibrous band (shown here as transparent) uniting the tibial and fibular attachments of the muscle. It is deeply situated and surfaces only at the distal extremity of the leg on either side of the calcaneal tendon.

The other two muscles are biarticular, i.e. the two heads of the gastrocnemius. The **lateral head** (4) arises from the *lateral femoral condyle* and the lateral condylar plate and often contains a sesamoid bone. The **medial head** (5) likewise originates from the *medial condyle and the medial condylar plate*. These two muscle bellies converge towards the midline and form the lower V of the diamond-shaped popliteal fossa (10). On both sides they are held in place by the tendons of the hamstring muscles, which diverge above to form the upper inverted V of the popliteal fossa, i.e. laterally by the **biceps femoris** (6) and medially by the **anserine muscles** (7). The gliding of the gastrocnemius over the hamstring tendons is facilitated by **two intervening synovial bursae:** one bursa between the semitendino-sus and the medial head of gastrocnemius (8) (always present) and the other bursa (occasionally present) between the biceps and the lateral head of the gastrocnemius (9); these bursae can give rise to *popliteal cysts*. The gastrocnemius and the soleus terminate in a *complex aponeurosis* (described on the next page) that gives rise to the calcaneal tendon proper.

The excursions during contraction of these components of the triceps surae (**Fig. 113**, seen in profile) are *obviously different*: the excursion of the soleus (Cs) is 44 mm, and that of the gastrocnemius (Cg) is 39 mm. This is due to the fact that the efficiency of the biarticular gastrocnemius depends *closely on the degree of knee flexion* (**Fig. 114**: seen in profile, knee flexed): between the extreme positions of flexion and extension the displacement of the origins of the gastrocnemius produces a relative elongation or shortening (e), which is equal to or exceeds its excursion (Cg). Thus, when the knee is extended (**Fig. 115**), the passively stretched gastrocnemius can generate maximal power, as this allows some of the power of the quadriceps to be transmitted to the ankle. On the other hand, when the knee is flexed (**Fig. 117**), the gastrocnemius is completely slackened with e greater than Cg and thus loses all its efficiency. The soleus then remains the *only active muscle*, but its power would be inadequate to allow walking, riding or jumping if knee extension was not an essential part of these activities. Note that the gastrocnemius is nonetheless not a knee flexor.

Any movement combining ankle extension and knee extension, i.e. climbing (**Fig. 116**) or running (**Figs 118 and 119**) activates the gastrocnemius. The triceps surae achieves **maximal efficiency** when, starting from the flexed ankle-extended knee position (**Fig. 118**), it contracts to extend the ankle (**Fig. 119**) and provides the **propulsive force** during the last phase of the step.

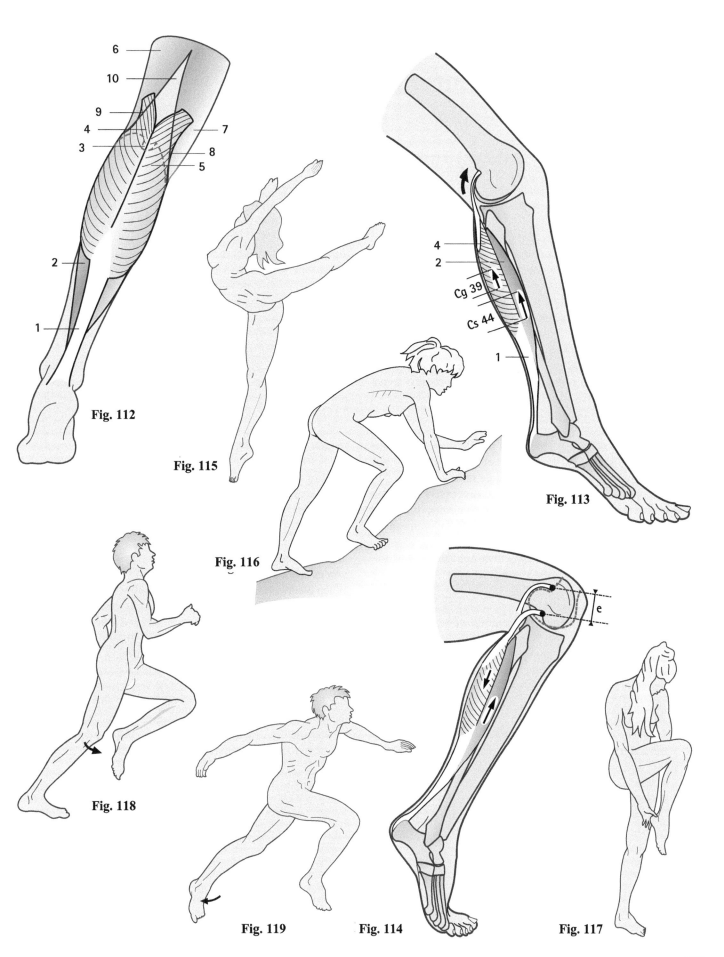

Fig. 112

Fig. 115

Fig. 116

Fig. 113

Fig. 118

Fig. 119

Fig. 114

Fig. 117

The triceps surae (*continued*)

The **triceps surae has a very complex aponeurotic system** (**Fig. 120**: anterior view with tibia removed, showing the deep aspect of the muscle from the front) comprising an **aponeurotic origin** and an **aponeurotic termination** that culminates in the **calcaneal tendon.**

Its origin consists of **three aponeuroses:**

- The **two tendons of the medial (1) and lateral (2) heads** of the gastrocnemius are attached just above the femoral condyles and form the lateral boundaries of its site of origin.
- The **thick tendinous sheet of the soleus** (3) arises from the tibia, the fibula and the soleal arch, and its inferior portion is deeply indented in the shape of a horseshoe with a medial (4) and a lateral (5) border.

Its termination consists of **two aponeuroses:**

- **The thick common terminal sheet** (6) runs parallel to the soleus and gives rise to the calcaneal tendon (7) before its insertion into the calcaneus (8).
- The **sagittal sheet** (9) is perpendicular to the former and blends with its anterior surface. It is peculiar in that it tapers upwards behind the posterior surface of the soleal attachment site after passing through its horseshoe indentation.

There are thus anteroposteriorly **three successive aponeurotic planes:** that of the two gastrocnemius tendons; that of the common terminal sheet and that of the soleal tendinous sheet, which is straddled posteriorly by the sagittal sheet.

The **muscular fibres of the triceps surae** are arranged as follows relative to this aponeurotic system:

- The muscular fibres of the **medial** (10, red) and of the **lateral heads of the gastrocnemius** (11, green) (**Fig. 121**: anteromedial view in perspective after removal of the medial half of the soleal sheet) originate directly from the tent-like supracondylar surface of the femur and from the anterior surfaces of their tendons of origin and descend medially towards the axis of the leg before inserting into the anterior aspect of the terminal sheet;
- The **muscular fibres of the soleus** (**Fig. 122**: same as above with the soleal sheet intact) are organized in two layers:
  - the **anterior layer** (12) with its fibres (dark red) inserting into the anterior aspect of the terminal sheet (only the medial fibres are shown here) and to a lesser degree into its medial and lateral margins
  - the **posterior layer** (13) with its fibres (dark blue) inserting into the two sides of the sagittal sheet.

This diagram also illustrates the spiral structure (14) (red and blue fibres) of the calcaneal tendon, which is responsible for its elasticity.

The **force of the calcaneal tendon** is applied to the posterior extremity of the calcaneus (**Fig. 123**) at a very wide angle to its lever arm AO. Decomposition of this force AT (green vector) shows that the **effective component T1** (red vector) perpendicular to the lever arm is greater than the centripetal component T2. Thus the muscle works at a high mechanical advantage.

The effective component T1 always exceeds T2, whatever the degree of ankle flexion or extension. This is due to the mode of insertion of the tendon (**Fig. 124**) into the lower part of the posterior calcaneal surface (k), while separated from the upper part by a bursa. Therefore the muscular pull is applied not at the insertion point k but at the point of contact a between the tendon and the posterior calcaneal surface. With the ankle flexed I (**Fig. 124**) this point a lies relatively far up on the posterior calcaneal surface. With the ankle extended II (**Fig. 124**) the tendon 'rolls out' and moves away from the posterior calcaneal surface so that its contact point a' 'descends' on the bone, while the direction of the lever arm a' O stays more or less horizontal, maintaining a constant angle with the direction of the tendon. This mode of insertion of the tendon allows it to '**roll out**' on the segment of a pulley provided by the posterior calcaneal surface and thus increases its efficiency during extension. It is *identical to the mode of insertion of the triceps brachii into the olecranon process* (see Volume 1).

When the triceps surae is maximally contracted (**Fig. 125**), extension is combined with a **movement of adduction-supination**, which directs the sole of the foot to face *posteriorly and medially* (red arrow Add+Sup). This terminal component of adduction-supination is due to the fact that the triceps acts on the ankle joint through the subtalar joint (**Fig. 126**). It mobilizes these two joints in sequence (**Fig. 127**): first, it extends the ankle joint 30° around the transverse axis XX", and then it extends the subtalar joint and tilts the calcaneus about Henke's axis mn so that the foot is adducted 13° (Ad) and supinated 12° (Su) (Biesalski and Mayer).

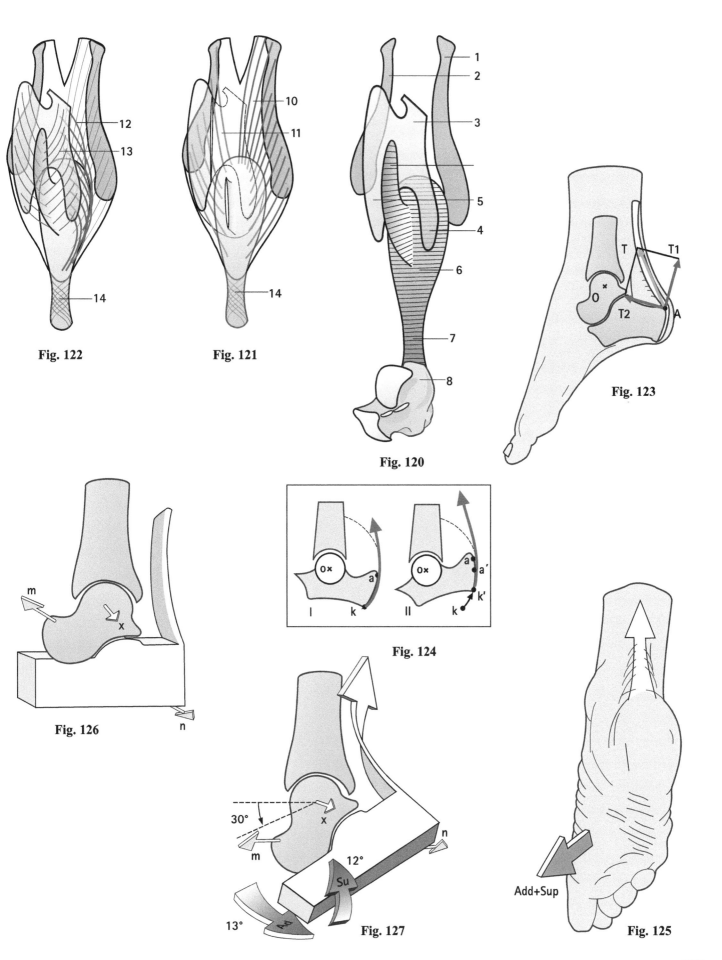

Fig. 122

12
13
14

Fig. 121

10
11
14

Fig. 120

1
2
3
5
4
6
7
8

Fig. 123

T
T1
O ×
T2
A

Fig. 126

m
x
n

Fig. 124

O ×
a
k
I

O ×
a
a'
k
k'
II

Fig. 127

30°
x
m
12°
Su
13°
Ad
n

Fig. 125

Add+Sup

The other extensor muscles of the ankle

All the muscles running posterior to the transverse axis XX' of flexion-extension (**Fig. 128**) are **ankle extensors.** In addition to the triceps surae (1), there are five other ankle extensors. The plantaris (not described here) is so weak as to be negligible and is only important in providing a ready tendon for transplantation; unfortunately it is not always present.

Laterally (**Fig. 129**: lateral view of the ankle) the extensors include the **fibularis brevis** (2) and the **fibularis longus** (3), which lie lateral to Henke's axis UU' (**Fig. 104**) and are thus also *simultaneous abductors and pronators* (see next page).

Medially (**Fig. 130**: medial view of the ankle), the extensors are the **tibialis posterior** (4), the **flexor digitorum longus** (5) and the **flexor hallucis longus** (6); since they lie medial to Henke's axis UU' (**Fig. 104**) they are *simultaneous adductors and supinators.*

Therefore, pure ankle extension can result only from the **synergistic-antagonistic** action of these two muscle groups, i.e. one lateral and the other medial. Nevertheless, the extensor action of these muscles, which can be called *accessory extensors*, is quite small compared with that of the triceps surae (**Fig. 131**: diagram showing the relative power of the extensors). In fact, the **force of triceps surae is equivalent to 6.5 kg** (left side), and since it combines the force of the soleus (Sol) and that of the gastrocnemius (Gc), it is considerable compared with that of the other extensors (right side), i.e. **0.5 kg** or *one-fourteenth of the total power of the extensors.* It is well known that the force of a muscle is proportional to its cross-sectional surface and to its excursion, and so can be represented diagrammatically by a three-dimensional figure whose base and height correspond to the cross-sectional area and the excursion of the muscle, respectively.

Thus the soleus (Sol) with a cross-sectional surface 20.2 cm² and an excursion of 44 mm is slightly less powerful (880 kg/cm²) than the gastrocnemius (Gc) (897 kg/cm²) with an overall cross-sectional area of 23 cm² and an excursion of 39 mm. On the other hand, the power of the **fibular** muscles (Fib), i.e. the **fibularis longus** (FL, green) and the **fibularis brevis** (FB, orange), is half of the total force of the accessory extensors, represented by the three-dimensional figure AE (blue). The fibularis longus itself is twice as strong as the fibularis brevis.

After rupture of the calcaneal tendon, the accessory extensors can *actively extend the ankle when the foot is free* and not pressing on any surface, but they cannot raise the body on tiptoe. The loss of this active movement serves as a **test for calcaneal tendon rupture.**

The structure of the triceps tendon not only favours the transmission of the force exerted by the muscle during ankle extension but also the absorption of the impact generated by jumping on to the tips of the toes. In fact (**Fig. 131bis**) its fibres run lengthwise in the centre while spiralling and crisscrossing one another at the periphery. As the tendon is passively stretched **A**, its spiral peripheral fibres tighten up, move towards the centre and strongly compress (outer arrows) the central fibres, with the result that their resistance to crushing (inner arrows) and their return to their initial volume **B** account for the elasticity of the tendon. In short, as the tendon is stretched (**arrow T**) the length of the tendon increases, while its diameter decreases, especially centrally. This generates the elastic resistance that absorbs the stress. When the stress is removed, the tendon regains its normal diameter and becomes shorter (**arrow R**). All elastic structures in the body have this same spiralling structure because their elasticity depends on the compression of their central fibres.

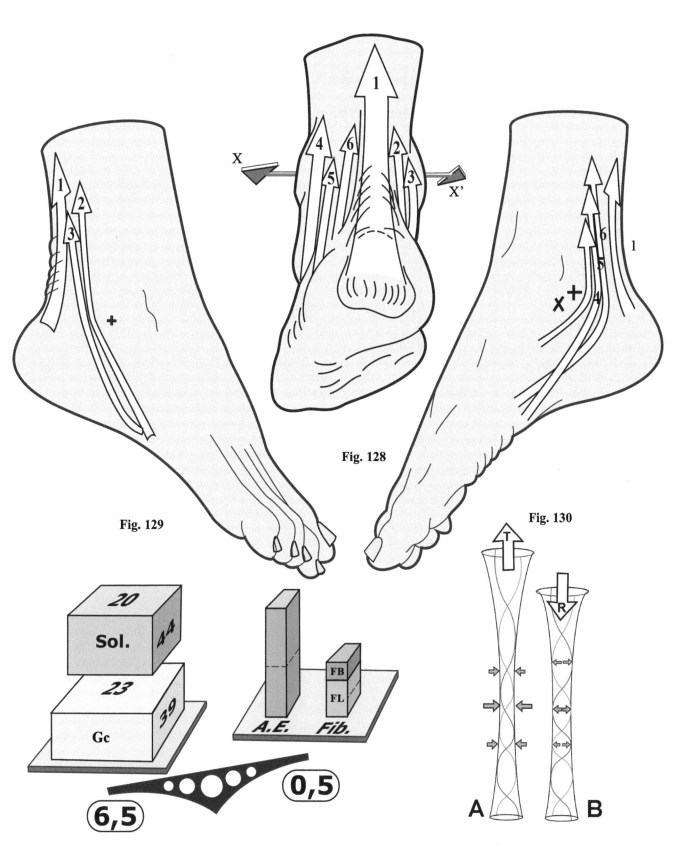

Fig. 128

Fig. 129

Fig. 130

Fig. 131

Fig. 131bis

227

The abductor-pronator muscles: the fibularis muscles fibulaires

The **fibularis muscles** run posterior to the transverse axis XX' and lateral to Henke's axis UU' (see **Fig. 104**, p. 221) and so are simultaneously **(Fig. 132)**:

- extensors (blue arrow)
- abductors (red arrow) that shift the axis ZZ' laterally
- pronators (yellow arrow) that laterally orient the plane of the sole of the foot to face laterally (orange plane).

The **fibularis brevis** (1), inserted **(Fig. 133)** into the lateral tuberosity of the fifth metatarsal, is essentially an abductor of the foot: according to Duchenne de Boulogne, it is in fact the only direct abductor of the foot **(Fig. 100**, p. 219). Certainly it is a more efficient abductor than the fibularis longus. It also **pronates (Fig. 134**: red arrow) the forefoot by elevating the lateral metatarsal rays (green arrow) and is assisted by the **fibularis tertius** (3) and the extensor digitorum longus (not shown here), which are also abductors-pronators as well as ankle flexors. **Pure abduction-pronation** therefore results from the synergistic-antagonistic action of the three fibularis muscles on the one hand, and of the extensor digitorum longus on the other.

The **fibularis longus** (2) **(Figs 133 and 135)** plays a key role in movements of the foot and in the statics and dynamics of the plantar arch:

1. It is an **abductor** like the fibularis brevis, and its contracture causes the forefoot to bend out of shape laterally **(Fig. 137)** and the medial malleolus to jut out more prominently.

2. It produces **extension** directly and indirectly:
- directly by lowering the head of the first metatarsal **(Fig. 134**, blue arrow and **Fig. 135**, green arrow);
- indirectly and more strongly by dragging the first metatarsal laterally **(Fig. 135**, blue arrow) and locking together the medial and lateral metatarsals **(Fig. 136)**. On the other hand, the **triceps surae** (4) directly extends only the lateral metatarsals (shown diagrammatically as a single beam): thus by '**coupling**' the medial and the lateral metatarsals the fibularis longus allows the triceps to pull on all the rays of the sole of the foot. This action is confirmed by instances of fibularis longus paralysis, when only the lateral arch is extended by the triceps and the foot is rotated into **supination**. Therefore **pure foot extension** results from the **synergistic-antagonistic contraction** of the triceps and of the fibularis longus: synergistic in extension and antagonistic in pronation-supination.

3. It is also a **pronator (Fig. 134)** as it lowers (blue arrow) the head of the first metatarsal when the foot is off the ground. Pronation (red arrow) is the result of elevation of the lateral arch (green arrow) along with depression of the middle arch (blue arrow).

We shall see later (p. 241) how the fibularis longus accentuates the curvatures of the three arches of the foot and constitutes their **main muscular support**.

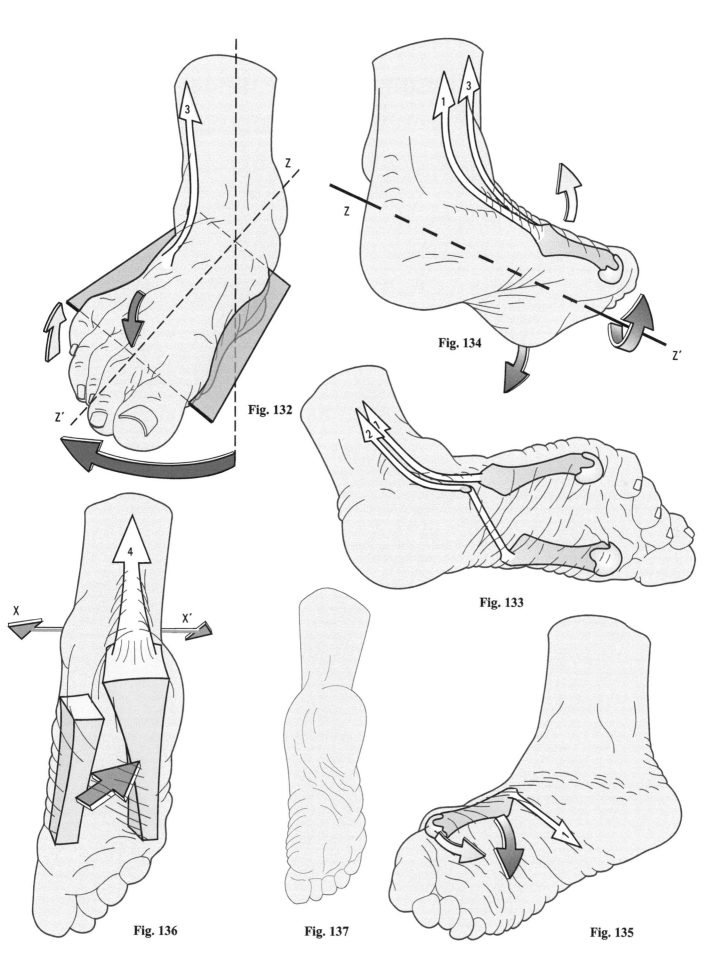

Fig. 132

Fig. 134

Fig. 133

Fig. 136

Fig. 137

Fig. 135

229

The adductor-supinator muscles: the tibialis muscles

The **three medial retromalleolar muscles,** located posterior to the axis XX' and medial to the axis UU' (see **Fig. 104,** p. 221), are simultaneously **(Fig. 138)**:

- extensors (blue arrow)
- adductors (green arrow) that shift the long axis of the foot medially
- supinators (yellow arrow) that orient the plane of the sole of the foot to face medially.

The **tibialis posterior** (1), the most important of these three muscles, is inserted **(Fig. 139)** into the tuberosity of the navicular (yellow). Since it crosses the ankle, the subtalar and the transverse tarsal joints, it acts simultaneously on all three:

- By pulling the navicular medially **(Fig. 140)** it is a very powerful **adductor** and rotates the entire posterior tarsus. (For Duchenne de Boulogne it is more an adductor than a supinator.) It is thus a direct antagonist of the fibularis brevis (2), which pulls the anterior tarsus laterally **(Fig. 141)** by acting on the fifth metatarsal and produces the inverse rotation of the posterior tarsus.
- It is a **supinator** because of its plantar expansions attached to the tarsal and metatarsal bones (see **Fig. 100,** p. 219). It plays a crucial role in the support and orientation of the plantar vault. The congenital absence of these expansions of the tibialis posterior has been cited as one of the causes of pes planus valgus. The range of supination is 52° with 34° occurring at the subtalar joint and 18° at the transverse tarsal joint (Biesalski and Mayer).
- It is an **extensor (Fig. 142)** of both the ankle (green arrow) and transverse tarsal joints (red arrow) by lowering the navicular: the ankle movement is continued into the forefoot (see p. 161, **Fig. 5**).

As an extensor and an adductor it is assisted by the flexor hallucis longus and the flexor digitorum longus.

The tibialis anterior (1) and the extensor hallucis longus **(Fig. 142:** only the tibialis anterior is shown) run anterior to the transverse axis XX' and medial to Henke's axis UU' **(Fig. 104)** and are therefore **ankle flexors and at the same time adductors and supinators of the foot.**

The **tibialis anterior (Fig. 138,** 3) is **more of a supinator than an adductor** and acts by *elevating all the structures of the medial arch* **(Fig. 142)**:

- It elevates the base of the first metatarsal above the medial cuneiform (arrow a), causing the head of the first metatarsal to rise
- It elevates the medial cuneiform above the navicular (arrow b) and the navicular over the talus (arrow c) before flexing the ankle joint (arrow d)
- By flattening the medial arch it supinates the foot, and thus is the direct antagonist of the fibularis longus
- It is a less strong **adductor** than the posterior tibialis
- It **flexes the ankle** and in conjunction with its synergist-antagonist, i.e. the tibialis posterior, it produces pure adduction-supination without any flexion or extension
- Its **contracture** causes a pes talovarus with flexion deformity of the toes **(Fig. 144)**, especially of the big toe.

The **extensor hallucis longus** (4) **(Fig. 143)** is less powerful than the tibialis anterior in producing adduction-supination. It can replace the latter as an ankle flexor, but there is often some residual clawing deformity of the big toe.

The **strength of the supinators** (2.82 kg) *exceeds that of the pronators* (1.16 kg). When the foot is not resting on the ground, it spontaneously rotates into supination. This imbalance offsets beforehand the natural tendency of the foot to rotate into pronation (see p. 242) when it supports the body weight on the ground.

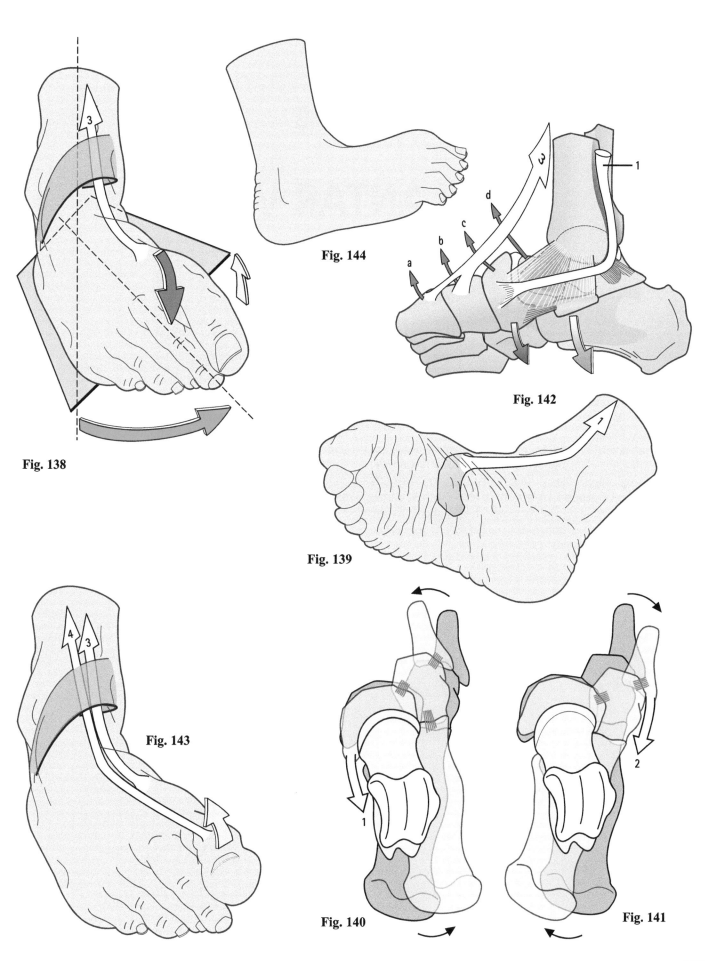

Fig. 138

Fig. 144

Fig. 142

Fig. 139

Fig. 143

Fig. 140

Fig. 141

231

Chapter 5

THE PLANTAR VAULT

The plantar vault is an architectural complex blending harmoniously all the osteoarticular, ligamentous and muscular components of the foot.

It is the equivalent, in the foot, of the palm of the hand, but during evolutionary adaptation it has assumed a new function, in line with bipedalism, i.e. the **optimal transmission of the body weight towards the ground**, despite all its irregularities, during standing, walking, running and jumping. This is achieved at the expense of the ability to climb trees (so necessary for monkeys, which can be quadrimanual).

Thanks to its changes of curvature and its elasticity, the plantar vault can adapt to all irregularities of the ground and can transmit to the ground the loads and stresses imposed by the *earth's gravity* under all possible conditions and with the best mechanical advantage. (One might ask how the plantar vault would have evolved if subjected to the gravitational fields of the Moon or Jupiter.) It acts as a **shock absorber, essential for the elasticity of the gait.** Any lesions that accentuate or flatten its curvatures will seriously compromise the way the body is supported on the ground and inevitably interfere with walking, running, jumping and standing still.

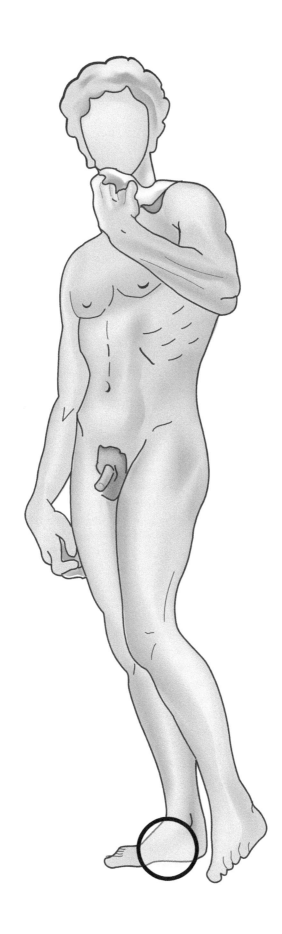

Overview of the plantar vault

Viewed as a whole, the architecture of the plantar vault can be defined as a **vault supported by three arches.** Such a vault has been built by architects and engineers (Fig. 1: Centre for New Industries and Technologies, in La Défense, near Paris): it rests on the ground at **three points A, B and C**, which (Fig. 2, flat view) lie at the corners of an *equilateral triangle*. Between each of the adjacent supports **AB**, **BC** and **CA** there is an **arch** that *constitutes one of the sides of the vault*. The weight of the vault (Fig. 3: the classic vault) is applied at the **keystone** (arrow) and is then distributed by two buttresses to the support points A and B, also known as the abutment piers of the arch.

Following Lapidus's lead, some authors, e.g. De Doncker and Kowalski, find fault with this view of the plantar vault as too static, and they consider, undoubtedly with some justification, that the medial, lateral and anterior arches are purely hypothetical. They prefer to compare the foot to a 'truss' (Fig. 4: roof truss) consisting of **two rafters** SA and SB, joined at the rooftop S and kept together by a **tie beam** AB, which, as a result of traction, prevents the collapse of the triangle under a load applied to the rooftop. Thus the foot would consist only of a *single axial truss* with a *main tie beam*, formed by the powerful plantar ligaments and the *plantar muscles*, and *two secondary lateral tie beams* corresponding to the traditional medial and lateral arches.

This notion is more in keeping with the anatomical reality, especially as regards the ligaments and the muscles that constitute the chords of the arches, which are subjected to elongation stresses and can be compared to tie beams. The terms *vault* and *arches*, however, are so evocative and so entrenched in usage that it is preferable to continue using them along with *truss* and *tie beams*. As is *often the case in biomechanics, two ideas that at first appear contradictory are not mutually exclusive*, and *contribute to a synthetic approach to a problem*. We shall therefore go on using *plantar vault* and *arches*.

The **plantar vault** (Fig. 5: medial view, structures shown as transparent) does not form an equilateral triangle but, as it contains **three arches and three support points**, its structure is comparable to a triangle, despite its asymmetry. Its support points (Fig. 6: foot seen from above, taken as transparent) lie within the zone of contact with the ground, i.e. the **footprint** (green zone) and correspond to the head of the first metatarsal A, the head of the fifth metatarsal B and the medial and lateral processes of the calcaneal tuberosity C. Each support point is shared by two adjacent arches.

The **anterior arch**, the shortest and the lowest, stretches between the **two anterior supports A and B.** The **lateral arch**, of intermediate length and height, stretches between the **two lateral supports B and C.** Finally, the **medial arch**, the longest and the highest, stretches between the **two medial support points C and A** and is also the most important of the three arches in the statics and dynamics of the foot.

The shape of the plantar vault (Fig. 5: bottom part) therefore resembles that of a *jib swollen by the wind*. Its top is clearly displaced posteriorly, and the body weight (green arrow) is applied on its posterior slope (red arrow) at a point (Fig. 6, black cross) located at the **centre of the instep.**

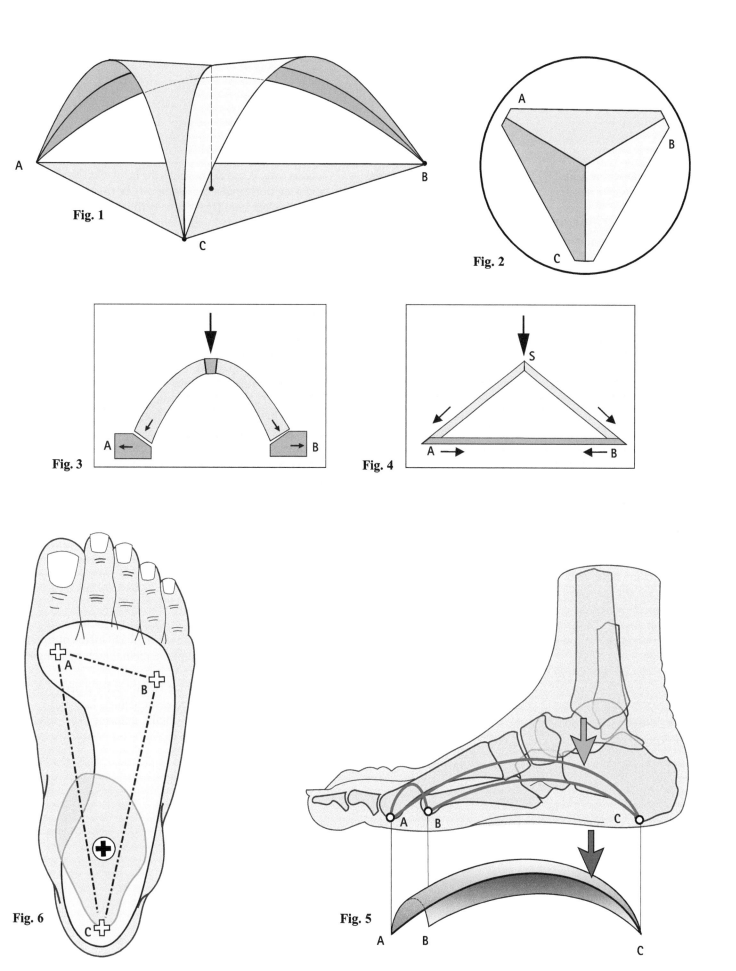

Fig. 1

Fig. 2

Fig. 3

Fig. 4

Fig. 5

Fig. 6

The medial arch

Between its **anterior A and its posterior C support points** the anterior arch comprises five bones arranged anteroposteriorly (Fig. 7):

- the **first metatarsal (M1)**, whose head touches the ground
- the **medial cuneiform (C1)**, totally clear of the ground
- the **navicular (Nav)**, which is the keystone of the arch (shown as a green trapezium) and hovers 15-18 mm above the ground
- the **talus (Tal)**, which receives the stresses transmitted by the leg and distributes them over the vault (see Fig. 15, p. 187)
- the **calcaneus (Cal)**, which is in contact with the ground only at its posterior extremity.

The **transmission of the mechanical stresses** (Fig. 8) is reflected in the disposition of the bony trabeculae:

- The trabeculae arising from the anterior cortex of the tibia run obliquely inferiorly and posteriorly through the posterior buttress of the arch. They traverse the body of the talus to fan out below the posterior talar facet of the calcaneus towards the posterior abutment of the arch at the point of contact between the calcaneus and the ground.
- The trabeculae arising from the posterior cortex of the tibia run obliquely inferiorly and anteriorly through the neck and head of the talus and the navicular to reach the anterior buttress of the arch, i.e. the medial cuneiform and the metatarsal.

The medial arch maintains its **curvature** with the help of ligaments and muscles (Fig. 7).

Many **plantar ligaments** unite these five bones, i.e. the cuneometatarsal, the naviculocuneiform and especially the **plantar calcaneonavicular** ligament (1) and the **interosseous talocalcaneal ligament** (2). These ligaments resist violent but short-lived stresses in contrast to the muscles, which oppose long-lasting distortions.

Each of these muscles connects two points lying at varying distances along the arch and forms chords that span part or the whole of the arch. They act as veritable **tighteners.**

- The **tibialis posterior** (4) *spans part of the arch* (Fig. 10) near its dome, but it is of vital importance. In fact, its strong tendon (Fig. 9, red arrow) pulls the navicular (Nav) inferiorly and posteriorly under the talar head (Tal) along a circle drawn with a broken line. This relatively trivial shortening (e) of the tendon is associated with a **change in the direction of the navicular** that leads to a lowering of the anterior buttress. Moreover, the plantar expansions of the tendon 3 (Fig. 7) blend with the plantar ligaments and act on the three middle metatarsals.
- The **fibularis longus** (5) also acts on the medial arch and accentuates its curvature (Fig. 11) by flexing the first metatarsal (M1) on the medial cuneiform (C1) and the latter on the navicular (Nav) (Fig. 9) (see also its action on the transverse arch, p. 240).
- The **flexor hallucis longus** (6) spans most of the medial arch (Fig. 12) and so acts strongly on its curvature with the help of the **flexor digitorum longus** (7), which crosses its deep surface (Fig. 13). It also *stabilizes the talus* and the calcaneus: as it courses between the two talar tubercles it prevents (Fig. 14) the talus from receding (white arrow). When the navicular is pushed posteriorly (white arrow), the interosseous talocalcaneal ligament (2) is tightened first, and the talus is restored to its anterior position by the tendon, which propels it forwards, *just as a bowstring propels an arrow.* As it runs beneath the sustentaculum tali (Fig. 15), the tendon of the flexor hallucis longus is subjected to a similar boosting effect and *raises the anterior extremity of the calcaneus* (blue arrow), which accommodates the vertical force (white arrow) exerted by the talar head.
- The **abductor hallucis** (8) *spans the entire medial arch* (Fig. 16) and is therefore a particularly efficient tightener: it increases the curvature of the medial arch by bringing its two ends closer.

On the other hand (Fig. 17), the two muscles inserted into the convexity of the arch, i.e. the extensor hallucis longus (9) - under certain conditions - and the tibialis anterior (10), reduce its curvature and flatten the arch.

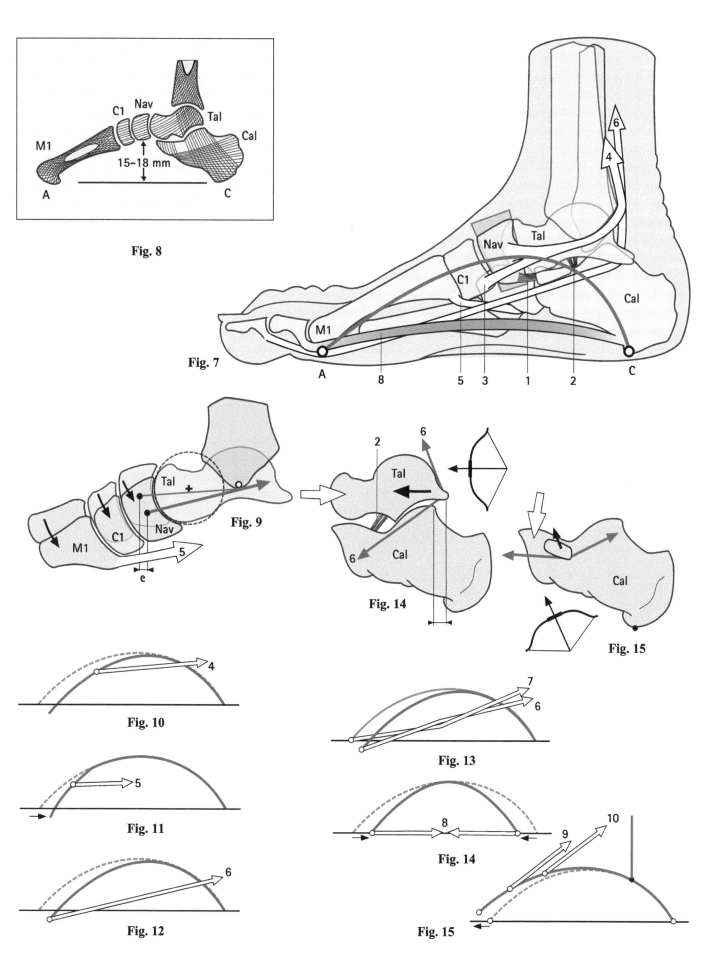

Fig. 8

Fig. 7

Fig. 9

Fig. 10

Fig. 11

Fig. 12

Fig. 13

Fig. 14

Fig. 14

Fig. 15

Fig. 15

15–18 mm

The lateral arch

The lateral arch comprises only **three bones** (Fig. 18: the lateral arch viewed in profile):
- the **fifth metatarsal (M5)**, whose head is the anterior support point (B) of the lateral arch
- the **cuboid (Cub)**, totally clear of the ground
- the **calcaneus (Cal)**, whose medial and lateral processes act as the posterior support point (C) of the arch.

Unlike the medial arch, which is suspended above the ground, the lateral arch is only *slightly elevated* (3-5 mm) and only *makes contact with the ground through the soft tissues.*

The **transmission of mechanical stresses** (Fig. 19) occurs through the talus and the underlying calcaneus via two trabecular systems:
- the **posterior trabeculae** arise from the anterior cortex of the tibia and fan out below the posterior talar facet of the calcaneus
- the **anterior trabeculae**, arising from the posterior cortex of the tibia, first of all traverse the talar head where it rests on the anterior calcaneal process and then run through the cuboid to reach the fifth metatarsal and the anterior support of the arch.
- In addition to the above-mentioned trabeculae, the calcaneus also harbours two **main trabecular systems:**
- a **superior arcuate system**, concave interiorly, converges into a dense lamella in the floor of the sinus tarsi and responds to *compressive stresses*
- an **inferior arcuate system**, concave superiorly, converges towards the plantar cortex of the calcaneus and responds to *elongation stresses.*

Between the two systems, there is a **point of weakness**, marked by a cross (+).

While the medial arch is eminently flexible because of the mobility of the talus on the calcaneus, the lateral arch is much more rigid in order to **transmit the propulsive thrust of the triceps surae** (Fig. 127, p. 225) Its rigidity is due to the strength of the **long plantar ligament**, whose deep (4) and superficial (5) fibres prevent the calcaneocuboid and the cubometatarsal joints

(Fig. 20) from gapping inferiorly under the weight of the body (white arrow). The keystone of the arch is the anterior calcaneal process D, which is the meeting point of the opposing stresses emanating from the posterior buttress CD and the anterior buttress BD. When an excessively violent stress is applied vertically to the arch across the talus, e.g. a fall on the foot from a great height, two types of injury can ensue:
- The long plantar calcaneocuboid ligament resists the shock, but the arch snaps at the level of its keystone and the **anterior process of the calcaneus is fractured** along a vertical split passing through the point of weakness.
- The **posterior talar facet of the calcaneus** is driven into the body of the calcaneus, and the normally obtuse angle of Boehler is straightened out or even inverted (Fig. 21, PT'D).
- On the medial side, the sustentaculum tali is often detached along a split running sagittally (not shown here).

Such calcaneal fractures are not easily reduced, since not only must the posterior talar facet of the calcaneus be re-elevated, but its anterior process must also be re-straightened; otherwise the medial arch stays collapsed.

Three muscles behave as **active tighteners** of the lateral arch:

1. The **fibularis brevis** (1) spans part of the arch (Fig. 22) but, just like the dorsal calcaneocuboid ligament, it prevents the foot joints from gapping **e** inferiorly (Fig. 23).

2. The **fibularis longus** (2), which runs parallel to the former as far as the cuboid, plays a similar role but, because it is hooked to the calcaneus by the **fibular trochlea** (6), it also props up the anterior end of the calcaneus (Fig. 24, calcaneus 'suspended') by its own elasticity, just as the flexor hallucis longus props it up medially in the manner of a bowstring.

3. The **abductor digiti minimi** (3) spans the whole length of the lateral arch (Fig. 25) and has a similar action to that of its counterpart, the abductor hallucis.

Acting as they do on the *convexity of the lateral arch* (Fig. 26) the fibularis tertius (7) and the extensor digitorum longus (8) as well as the triceps surae (9) decrease its curvature under certain conditions.

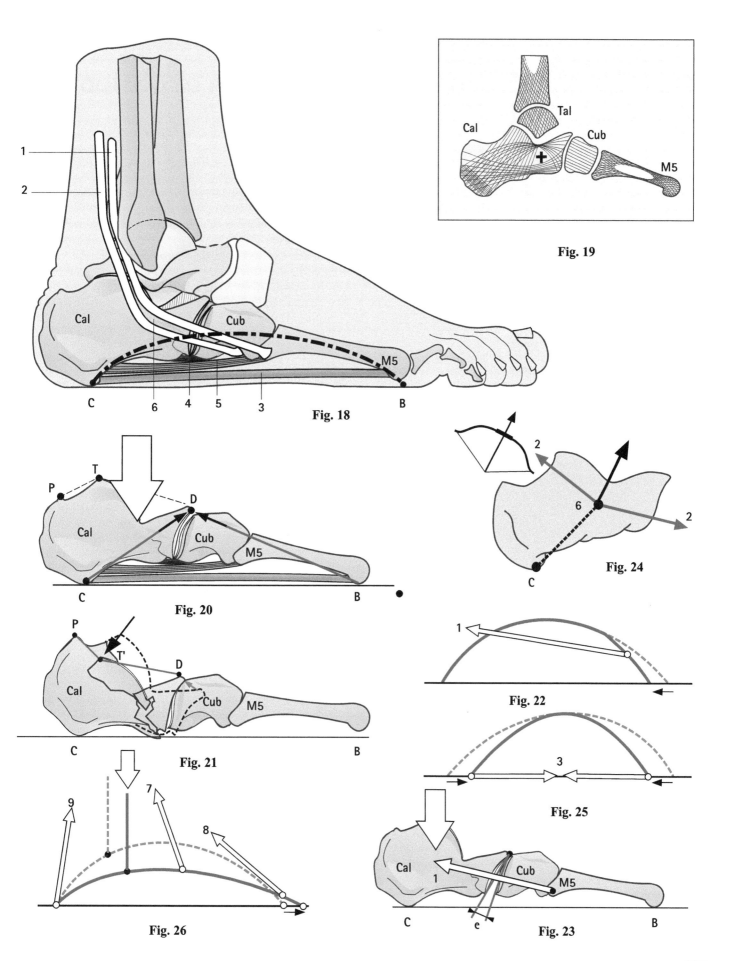

Fig. 18

Fig. 19

Fig. 20

Fig. 21

Fig. 22

Fig. 23

Fig. 24

Fig. 25

Fig. 26

The anterior arch and the transverse arch of the foot

The **anterior arch** (Fig. 27, cross-section I) stretches from the head of the first metatarsal, which rests on two sesamoid bones 6 mm above the ground A, to the head of the fifth metatarsal B, which also lies 6 mm above the ground. It passes through the heads of the other metatarsals, with the head of the highest, the second metatarsal (9 mm above ground), acting as the *keystone of the arch*. The head of the third (8.5 mm above ground) and that of the first metatarsal (7 mm above ground) occupy intermediate positions.

This arch has a relatively **low curvature** and rests on the ground cushioned by soft tissues, which constitute what some authors have called the '**anterior heel**' of the foot. It is subtended by the weak plantar metatarsal ligaments and by only one muscle, i.e. the transverse head of the adductor hallucis 1, which spans part or the whole of the arch as it courses over the heads of the metatarsals from the fifth to the second on its way to the big toe. It is a relatively weak and easily overloaded muscle. The anterior arch is often collapsed, i.e. **flat forefoot**, or even *inverted*, i.e. **convex forefoot**, leading to the formation of **calluses on the depressed metatarsal heads** (Figs 89 and 90, p. 259).

The anterior arch is the *site of culmination of the five metatarsal rays*. The first ray (Fig. 29) is the highest and forms (according to Fick) an angle of 18-20° with the ground. This angle between metatarsal and ground decreases regularly, being 15° for the second (Fig. 30), 10° for the third (Fig. 31), 8° for the fourth (Fig. 32) and only 5° for the fifth metatarsal (Fig. 33), which is nearly parallel to the ground.

The **transverse curvature of the vault** extends anteroposteriorly at the level of the **cuneiforms** (Fig. 27, cross-section II), comprises only four bones and rests on the ground only at its lateral extremity, i.e. the cuboid (Cub). The medial cuneiform (C1) is entirely clear of the ground; the intermediate cuneiform (C2) is the keystone (light green) and forms the *ridgeline of the arch* along the axis of the foot in conjunction with the collinear second metatarsal. This arch is subtended by the fibularis longus tendon 2, which therefore acts powerfully on the transverse arch.

At the level of the **navicular-cuboid couple** (Fig. 27, cross-section III) the transverse arch rests only on its lateral extremity, i.e. the cuboid (Cub). The navicular (Nav) is slung above the ground and cantilevered on the cuboid by its lateral margin. The curvature of this arch is maintained by the plantar expansions of the tibialis posterior 3.

A plantar view of the left foot (taken as transparent) shows (Fig. 28) how the *transverse arch of the vault is maintained by three muscles*, which are sequentially from front to back:

- The adductor hallucis 1 runs transversely.
- The fibularis longus 2, the most important muscle in the dynamics of the foot, runs obliquely and medially and *acts on the three arches of the foot.*
- The plantar expansion of the tibialis posterior 3, especially important in the statics of the foot, acts as a tightener, coursing obliquely anteriorly and laterally.

The **longitudinal curvature** of the entire plantar vault is controlled as follows:

- medially by the abductor hallucis 4 and the flexor hallucis longus (not shown here)
- laterally by the abductor digiti minimi 5

Between these two extreme tighteners, the **flexor digitorum longus** (not shown) and its companion, the **flexor digitorum brevis** (6), maintain the longitudinal curvature of the three intermediate rays as well as that of the fifth ray.

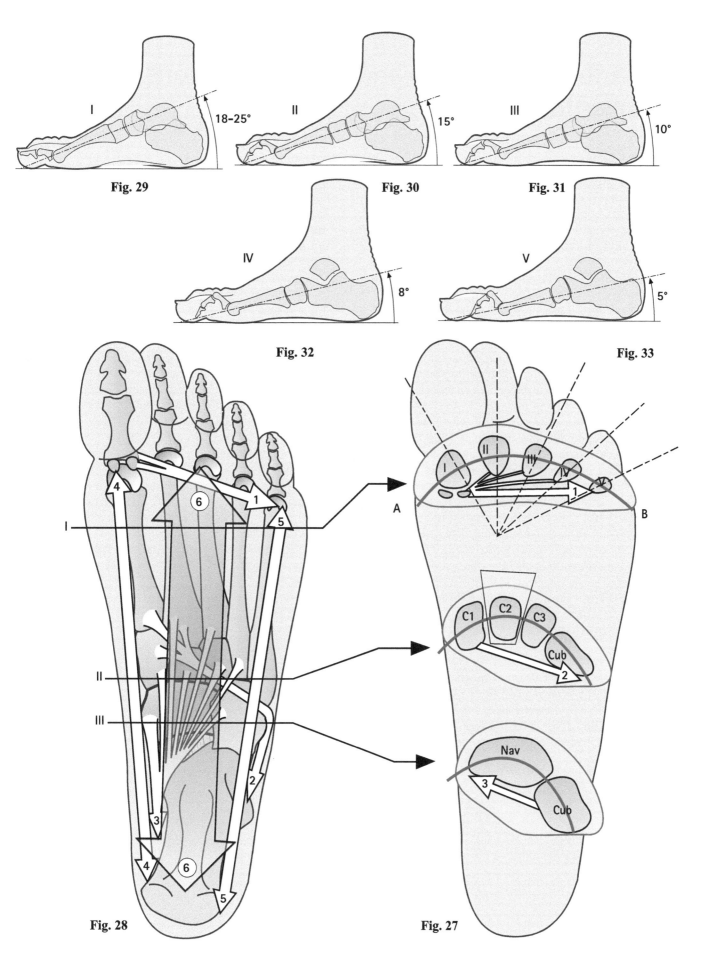

I

18–25°

Fig. 29

II

15°

Fig. 30

III

10°

Fig. 31

IV

8°

Fig. 32

V

5°

Fig. 33

Fig. 28

Fig. 27

The distribution of loads and static distortions of the plantar vault

The **body weight**, transmitted by the lower limb, is applied on the posterior tarsus (Fig. 34: superior view of the bony skeleton of the foot) at the **talar trochlea** (black cross) and **through the ankle joint**. From there the loads are distributed in **three directions** towards the three support (red crosses) points of the plantar vault (Seitz 1997):

- **towards the antero-medial support point A**, via the talar neck, located in the anterior buttress of the medial arch
- **towards the antero-lateral support point B** via the talar head and the anterior process of the calcaneus, located in the anterior buttress of the lateral arch. As these two lines of force diverge towards A and B, they form an acute angle of 35-40°, which is open anteriorly and corresponds more or less to the angle between the axis of the talar neck and that of the body of the talus
- **towards the posterior support point C**, via the talar body, the subtalar joint and the bony trabeculae lying under the posterior talar facet of the calcaneus, located in the common posterior buttress of the medial and lateral arches.

The relative distribution of these loads to each of these support points (Fig. 35) is easily remembered as follows: if a 6-kg weight is applied to the talus, then **1** kg is distributed to the antero-lateral support (B); **2** kg to the antero-medial support (A) and **3** kg to the posterior support (C) (Morton 1935). In the erect, vertical and stationary position, the heel bears the brunt of the load, i.e, one half of the body weight. This explains why a plastic surface is perforated when this load is applied through a stiletto heel over a half-centimetre square.

When loaded, each arch of the foot is flattened and elongated thus:

- In the **medial arch** (Fig. 36, medial view) the **medial and lateral processes of the calcaneal tuberosity**, which lie 7-10 mm above the ground, are lowered by 1.5 cm, and the sustentaculum tali of the calcaneus by 4 mm; the talus recedes on the calcaneus; the navicular climbs on the talar head while moving closer to the ground; the cuneonavicular

and the cuneometatarsal joints gap open inferiorly; the angle between the first metatarsal and the ground decreases; the **heel recedes and the hallucal sesamoid bones advance slightly.**

- In the **lateral arch** (Fig. 37) there are similar vertical displacements of the calcaneus; the cuboid is lowered by 4 mm and the tuberosity of the fifth metatarsal by 3.5 mm; the calcaneocuboid and the cuneometatarsal joints gap inferiorly; the **heel recedes and the head of the fifth metatarsal moves forwards.**
- In the **anterior arch** (Fig. 38. cross-section of the metatarsals) the arch is flattened and splayed out on either side of the second metatarsal; the distance between the first and second metatarsals increases by 5 mm; that between the second and third by 2 mm; that between the third and fourth by 4 mm; and that between the fourth and fifth by 1.5 mm - the **forefoot is widened by 12.5 mm.** During the heel-off stage of gait, the curvature of the anterior arch disappears and all the metatarsal heads touch the ground as they are subjected to varying pressures.

The **transverse curvature** of the foot is decreased also at the level of the cuneiforms (Fig. 39: cross-section of the cuneiforms) and of the navicular (Fig. 40: navicular-cuboid couple), as these two transverse arches are tilted at their lateral supports by an angle of x, which is proportional to the degree of flattening of the medial arch.

In addition (Fig. 41: superior view of the right foot) the talar head is displaced medially by 2-6 mm and the anterior process of the calcaneus by 2-4 mm. This causes **the foot to split and twist at the transverse tarsal joint**: the axis of the hindfoot is *shifted medially*, while the axis of the forefoot is *shifted laterally*, forming an angle y with that of the hindfoot. Thus, the hindfoot turns into **adduction-pronation** (arrow 1) and **slight extension**, while the forefoot undergoes a relative movement of **flexion-abduction-supination** (arrow 2). This phenomenon is particularly conspicuous in the **pes planus valgus** (see p. 255).

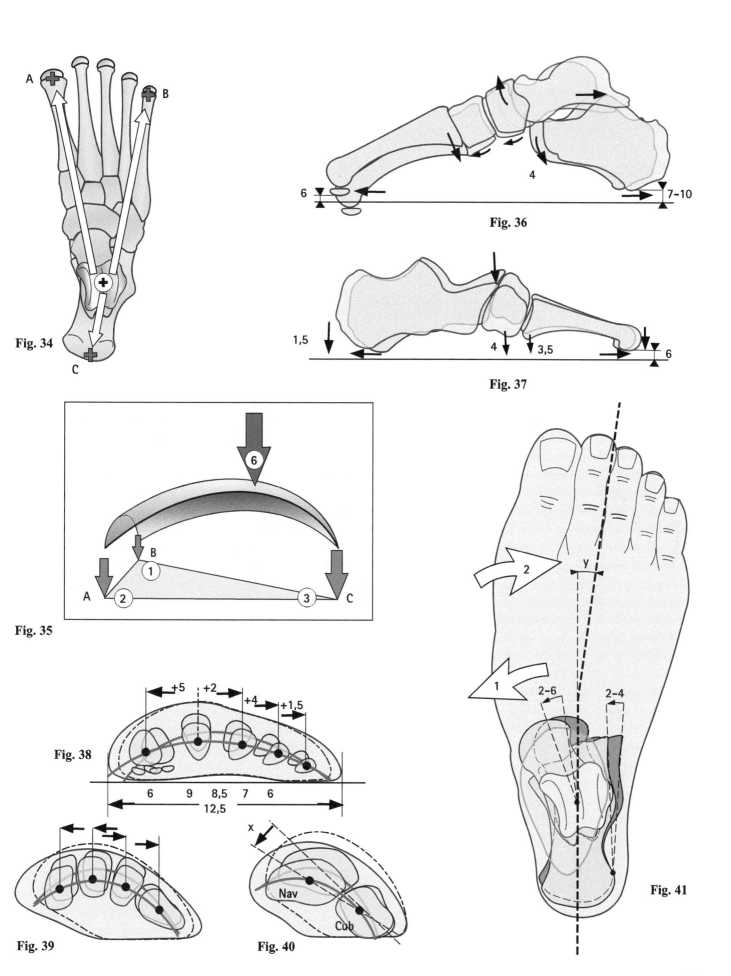

Fig. 34

Fig. 36

6   7–10

Fig. 37

1,5   4   3,5   6

Fig. 35

6

B
1
A 2   3 C

Fig. 38

+5   +2   +4   +1,5

6   9   8,5   7   6

12,5

Fig. 39

Fig. 40

x

Nav

Cub

Fig. 41

2

1

y

2–6   2–4

Architectural equilibrium of the foot

The foot is a **triangular structure** (Fig. 42) with:

- an **inferior surface A**, the base of the **plantar vault**, subtended by muscles and plantar ligaments
- an **anterosuperior surface B** containing the ankle flexors and the toe extensors
- a **posterior surface C** containing the ankle extensors and the toe flexors.

The normal shape of the sole of the foot controls its ability to adapt properly to the ground and is the **result of an equilibrium among the individual forces acting along these three sides of the triangle** (Fig. 43), which consist of three bony rays articulating with one another at the ankle and at the articular complex of the posterior tarsus.

Thus the **pes cavus**, secondary to an **increased curvature of the plantar vault**, can result from shortening of the plantar ligaments and contracture of the plantar muscles as well as from insufficiency of the ankle flexors.

The **pes planus**, due to **flattening of the plantar vault**, can result from insufficiency of the plantar ligaments or plantar muscles, as well as from hypertonicity of the anterior or posterior muscles of the foot.

This is yet another instance of the concept of **trilateral equilibrium** (Fig. 44), illustrated by the surfboard, which allowed us to explain the dynamic equilibrium of the knee. Stability results from a continuous dynamic equilibrium among three factors:

1. Flotation due to the buoyant force or the Archimedes thrust
2. The propulsive force provided by the wind in the sail
3. The instantaneous adjustments that take place as the surfer's body weight is variably applied to the sail and the board.

Our 'Cartesian' minds are used to bifactorial equilibria, but find it **harder to grasp intuitively trifactorial or multifactorial equilibria.** In certain cases, multifactorial equilibria exist, as in the *mobiles of Alexander Calder*, the painter and sculptor who invented these multifactorial equilibria.

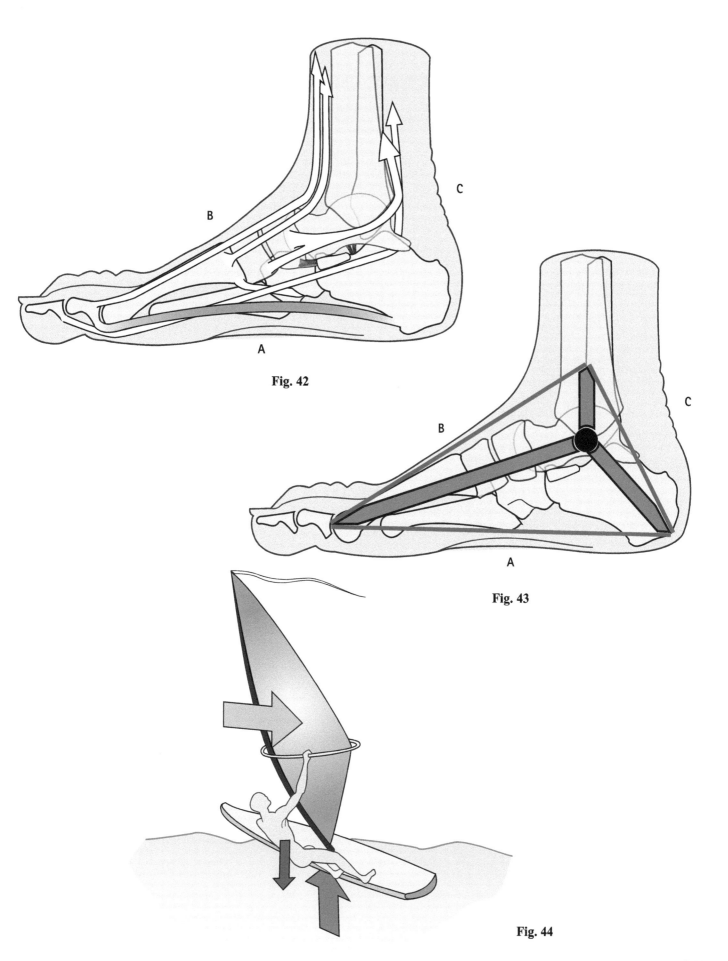

Fig. 42

Fig. 43

Fig. 44

Dynamic distortions of the plantar vault during walking

During walking, the stance phase subjects the vault to stresses and deformations that highlight its role as an elastic shock absorber. It has four periods:

First period: Heel strike or contact with the ground (Fig. 45)

When the swinging limb is about to hit the ground the ankle is straight or even **slightly flexed** by the ankle joint flexors (F). The foot then touches the ground at *the heel*, i.e. the posterior point of support of the plantar vault (C). Straight away under the *thrust of the leg* (red arrow) the rest of the foot contacts the ground (arrow 1), while the ankle is passively extended.

Second period: Maximal contact (Fig. 46)

The sole of the foot rests on the ground **over its entire bearing surface** (Fig. 46), corresponding to the footprint. The body, propelled by the contralateral foot, passes first vertically over the supporting limb and then moves in front of it: this is the **phase of single limb support.** Thus the ankle shifts passively from the previous position of extension **to the new position of flexion** (arrow 2). Simultaneously the weight of the body (red arrow) is applied to the plantar vault and flattens it. At the same time, the contraction of the plantar tighteners (P) counteracts this flattening of the vault: this is the **first stage of shock absorption.** As the vault flattens, it is slightly elongated. At the start of this movement the anterior support A *advances slightly*, but at the end of the movement, when the anterior support becomes more and more fixed on the ground, it is the posterior support C, i.e. the heel, that recedes. Women who wear high heels feel this acutely. The footprint is **maximal when the leg passes vertically above the foot.**

Third period: First stage of active propulsion (Fig. 47)

The weight of the body is now in front of the supporting limb and **contraction of the ankle extensors (T)**, especially the triceps surae, *raises the heel* (arrow 3). While the ankle joint is being actively **extended**, the entire plantar **vault rotates around its anterior support A.** The body is *lifted and carried forwards*: this is the first and more important stage of propulsion, since it calls powerful muscles into action. Meanwhile, the plantar vault is caught between the ground anteriorly, the muscular force posteriorly and the weight of the body centrally in the manner of a second-class lever and would be flattened without the intervention of the plantar tighteners (P); this is the *second stage of shock absorption*, which allows some of the force of the triceps surae to be stored for release at the end of the propulsive movement. On the other hand, it is at the moment when the body is supported anteriorly that the *anterior arch is flattened* in its turn (Fig. 48) and the *forefoot spreads out on the ground* (Fig. 49).

Fourth period: Second stage of active propulsion (Fig. 50)

The propulsive force supplied by the triceps surae is prolonged by a second propulsive force (arrow 4) generated by **contraction of the toe flexors (f)**, especially the sesamoid muscles and the flexor hallucis longus. The foot is again lifted farther forward, *loses the support of the anterior heel and now rests entirely on the first three toes* (Fig. 51), especially the big toe, during the final phase of support. During this second propulsive phase, the *plantar vault resists flattening* once more thanks to the plantar tighteners, including the toe flexors. It is at the end of this phase that the energy stored by the tighteners is released. The *foot then leaves the ground while the other foot goes through its stance phase.* Thus both feet have been simultaneously in contact with the ground for a short time, i.e. the **double-limb support phase.** In the next phase, i.e. of single-limb support, the plantar vault of the swinging foot, i.e. the one that has just left the ground, regains its original state and curvature thanks to its own elasticity.

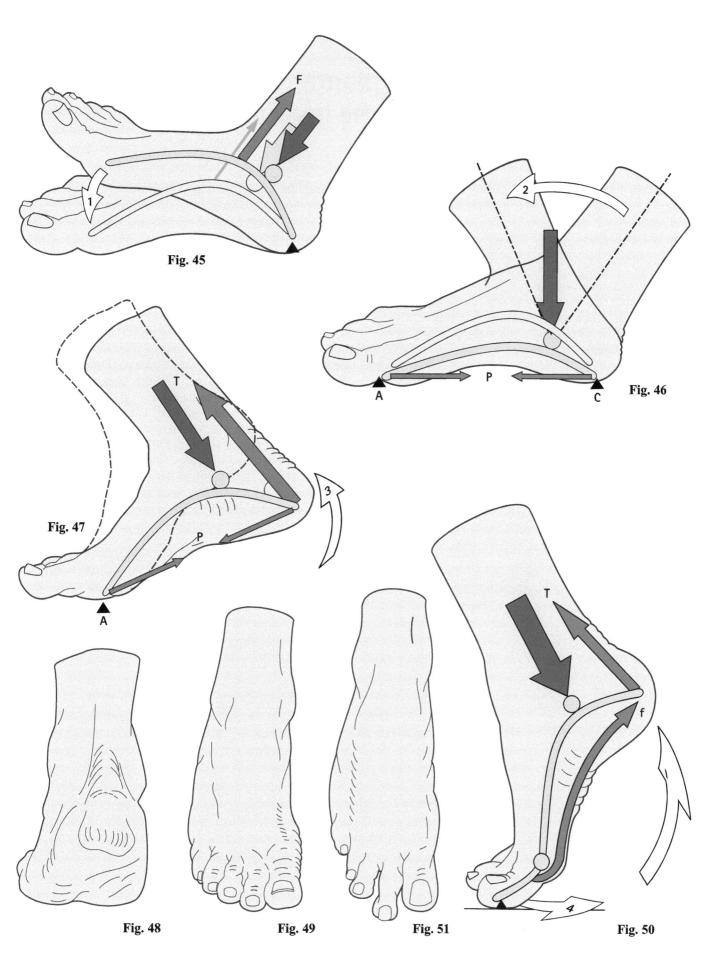

Fig. 45

Fig. 46

Fig. 47

Fig. 48

Fig. 49

Fig. 51

Fig. 50

Dynamic distortions of the plantar vault secondary to inclination of the leg on the inverted foot

So far, we have examined the changes in the plantar vault during walking, i.e. when the leg is variably inclined on the foot in the sagittal plane.

Nonetheless, during walking or running along a curved path or uneven ground, the leg *must be able to bend on the foot in the coronal plane, i.e. laterally or medially relative to the footprint*. These side-to-side inclination movements occur at the subtalar and the transverse talar joints and lead to changes in the shape of the plantar vault. The ankle joint, however, is not involved, while the talus, gripped between the two malleoli, moves relative to the other tarsal bones.

Medial inclination of the leg relative to the foot resting on the ground and taken to be stationary **corresponds to inversion** (Fig. 52), with **four consequences:**

1. Lateral rotation of the leg on the foot (arrow 1) takes place only when the sole of the foot is firmly fixed to the ground. It is clearly recognized as a *posterior displacement of the lateral malleolus* relative to its position when the foot, perpendicular to the leg, touches the ground initially only on its medial border (Fig. 53: frontal view of the foot in its normal position). This lateral rotation of the bimalleolar pincers causes the *talus to slide laterally*, especially its head lodged in the concavity of the navicular.

2. Abduction-supination of the hindfoot (Fig. 54) The abduction is the result of an uncompensated component of lateral rotation; the supination is due to the medial displacement of the calcaneus, which is indicated on this posterior view as the angle x between the axis of the heel and the axis of the leg in comparison with a foot clear of the ground (Fig. 55: posterior view of foot in normal position). This 'varus' displacement of the calcaneus is indicated by the **bending of the medial border of the calcaneal tendon** (**Fig. 54**: posterolateral view of the foot resting in a varus position).

3. Adduction-pronation of the forefoot (Fig. 52) For the anterior arch to touch the ground the forefoot must be displaced medially while the sagittal plane P running through the axis of the forefoot, i.e. the second metatarsal, rotates medially to reach the final position P'. The angle **m** between the two points P and P' is a measure of this movement of **adduction**. Moreover, the forefoot is **pronated**. It is clear, however, that these movements of adduction-pronation are only *relative* to those of the hindfoot and occur at the transverse tarsal joint.

4. Hollowing of the medial arch (Fig. 52) This increase in the curvature of the medial arch (arrow 2) is itself the result of movements of the forefoot relative to the hindfoot. It is indicated by the elevation of the navicular relative to the ground, which is both *passive* because of the lateral displacement of the talar head and *active* secondary to contraction of the posterior tibialis. The overall hollowing of the plantar vault is reflected by a *widening of the indentation* in the footprint, as in the **pes cavus varus**.

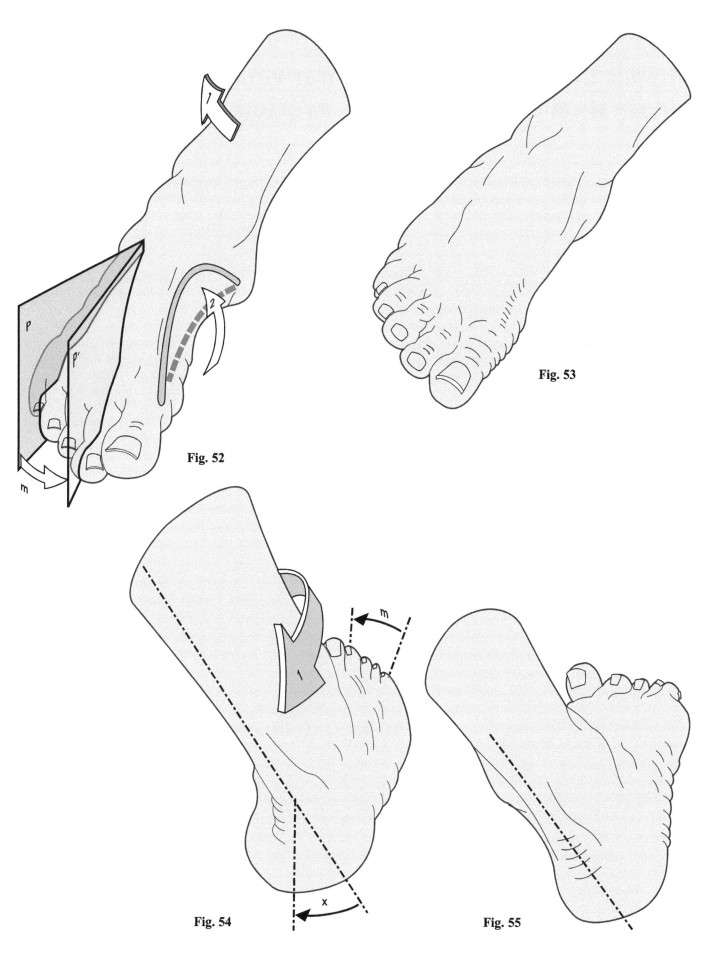

Fig. 52

Fig. 53

Fig. 54

Fig. 55

249

Dynamic distortions of the plantar vault secondary to inclination of the leg on the everted foot

When one is walking on sloping terrain along a straight path running perpendicular to that of the slope (see Fig. 62, p. 253) one foot must be inverted and the other everted for the lower limb and the body as a whole to be vertical. In the diagram the right foot is inverted and the left everted.

When the leg is inclined laterally with respect to the stationary foot resting on the ground, the **foot is in the everted position** (Fig. 56: anteromedial view of the everted foot) with the following **four consequences, which are the symmetrical opposites of those for the inverted foot.**

1. **Medial rotation of the leg on the foot (arrow 3)** The medial malleolus recedes as compared to its position when the foot rests only on its lateral border (Fig. 57) without being applied to the ground; the talus shifts medially so that its head projects on the medial border of the foot.

2. **Adduction-pronation of the hindfoot** (Fig. 58: posteromedial view of the everted foot) The hindfoot is adducted as a result of an incompletely compensated medial rotation and is pronated by the valgus displacement of the calcaneus with the formation of an angle y open laterally and lying between the axis of the heel and the axis of the leg as compared with the unconstrained position of the foot (Fig. 59).

3. **Abduction-supination of the forefoot** (Fig. 56) is reflected, as for inversion, by the abduction angle n between the two planes P and P'.

4. **Flattening of the medial arch (arrow 4)** The surface area of the footprint is increased with a decrease in the size of its medial indentation, as in the **pes planus valgus.**

These positions of the foot during adaptation to sloping terrain or during turns depend on the functionality of the subtalar and transverse tarsal joints, which are **indispensable for normal walking on bumpy ground.**

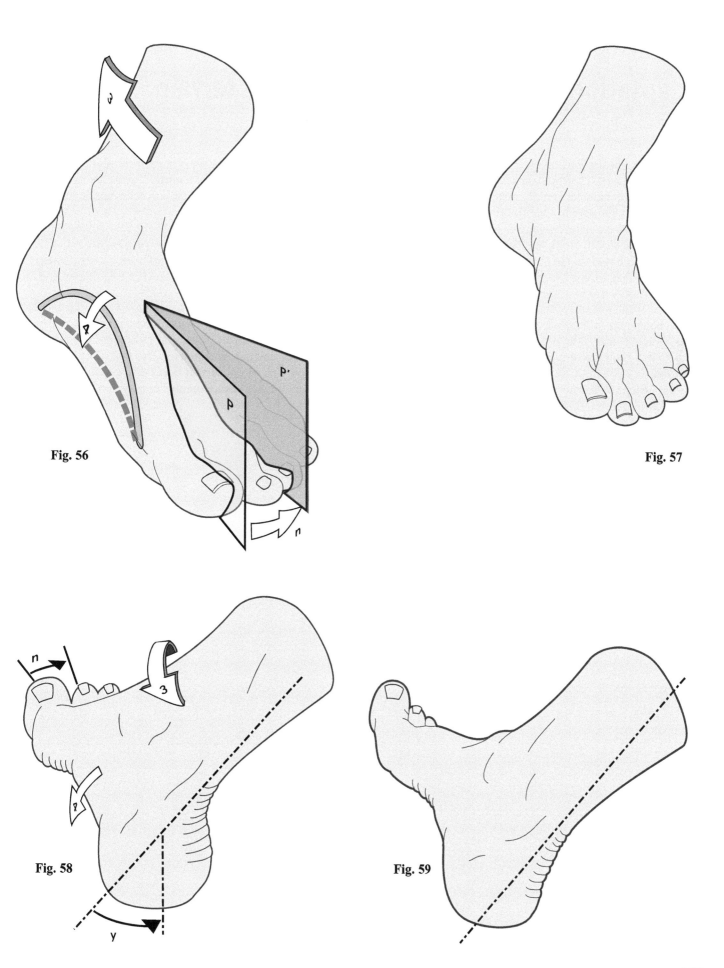

Fig. 56

Fig. 57

Fig. 58

Fig. 59

Adaptation of the plantar vault to the terrain

City dwellers always walk on even and firm ground with feet protected by shoes. Their plantar vaults have little incentive to adapt and the muscles mainly responsible for their maintenance eventually atrophy: the flat foot is the price paid for progress and some anthropologists go so far as to say that some day humans will 'walk' on feet reduced to mere stumps. This theory is based on the atrophic state of the toes and the absence of opposition of the big toe (which still persists in monkeys).

This is still far ahead in the future and even citydwelling human beings are still able to walk barefoot on a beach or on rocks. This 'return to the primitive state' is extremely beneficial to the plantar vault, which thus retrieves its **adaptive potential:**

- **Adaptation to the uneven features of the terrain,** to which the foot is able to cling (Fig. 60) thanks to the hollowing of the plantar vault
- **Adaptation to sloping terrains relative to the verticality of the body:**
  - The **anterior support** of the foot is wider when the ground slopes laterally (Fig. 61) because of the decreasing lengths of the metatarsal rays mediolaterally.

- **During standing on a transverse slope** (Fig. 62), the foot 'downstream' is supinated, while the foot 'upstream' is everted or in talus valgus (as described on the preceding page).
- **During climbing** (Fig. 63), the foot downstream needs to be anchored to the ground perpendicular to the slope, i.e. in the position of the pes planus varus, whereas the foot upstream hits the ground in full flexion and along the axis of the slope.
- **During descent on a slope** (Fig. 64), the feet must often be inverted in order to maximize their grip on the ground.

Thus, just as the palm of the hand allows prehension by changing its curvature and its orientation in space (see Volume 1), the sole of the foot can within certain limits *adapt to the bumps on the ground* in order to ensure optimal attachment to it.

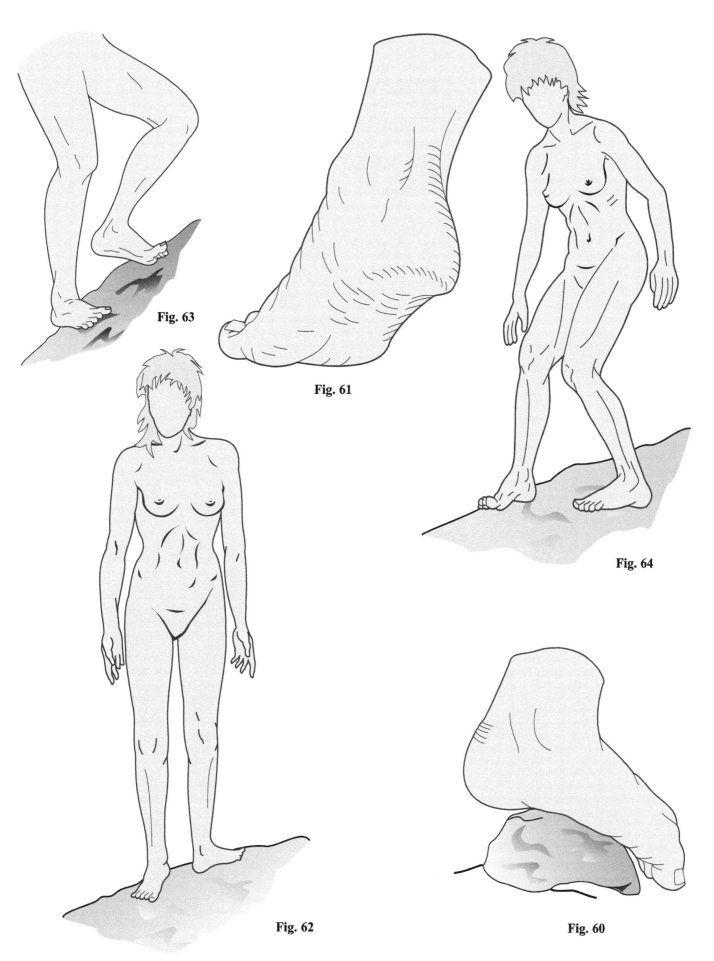

Fig. 63

Fig. 61

Fig. 64

Fig. 62

Fig. 60

The various types of pes cavus

The curvature and orientation of the plantar vault depend on an extremely delicate balance of muscular interaction, which can be studied with the help of Ombrédanne's model (Fig. 65: diagram of the bones and muscles of the foot):

- **The vault is flattened by the weight of the body** (blue arrow) and by contracture of the muscles inserted into its convex aspect, i.e. the triceps surae 1, the tibialis anterior and the fibularis tertius 2, the extensor digitorum longus and the extensor hallucis longus 3. The last two muscles are effective only if the proximal phalanges are stabilized by the interossei (7).
- **The vault is raised** by contracture of the muscles inserted into its concave aspect: the tibialis posterior (4), the fibularis longus and the fibularis brevis (5), the plantar muscles (6) and the toe flexors (8). It can also be raised by *relaxation of the muscles inserted into its convex aspect*. Conversely, relaxation of the muscles inserted into its concave aspect leads to flattening of the vault.

Insufficiency or contracture of a single one of those muscles disrupts the overall equilibrium and leads to some deformity. According to Duchenne de Boulogne, it is better from this viewpoint to have all the muscles paralysed than just a single one, since then the foot retains a fairly normal shape and orientation. There are **three types of pes cavus:**

1. The 'posterior' type (Fig. 66), so called because the lesion involves the posterior buttress, i.e. insufficiency of the triceps surae (1). The muscles on the concave aspect of the vault predominate (6), and the sole of the foot is hollowed further; the ankle flexors (2) tilt the foot into flexion. This leads to the pes cavus posterior (Fig. 67), which is often combined with a lateral inclination in *valgus* (Fig. 68) because of contracture of the abductor muscles (long extensors of the toes and the fibular muscles).

2. The 'midfoot' type (Fig. 69), relatively rare, results from contracture of the plantar muscles 6 caused by the use of shoes with excessively rigid soles or by shortening of the plantar aponeurosis (Ledderhose disease).

3. The 'anterior' type can be further subdivided into subgroups, which all share the equinus deformity (Fig. 70) with these two features:

- the equinus deformity of the forefoot e caused by the depression of the anterior buttresses
- the misalignment between the heel and the anterior tarsus d, which can be partially reduced when the body weight is being supported.

Depending on the mechanism involved, the following types of anterior pes cavus are described:

- Contracture of the tibialis posterior (4) and of the fibularis muscles (5) **depresses the forefoot** (Fig. 71). **Contracture of the fibularis muscles** alone can cause the pes cavus (Fig. 72) combined with a valgus inclination, i.e. **pes cavus equinovalgus.**
- **An imbalance at the metatarsophalangeal joints** (Fig. 73) is a very common cause of pes cavus: insufficiency of the interossei (7) tips the balance in favour of the toe extensors (3), and *hyperextension* of the proximal phalanges follows. Next the metatarsal heads are lowered b with lowering of the forefoot; hence the **pes cavus with claw toes.**
- **Lowering of the metatarsal heads** (Fig. 74) can also be due to insufficiency of the tibialis anterior (2): the extensor muscles (3) try to compensate and tilt the proximal phalanges backwards; the plantar muscles (6), now unbalanced, accentuate the curvature of the vault, and the triceps (1) causes a mild form of equinus deformity; a lateral inclination in valgus (Fig. 75) results from the slight predominance of the extensor digitorum longus. This is the **pes cavus equinovalgus.**
- A common cause of pes cavus is the **wearing of shoes that are too short or have high heels** (Fig. 76): the toes hit the tips of the shoes and are hyperextended a, depressing the metatarsal heads b. Under the weight of the body (Fig. 77) the *foot slides* down the slope of the shoe, and the *heel moves closer to the toes*, thus increasing the curvature of the plantar vault.

The diagnosis of pes cavus is made easier by examination of the **footprint** (Fig. 78). In comparison with the normal footprint (I) the early stage of pes cavus (II) is characterized by a convex projection on its lateral border m and a deepening of the indentation on its medial border n. In the next stage (III) the deepening of the indentation blends with the lateral border p and divides the footprint into two parts. Finally, in **chronic cases of pes cavus (IV)**, there is the additional loss of the toeprints q, secondary to the development of **claw toes.**

One must be aware that the pes cavus footprint with loss of the lateral zone of support can also be seen with the **talipes planovalgus of children and adolescents:** the valgus of the calcaneus and the lowering of the medial arch can cause the lateral arch to rise slightly and lose contact with the ground in its middle part. These findings can lead to misdiagnosis, but it is easy to detect *this mimic of the flatfoot imprint* as follows: all the toes lie flat on the ground and, when the medial arch is raised or, better still, when the leg is made to rotate laterally with the foot on the ground, the lateral border of the footprint reappears, while the medial arch hollows once more.

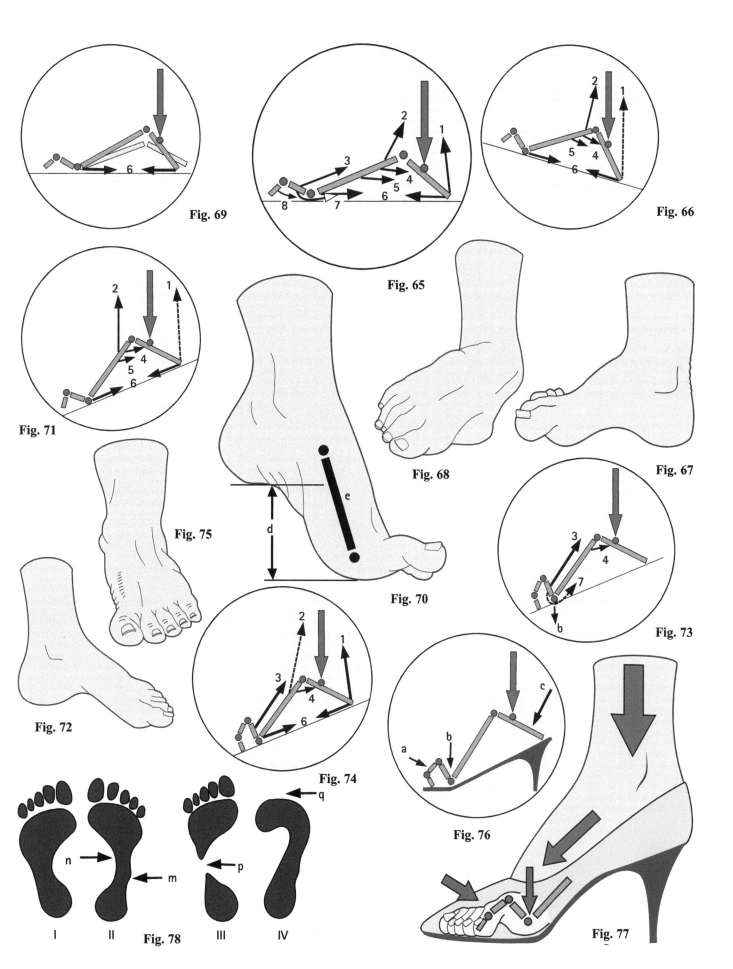

Fig. 69

Fig. 65

Fig. 66

Fig. 71

Fig. 68

Fig. 67

Fig. 75

Fig. 70

Fig. 73

Fig. 72

Fig. 74

Fig. 76

Fig. 78

Fig. 77

The various types of pes planus

The collapse of the plantar vault is due to the **breakdown of its natural muscular and ligamentous support systems.** The ligaments alone can maintain the curvature of the plantar vault for a short period of time, since the footprint of an amputated leg is normal, except if the ligaments have been previously cut. In life, however, **if the muscular supports fail, the ligaments become stretched eventually and the vault collapses for good.** The pes planus is therefore due mainly to muscular insufficiency (Fig. 79), i.e. insufficiency of the tibialis posterior (4) or more often of the fibularis longus (5). If the foot is off the ground, it lies in a **varus position** (Fig. 80) because the fibularis is an abductor. On the other hand, as soon as the weight of the body is applied to the vault, the *medial arch collapses*, as illustrated in the diagram (Fig. 81), where the collapsed arch is shown as red and the *foot is 'rotated' into valgus.* This valgus is due to two factors:

1. The **transverse curvature of the vault**, normally supported (Fig. 82) by the fibularis longus tendon (white arrow), becomes flattened (Fig. 83); at the same time, the medial arch is lowered. As a result, the arch is elongated (3), the forefoot is rotated (e) on its long axis so that the whole surface of the sole of the foot touches the ground while the forefoot is also deviated (d) laterally.

2. The **calcaneus rotates into pronation** (Fig. 84) on its long axis and tends to lie flat on its medial surface. This valgus, visible and measurable by the angle (f) between the axis of the heel and the calcaneal tendon, exceeds the physiological limits of 5° and attains 20° in certain flat feet. According to some authors, this valgus would be due primarily to a malformation of the subtalar articular surfaces and to an abnormal degree of laxity of the interosseous ligament; other authors believe that these lesions are secondary.

Whatever the cause, the valgus displaces the centre of pressure *towards the medial border of the foot and the talar head dips inferiorly and medially.* The medial margin of the foot then displays **three more or less distinct projections** (Fig. 83).

- the medial malleolus, abnormally prominent (a)
- the medial part of the talar head (b)
- the tubercle of the navicular (c).

The projecting navicular tubercle represents the apex of the obtuse angle, open laterally, and formed by the axis of the hindfoot and that of the forefoot: *adduction-pronation of the hindfoot is offset by abduction-supination of the forefoot* resulting in the **loss of the vault curvature.** The mechanism behind these changes was worked out by such classical authors as Hohmann, Boehler, Hauser and Soeur.

This combination of deformities, although less severe, has already been described when *static loads are applied to the vault* (Fig. 41, p. 243). It is a relatively common condition, known as the **painful pes planus valgus or tarsalgia of adolescents,** and is easily recognized in a posterior view of the foot (Fig. 84) as a lateral valgus displacement of the calcaneus (f).

The diagnosis of pes planus is made easier with the use of the **footprint** (Fig. 85), which is easily obtained by placing the wet foot on top of a dark, dry surface. In comparison with the normal footprint I, the *evolving stages of pes planus* reveal a progressive decrease in the size of the medial indentation II and III, until in longstanding cases, the medial border may even become convex IV.

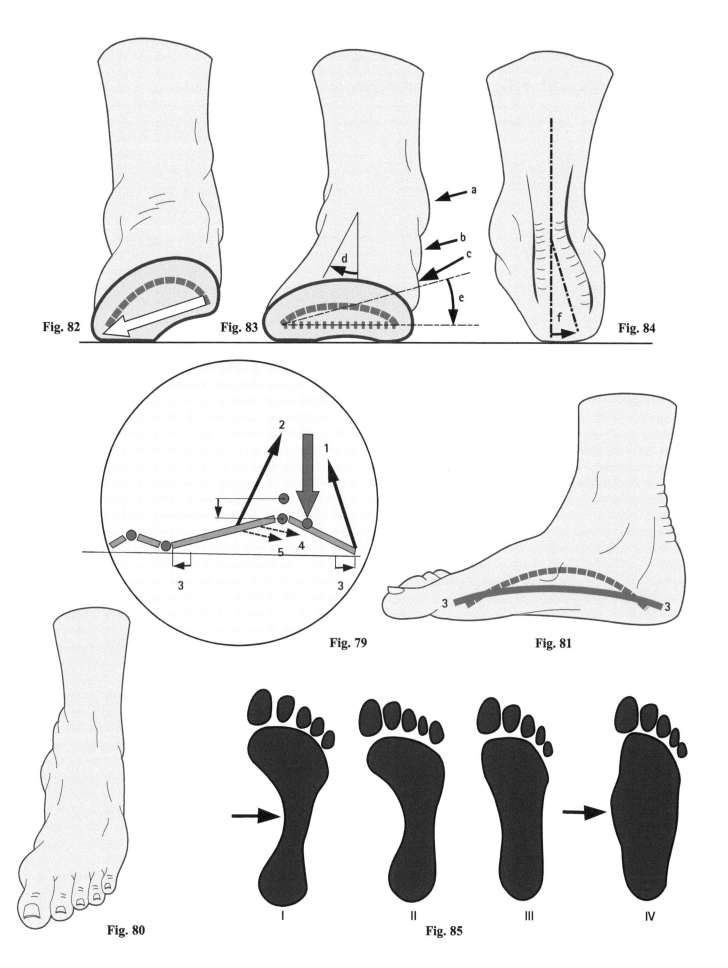

Fig. 82

Fig. 83

Fig. 84

Fig. 79

Fig. 81

Fig. 80

Fig. 85

Imbalances of the anterior arch

Whenever the plantar vault is warped, the anterior arch can be thrown into **imbalance at its points of support** or become **distorted in its curvature.**

The **imbalance** is generally secondary to an anterior type of pes cavus, since the equinus deformity of the forefoot increases the stresses applied to the anterior arch in the following three ways:

1. The equinus deformity of the forefoot is symmetrical (Fig. 86: cross-section at metatarsal level), without any pronation or supination, and the arch curvature is maintained. Under these circumstances, both points of support are overloaded and calluses* develop under the heads of the first and fifth metatarsals (arrows).

2. The equinus deformity of the forefoot is combined with pronation (Fig. 87) because of the predominant lowering of the medial ray secondary to contracture of the tibialis posterior or of the fibularis longus. Since the curvature of the arch is maintained, its medial point of support bears the brunt of the overload and a callus develops under the head of the first metatarsal (arrow).

3. The equinus deformity of the forefoot is combined with supination (Fig. 88): since the arch curvature is maintained, the overload is applied to its lateral point of support and a callus forms under the head of the fifth metatarsal (arrow).

In **deformations of the arch** associated with some anterior types of pes cavus the curvature of the arch can disappear or become inverted:

*   When the **curvature is simply straightened or obliterated:** this is an example of the flat forefoot (Fig. 89); the overload is distributed to all the metatarsal heads, and a callus forms under every metatarsal head (arrows).
*   When the **curvature is completely inverted** (Fig. 90), the condition is called the round forefoot or the *anterior convex foot*; the overload is applied to the heads of the three middle metatarsals, leading to the formation of three very painful calluses underneath.

These **calluses** are **hyperkeratotic thickenings** of the skin caused by excessive pressure applied locally (the superficial cells of the skin are called **keratinocytes**). They often **extend deep into the skin** and are **very painful** on the slightest pressure. These calluses provide a lucrative business for podiatrists, who remove them with special scalpels or graters, but the patient is regularly disappointed, since paring down a callus does not remove the cause, i.e. the overload. Hence, the only way to get rid of them permanently is to **restore the normal anatomy of the anterior arch** and the normal distribution of the loads on the arch often with the help of insoles made to measure.

---

* The presence of a callus or corn reflects an abnormal pressure point due to a deformation of the plantar arch.

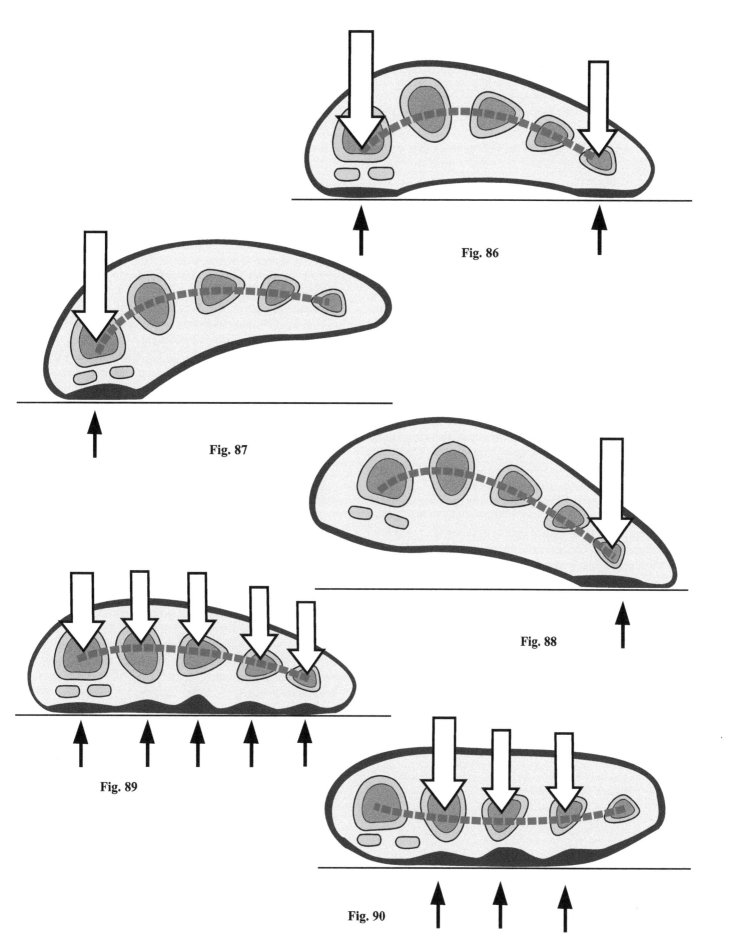

Fig. 86

Fig. 87

Fig. 88

Fig. 89

Fig. 90

Types of feet

The feet are certainly the parts of the human body that get the worst treatment from their owners, especially from women. In the natural state, the human foot could spread out free and happy without any constraints.

The **ancestral foot**, also called the pes antiquus (Fig. 91: view of the skeleton of the foot), reminiscent of the pre-human foot with the prehensile big toe, could have a wide contact with the ground thanks to its widely separated metatarsals and toes.

When in civilized societies it was enclosed inside more or less constraining shoes it *had to adapt*; with the advent of fashion, especially as regards women's *pointed shoes*, these constraints had a catastrophic effect (Fig. 92: skeleton of foot inside pointed shoe), resulting in the appearance of what now bears the barbaric name of '**hallux valgus**':

- The first metatarsal is widely separated from the second, i.e. **metatarsus varus or adductus,** and is displaced away from the midline causing the big toe to shift obliquely, anteriorly and laterally **a.**
- The result is an **abnormal prominence of the first metatarsal head**, where the constant friction with the shoe leads to the formation of an exostosis **b** and later of a callus, also called a bunion, which can become infected.
- The second metatarsal clearly overshoots the other metatarsals and therefore becomes the support point **at the end of the step**; this overload causes pain at its tarsometatarsal joint and at times a fatigue fracture (the tired foot).
- The fifth metatarsal is also displaced away from the midline (**metarsus quintus valgus or abductus**) and is pushed back medially **c** with the fifth toe.
- Soon the imbalance becomes permanent, frozen by the *retraction of the articular capsules* and the **lateral dislocation of the sesamoid bones d** and of the flexor tendons **e**, which worsens the imbalance.
- The obliquely set big toe **pushes away the middle toes** and may even lodge beneath the second toe (Fig. 93), i.e. the so-called '**hallux infraductus**'.
- On the lateral side of the foot, the fifth toe suffers the inverse deformity, i.e. **quintus varus**, thus reducing the space for the

middle toes and forcing them into the **hammer-toe** deformity (Fig. 94); calluses, also known as 'corns', form on the dorsal surface of the proximal interphalangeal joint.

- The claw of the median toes presses down on the metatarsal heads and depresses them causing the anterior arch to become convex, i.e. the **anterior convex forefoot.**

In the aggregate this very banal deformity combining hallux valgus, hammer-toes and anterior convex forefoot makes the wearing of shoes very awkward and can only be corrected **surgically.**

The **morphology of the foot** plays an important role in the development of these deformities. In reference to the graphic and plastic arts, **three types of feet** are recognized:

- The **Greek foot** (Fig. 95) as observed in classical Greek statues: the second toe is the longest x, followed by the big toe and the third toe of nearly equal length, the fourth toe and finally the fifth toe. This type of foot, the commonest, is conducive to the best distribution of loads on to the forefoot.
- The **Egyptian foot** (Fig. 96), seen on the statues of the Pharaohs, is characterized by the longest big toe y, with the others decreasing in length successively. This type of foot is the most prone to problems. The relatively long big toe is shifted inside the shoe (hallux valgus) and is unduly overloaded during the terminal stance or 'heel-off' phase of the step, leading to osteoarthritis of its metatarsophalangeal joint, i.e. **hallux rigidus.**
- The **Polynesian foot** (Fig. 97) or the '**square foot**', as seen in Gauguin's paintings, has toes of nearly equal length, at least the first three. It gives no problems.

In summary, one must avoid wearing – and this concerns women above all – shoes that are too small and heels that are too high (the latter being equivalent to the former), since the toes bump into one another and are folded over (Fig. 93). All these factors combine to produce the hallux valgus.

If one wanted to draw a lesson from these observations, a famous saying could be paraphrased as follows: '**the shoe is made for the foot and not the foot for the shoe**'.

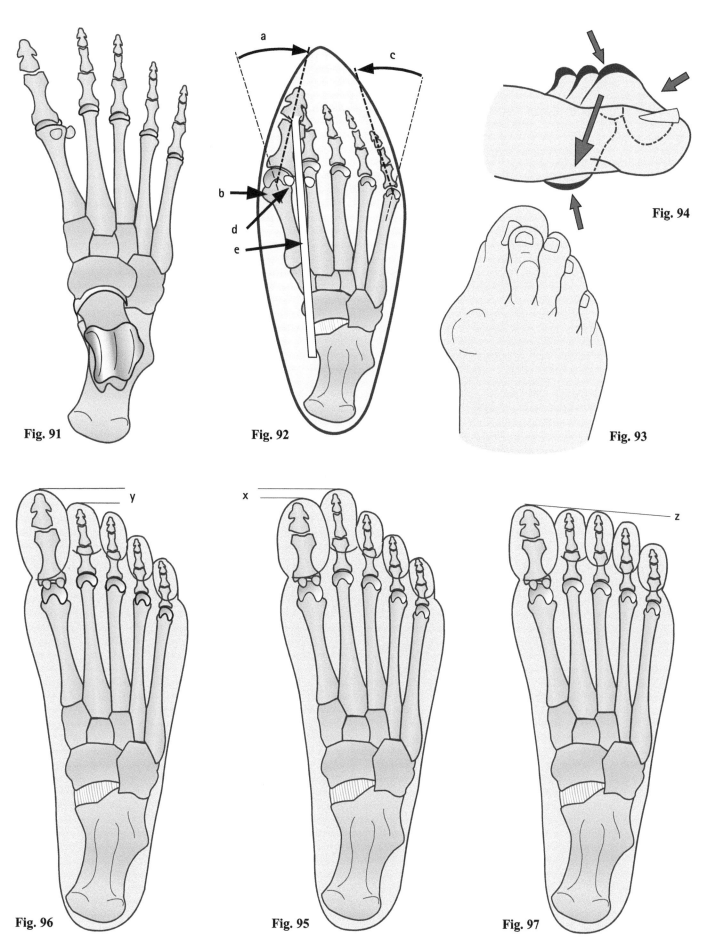

Fig. 91

Fig. 92

Fig. 94

Fig. 93

Fig. 96

Fig. 95

Fig. 97

Chapter 6

WALKING

Just like speech and writing, walking on two feet is a human characteristic. (Michelangelo initially drew his David walking with his slingshot in his left hand.) Other animals can rear themselves up on their hind legs and take a few steps in the erect position, but this is not their normal posture, even for the higher apes.

Humans have colonized the planet thanks to their ability to walk on two feet and also to break free of their ancestral environment, unlike the apes, which have failed to do so.

In contrast to the newborn gazelle, which is able to run after its mother from birth (an essential condition for survival) the human neonate has to go through a long and hard training of standing up and then of walking, punctuated by multiple, fortunately inconsequential, falls. It has to control its own unstable equilibrium on its two feet and then to accept the forward fall that accompanies every step. Walking means passing from an already statically unstable stance on two feet to a dynamically even more unstable position characterized by successive forward falls, which are offset at the last moment. It is like a continuously repeated miracle dependent on motor coordination controlled by the nervous system.

For human beings, walking on two feet is a requirement and a guarantee of their individual freedom; without the ability to walk they lose their autonomy and become dependent on others. Walking has allowed humans to conquer every environment, including the highest mountain peaks. Thanks to their intelligence they have been able to invent the wheel, which is unknown in Nature, and to create additional modes of locomotion on land, on water or under water, and even in the air by imitating birds. They even aspire to the conquest of space, but their favourite and indispensable mode of locomotion remains walking. This explains the significance of the riddle put to Oedipus by the Sphinx: 'What goes on four legs in the morning, on two legs at noon and on three legs in the evening?'*

---

* Find the answer, if you do not already know it, at the end of this book.

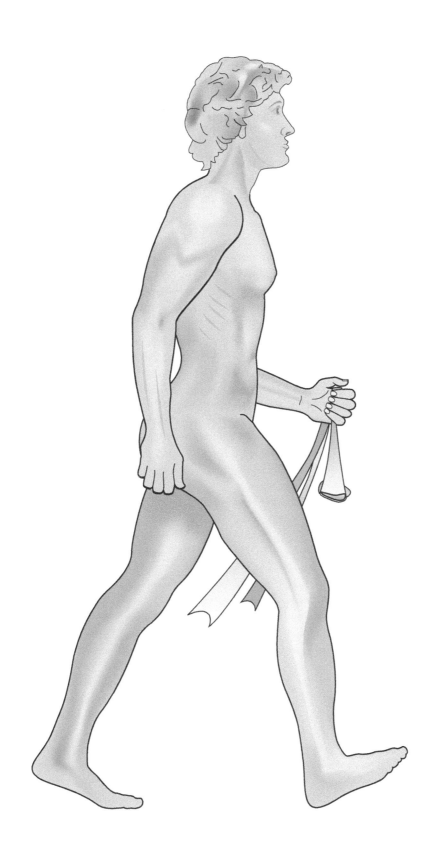

The move to bipedalism

When our remote ancestors, starting with the tetrapods, left the sea 300 million years ago, they were quadrupeds. All vertebrates are built from the same prototype; they have four limbs and walk horizontally on their four feet. Even the higher apes move on the ground as quadrupeds, but, since they live in trees, they have to use their anterior limbs to climb, an obligatory step in the transition to bipedalism.

The transition has been long and difficult, requiring profound changes in the structure of the body as a whole.

Starting from the quadruped position (Fig. 1), when the spine is globally convex upwards, the raising of the body (Figs 2 and 3) is associated with straightening of the lumbar spine (arrow 1) and verticalization of the sacrum (arrow 2). At the same time, the change of orientation of the head needed to maintain a horizontal gaze led to a forward migration of the foramen magnum (arrow 3).

The verticalization of the sacrum requires retroversion of the pelvis (Figs 4 and 5), which then causes forced extension of the hip, followed in turn by tightening of the anterior ligaments and a considerable alteration in the congruence of the articular surfaces. As a result, the femoral head becomes 'exposed' anteriorly (see Fig. 71, p. 31).

If the anterior hip ligaments (1) do not elongate adequately (Fig. 4), pelvic retroversion will be incomplete (blue arrow), and the sacrum (2) will stay at a 45° angle with the vertical, causing a lumbar hyperlordosis (3) with secondary effects on the other spinal curvatures. On the other hand, if the anterior ligaments elongate sufficiently (Fig. 5), pelvic retroversion will be complete (blue arrow) and the sacrum verticalized (5), leading to a flattening of the lumbar lordosis (6) and, secondarily, of the other spinal curvatures.

This transition has been extensively studied by A. Delmas (see Volume 3, Fig. 16, p. 15) and can be summarized with the help of three diagrams (Fig. 6) as follows:

- Pelvic retroversion is incomplete **a**, and the sacrum is horizontal: this accentuates the three spinal curvatures, i.e. lumbar hyperlordosis, thoracic kyphosis and cervical hyperlordosis
- At the other extreme **c** pelvic retroversion is complete, the sacrum is verticalized and the spinal curvatures are attenuated
- In the intermediate position (the commonest), the sacrum is at a 45° angle, and the spinal curvatures are of intermediate amplitudes.

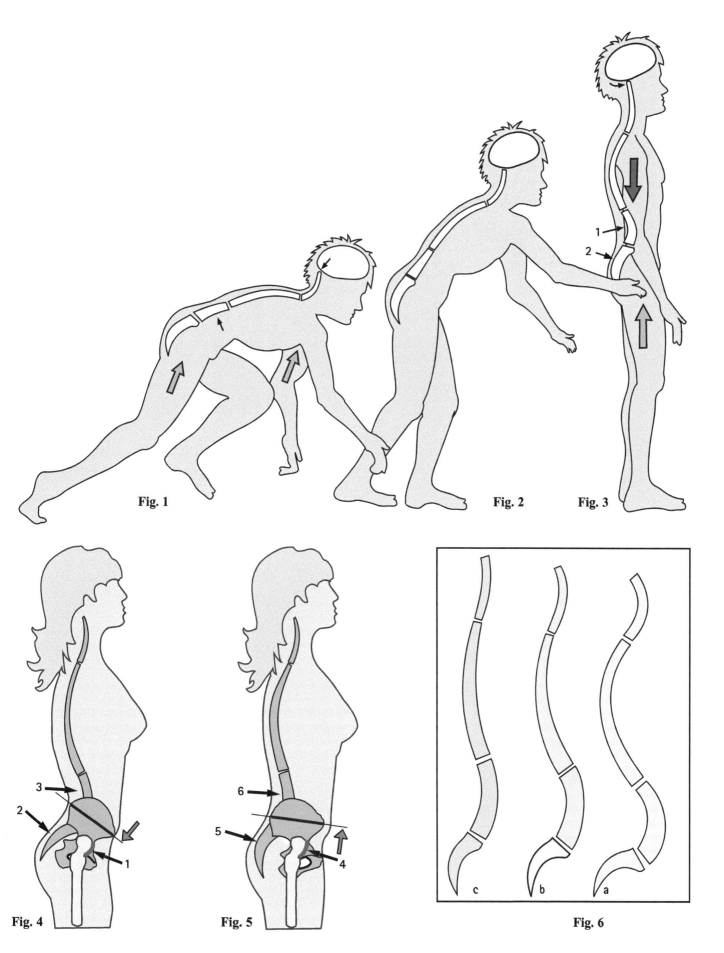

Fig. 1

Fig. 2

Fig. 3

Fig. 4

Fig. 5

Fig. 6

The miracle of bipedalism

Mechanically speaking, **the bipedal position is** totally abnormal and is close to a permanent miracle. In fact, the human body in the erect posture with double-limb support (Fig. 7: drawing of the KOUROS, taken from Greek art) is an **eminently unstable structure** for three reasons:

1. First, the surface area of its support base *is very small* compared with its overall height.

2. Then, the *upper part of the structure is longer and bulkier* than its lower part, like a truncated pyramid with its base located on top.

3. Finally, *its base is absolutely not anchored to the ground* (Fig. 8): no architect would build such a building, as it would collapse without fail. When a very high tower like a skyscraper is built, its foundations dig deep into the ground (Fig. 9). This is not the case for the human biped.

The human body is a stable structure (Fig. 10) only when the **perpendicular drawn from its centre of gravity falls within the body support area**, shown here as the green rectangle that contains the footprints.

The **centre of gravity** of a mass-containing object is the theoretical point where the total mass of the object is concentrated. It is also called the **barycentre**. For example it is easy on a diagram **(Fig. 10bis)** to calculate the common centre of gravity of three bodies **A**, **B** and **C** with weights of **P1**, **P2** and **P3**. Start by finding the common centre of gravity for **B** and **C**, which lies on the line joining the two centres at a point **O**, which divides the segment in an inverse ratio to the weight P3/P2 and thus lies closer to the heavier body. At this point **O** is applied the sum of the two weights **P2** and **P3**. Then proceed in the same way for the weights **A** and **B** to find the point **O'**, which is the barycentre for **A** and **B** and where the sum of P1 + P2 is applied. Finally, find between O and O' the common barycentre of the three weights **A**, **B** and **C**, where **M**, the sum of the three weights **A**, **B** and **C** is applied.

Each part of the human body has a barycentre, as if it were separate from the rest of the body. For example, the centre of gravity of the upper limb (green dot) lies a little below the elbow, that of the lower limb (violet dot) slightly above the knee and that of the trunk (blue dot) at the level of the epigastrium. The location of the barycentre depends on the geometry of the mass-containing volume, and if the upper limb is flexed its centre of gravity will come to lie outside it in front of the elbow. In the position of standing to attention the overall barycentre of the body (red dot) depends on the **mechanical composition of the segmental centres of gravity** and lies in the pelvis at the level of S2-S3, i.e. at about 55% of the height of the body. But depending on the various body positions, e.g. in a pole vault, this centre can be markedly displaced, but most often around a mean position in the pelvis; exceptionally it can lie outside the body. When the back is arched **(Fig. 9bis)**, the backward projection of the limbs displaces their barycentre backwards **(green arrow)** so that their partial barycentres **(white arrow)** are also displaced backwards, resulting in a displacement of the general barycentre of the body. This placement of the barycentre is very important, especially in **women** (Fig. 11: woman in profile), because it is in the pelvis around the barycentre that the fetus develops and is thus protected as much as possible from shocks. In fact **(Fig. 11bis)** the barycentre of the pregnant uterus **(black star)** simply causes the new barycentre of the body to move forward superoanteriorly **(blue star)** as compared with that of a non-pregnant woman (red star). The forward displacement of the barycentre in pregnancy causes a lumbar lordosis, but it still remains above the pelvic boundary.

The diagram also illustrates the **significance of the tonus of the postural muscles** (also known as **antigravity muscles**) in the erect posture. In fact, every segment of the body tends to collapse under the force of gravity, and this is averted by the postural muscles, i.e. the gluteus maximus (1), the lumbar (2) and thoracic (3) paravertebral muscles, the posterior neck muscles (4), the quadriceps (5) and the triceps surae (6).

The contraction and tonic activity of these muscles is constantly controlled by the nervous system, which takes into account the numerous bits of information emanating from the plantar support points, the position of the various body segments relative to the **body as a whole**, the **position of the head** supplied by the **cochlea** in the inner ear and from the **eyes** as they localize the horizon. The constant adjustments of the activity of these muscles in all positions and in all dynamic situations are an essential requirement for the bipedal posture: without the watchfulness of the nervous system the body would fall down and bipedalism would be impossible. This is what happens in diseases of the central nervous system and in myopathies.

As the tightrope walker **(Fig. 8bis)** walks on a wire stretched high up in the air, he uses a balancing pole curved downwards **(yellow arrow)** so that his general barycentre **(red arrow)** is also lowered, providing him with greater stability and improving his ability to control and correct any displacement of his own barycentre.

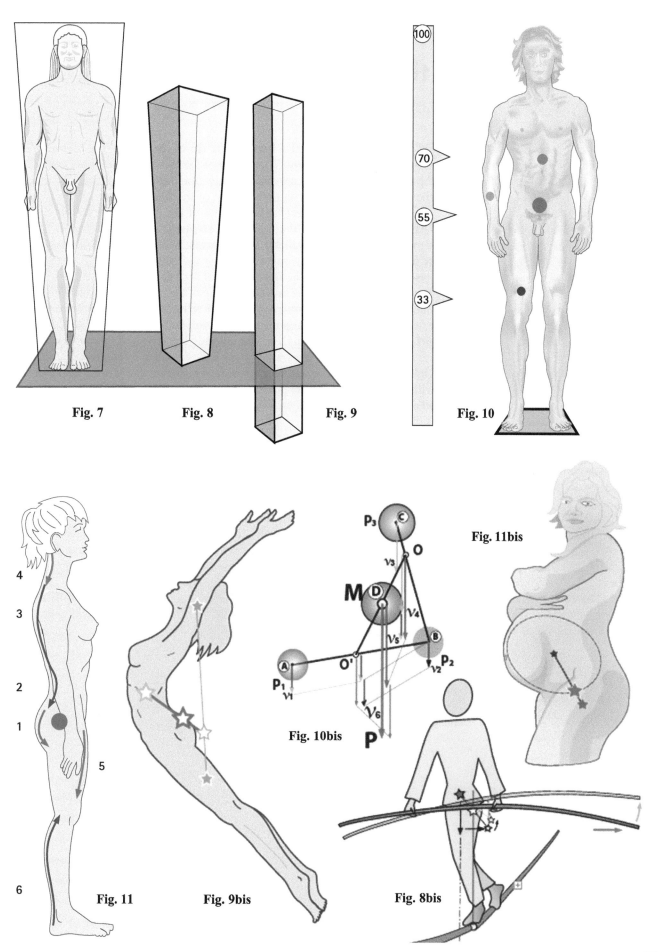

Fig. 7

Fig. 8

Fig. 9

Fig. 10

Fig. 11bis

Fig. 10bis

Fig. 11

Fig. 9bis

Fig. 8bis

267

The initial step and those that follow it

The **initial step**, or the **inaugural step,** should not be confused with the **first step** of the young child, which is rightly celebrated by the entire family, as it means the start of the whole period of bipedal life, until disease or death restores the human body to its definitive horizontal position.

When one of the parents lets go of the child's hand and the child takes its first step, the usual tendency to fall is miraculously prevented by the "initial step," i.e., **the step that signals the start of normal walking.** In fact, **when the body is symmetrically erect (Fig. 12),** the body weight is distributed equally on the two feet, making it impossible to raise one foot in order to advance the other. The start of the initial step therefore raises the problem of load distribution on the feet: **the body weight must be shifted on to one foot for the other to be lifted!**

In general, right-footed people advance the right foot first, just as right-footed soccer players kick the ball with the right foot. Under these conditions, the **preparatory period of the initial step (Fig. 12:** frontal view) consists of the lateral tilting of the pelvis towards the supporting limb, i.e., the left foot in this case. The **left adductors (red arrow)** contract to tilt the pelvis to the left **(blue arrow),** while simultaneously the glutei minimus and medius contract **(small red arrow)** to raise the right half of the pelvis **(black arrow).** Thus the barycentre of the body is displaced to the left **(white arrow),** while the body weight is lifted off the right foot. This marks the **start of the first period of the step (Fig. 12bis:** seen in profile), when the **contraction of the left hamstrings (blue arrow)** propels the pelvis forward and causes an anterior imbalance initiating a fall forward, which is checked as the triceps surae **(black arrow)** contract to restrict flexion of the left ankle. At the same time, the right hip flexors propel the right knee forward **(small black arrow)** and the **right ankle flexors**

raise further the tip of the toes of the already raised right foot. The raising of the tips of the toes is very important in that it prevents the toes from hitting the ground and thus interfering with the advance of the foot. Any loss of this movement **as a result of paralysis of the ankle flexors** gives rise to the condition known as **steppage or foot-drop gait.** Thus, in adults walking always begins with an initial fall forward induced by the initial step: it is the indispensable start of the gait cycle.

The **first period of forward progression (Fig. 13)** begins with the raising of the tip of the posterior foot due to the simultaneous **contraction of the triceps surae** and of the hamstrings, which propels the pelvis forward **(blue arrow).** At the same time, the thigh of the anterior leg is flexed, propelling the lower limb forward with its knee extended by contraction of the quadriceps and its ankle flexed to ensure that it is the heel that will contact the ground.

Then follows **midstance (Fig. 13bis),** when the heel of the anterior limb touches the ground **(A)** and its sole flattens on the ground; meantime the supporting limb **rotates forward** and the posterior limb, propelled forward by the hip flexors, overtakes the weight-bearing limb **(B)** so that with both knee and ankle flexed it undergoes another fall forward. Then follows the second period of forward progression, as already described **(Fig. 13).** It is initiated by flexion of the toes, especially the big toe, which will rotate the posterior limb forward on to its tip, while the heel of the anterior limb touches the ground. This corresponds to the very brief period of double limb support preceding the first period of forward progression.

In sum, normal walking is only a **series of falls forward** interrupted just in time by the anterior foot making contact with the ground.

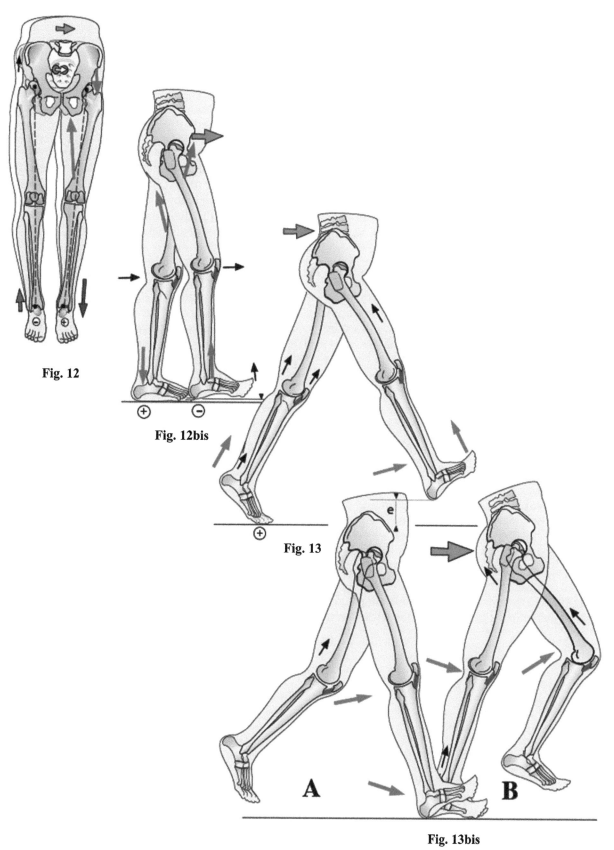

Fig. 12

Fig. 12bis

Fig. 13

A

B

Fig. 13bis

Swing phase of the gait cycle

The forward fall induced by the initial step in the gait cycle signals the start of the **single-limb support period,** when the trailing or swing limb moves ahead of the leading limb in order to prevent the fall from occurring. The **swing limb** is thus responsible for the **forward movement of the step.**

The French physiologist **Etienne Jules Marey** was the first at the end of the nineteenth century to subdivide the various periods of the gait cycle and to record them (Fig. 14: graph based on Marey's chronophotographic experiment) with the help of the 'photographic gun', which he invented and which became the precursor of the camera. Thus, he is **one of the pioneers of the cinema** and of chronophotography (also known as **stroboscopy**). The graph shows very clearly the **two stages of the gait cycle:**

- The **single-limb support period** of the stance phase (A) occurs when the leading limb hits the ground heel first and then tilts forwards on itself as a result of extension of the ankle and of the toes, especially of the big toe, thus producing the foot-flat or the loading response that precedes the *propulsive* movement.
- It also includes the **swing phase** (B) of the *non-weight-bearing limb as it advances as a result of hip flexion and shortens as a result of knee and ankle flexion* before hitting the ground with the heel and preventing a fall at the last minute.
- The **double-limb support period** is quite short and starts at the end of the propulsive phase, before the heel of the posterior weight-bearing limb leaves the ground.
- The wheel does not exist in Nature, but the lower limbs can be viewed as the radii of **two alternating wheels with variable radii:**
- The **leading limb** (Fig. 15: diagram of the leading limb) corresponds to the radius of a wheel that elongates first as

it rotates during the foot-flat or loading-response phase and finally during the propulsive phase.
- The **swing limb** corresponds to the radius of a wheel that shortens as it moves forward to become once more the weight-bearing limb.

An analysis of the diagram, in particular the three lines of coloured dots representing the hips, the shoulders and the head, shows the following:

1. The **first stage of the stance phase** (points 1-2), when the supporting limb rotates around the point of contact with the ground as it is propelled forward. The hip becomes vertical and attains the *first apex* of its arc of motion.

2. The **second stage of the stance phase,** when it is slightly flexed (point 3) setting the stage for extension of the knee (point 4) and of the ankle (point 5). The arc of motion of the hip then attains its highest point.

Thus the gait cycle is nothing but a succession of forward falls avoided and controlled.

These two alternating wheels have limited contact with the ground and the subtalar joint allows the foot to adapt to any slope in the terrain. These two wheels do not require smooth surfaces like roads and therefore allow humans to move in the bumpiest places and even up to the peaks of mountains!

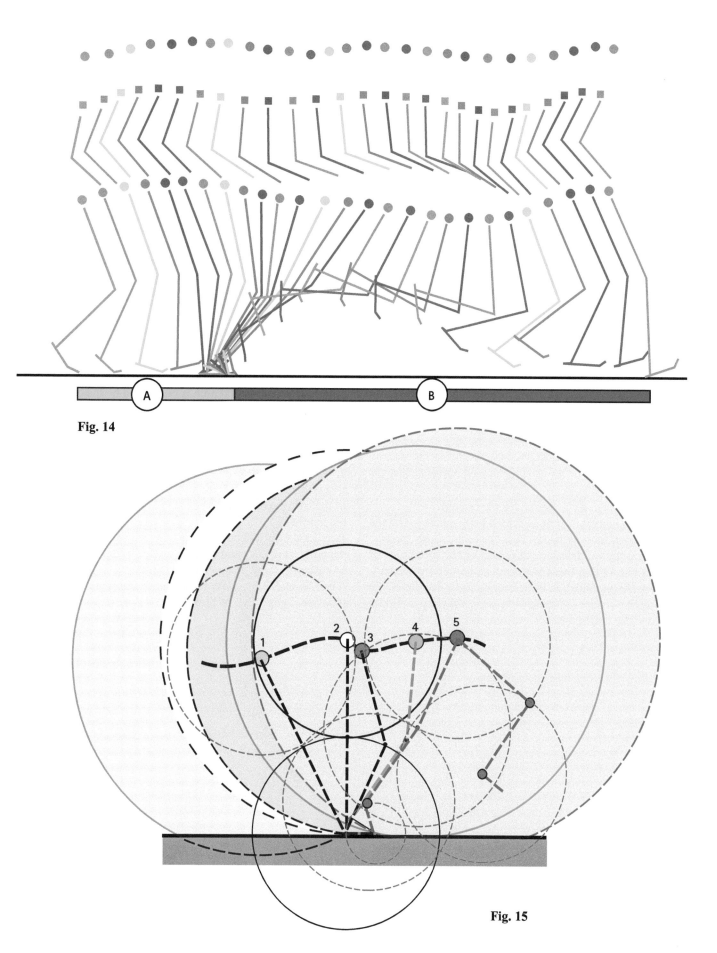

Fig. 14

Fig. 15

The stance phase of the gait cycle

While supported on the ground, the foot of the leading limb goes through what is conventionally known as the **stance phase with four periods.**

This process is summarized in the diagram (Fig. 16), which superimposes all the phases of this progression with the **three main points of the support** of the foot marked by black triangles:

1. The **initial posterior contact point**, where the heel touches the ground under the impulse of the kinetic energy of the body (red arrow)

2. The **anterior point of support** of the medial arch at the level of the head of the first metatarsal is recruited when the entire sole of the foot rests on the ground (green arrow) and receives the propulsive force generated by ankle extension (blue arrow)

3. The **extreme anterior point of support**, which is the point of application of the propulsive force generated by flexion of the big toe (yellow arrow).

Also shown in the diagram are **three arcs of a circle** whose centres lie on each of the support points:

- the arc of the head of the first metatarsal before it hits the ground
- the arc of the heel as it rises above the ground
- the arc of the metatarsal head, which loses contact with the ground under the impulsion of the final propulsive force.

Normally, **gravity and friction generated by the roughness of the ground** ensure that these points of support stay stationary in relation to the ground, but, if the friction force decreases, the heel *cannot be anchored to the ground and slides*, e.g. a fall on an icy surface. Note that **gravity plays a fundamental role** in maintaining this support; thus walking is seriously disrupted by a decrease in the force of gravity and becomes impossible in zero gravity, as in a spacecraft.

A more detailed analysis of these four periods reveals the following.

1. The **heel strike** (Fig. 17), checked by friction against the ground, is followed by extension of the initially flexed ankle, while the sole hits the ground. This movement is checked by the contraction of the ankle flexors, in particular the tibialis anterior TA.

2. Flattening of the sole of the foot (Fig. 18) (the foot-flat stage) equivalent to collapse of the plantar vault under the full weight of the body as the weight-bearing limb flattens forward on to its toes. The flexor muscles help in flexing the ankle. The flattening of the medial arch is cushioned by the contraction of the plantar muscles.

3. The **first propulsive force** (1) (Fig. 19) (the heel-offstage) is generated by the powerful contraction of the triceps surae (blue arrow) against the resistance of the plantar muscles.

4. The **second propulsive force** (2) (Fig. 20) (the pre-swing stage) is generated by contraction of the toe flexors, especially of the two flexors of the big toe (F), while the triceps (T) keep on contracting.

Here again the effectiveness of the second propulsive force 2 depends on gravity and friction on the ground and is decreased or cancelled when the ground is slippery.

It can be said that gravity plays an essential role in walking and likewise in the flight of birds.

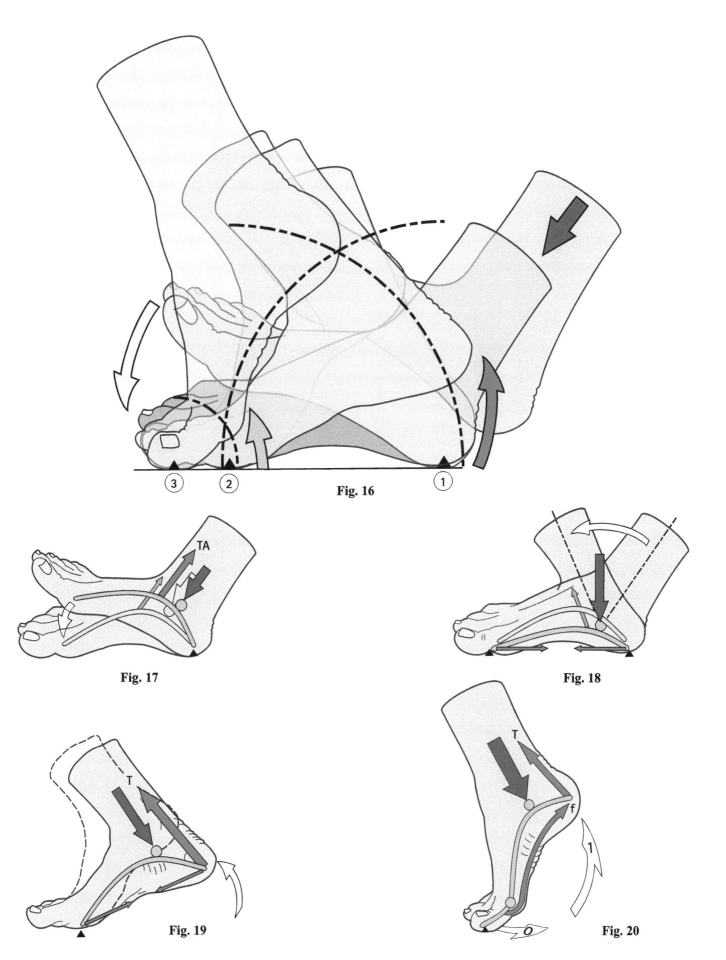

Fig. 16

Fig. 17

Fig. 18

Fig. 19

Fig. 20

The footprints

Footprints are readily seen when someone walks on a dry surface with wet feet or on the beach. In the latter case, the **depth of the footprint** reflects the weight of the subject and the depth of the deeper depressions anteriorly and posteriorly give an idea of the force of the heel strike or of the propulsive force.

Such a **sequence of footprints** (Fig. 21) allows one to define the gait cycle and to pick out its characteristics.

During **walking in a straight line** (SL)
- the **stride** S is defined as the distance between the prints of the same foot (in pink)
- the **step** (the half stride) (r and l) is the distance between the print of the right foot and that of the left.

Thus a stride includes a right step r and a left step l.

The axes of these footprints form **an angle of 15°** open laterally relative to the direction of locomotion, which is typical of normal walking. Some people, however, have an 'in-toe gait', especially young children during their growth period.

When walking takes place along a curved path (C), both lower limbs in their entirety are rotated at the hips. In the diagram, curving of the path to the right is initiated by the contraction of the lateral rotators of the right hip, followed by lateral rotation of the right foot (green footprint). If this curving of the path to the right persists, medial rotation of the left hip now produces medial rotation of the left foot. In two steps the **total rotation r** is measured by adding the lateral rotation of the right foot and the medial rotation of the left foot occurring at the hips.

The **characteristics of the stride** are typical of each individual. The **stride length** obviously depends on the **size** of the individual, which determines the length of his lower limbs, and also on his personality: people walk differently, and the ear can recognize certain footsteps. Likewise one can detect a limp associated with limbs of unequal length more easily by the ears than by the eyes.

The distance between the footprints relative to the axis of the direction of locomotion is normally 10-15 cm, but some people with balance problems or in a drunken state widen the distance between their footprints in an attempt to increase the body support area. Some walks are artificial, as on the catwalk at fashion shows, where the steps lie on the very direction of locomotion. Footprints reveal the stages of **the stance phase** (Fig. 22: each column corresponds to a stage in the progression):
- the rounded area located posteriorly **a** corresponds to the heel strike on the ground
- then the entire surface of the sole **b** and even the pads of the toes become imprinted on the ground
- the first propulsive force **c** is reflected in the support points of the forefoot and the toes
- the second propulsive force **d**, applied to the toes, is reflected initially by the imprint essentially on the medial aspect of the foot because of eversion of the forefoot
- it is applied to the big toe **e** in its final phase.

This footprint analysis is very useful in revealing muscular deficiencies responsible for abnormal gait.

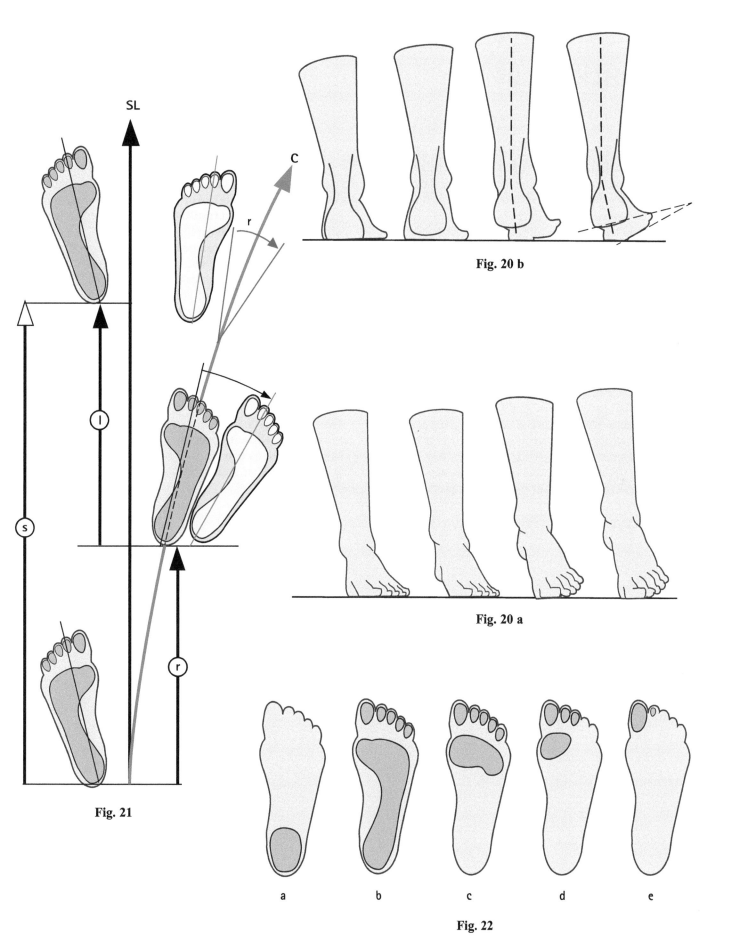

Fig. 20 b

Fig. 20 a

Fig. 21

Fig. 22

Pelvic oscillations

Movements of the lower limbs during walking are necessarily coupled with **oscillations of the pelvis.** With the help of telemetry, it is now possible to know very accurately the displacements of the body during walking, especially those of the pelvis and of the overall bary-centre of the body.

The pelvis oscillates in **two planes** (Fig. 23: 3-D diagrams contained within a parallelepiped), and the curves reflect the components of the movements of the centre of gravity:

- **side-to-side oscillations** (blue curve) in the horizontal plane
- **vertical oscillations** (red curve) in the sagittal plane.

To provide a visual representation, these curves have been drawn in a parallelepiped containing the two reference axes, the horizontal (pale yellow) and the vertical (light blue):

- In the **horizontal plane**, during each step, the pelvis shifts 2-2.5 cm towards each supporting side and these oscillations add up to 4-5 cm during the stride (blue curve).
- In the **vertical plane** the pelvis is at its highest point when the *weight-bearing limb* becomes vertical and at its lowest during movements of the swing limb. Therefore, there is a maximum (h) and a minimum (lo) for each step, indicating that **in the vertical plane the oscillation frequency is twice that in the horizontal plane.** The **vertical amplitude** of this curve is about **5 cm** between its highest and lowest points.

If an attempt is made to obtain a **real curve of the shifts of the centre of gravity** (Fig. 24) by combining the horizontal and vertical components, a **resultant curve** (deep blue) is obtained lying in the same parallelepiped.

The pelvic oscillations can be represented in space as follows:

- First in the **vertical plane** (Fig. 25): the left half of the diagram contains the curves of the pelvic oscillations during a stride; for the sake of greater clarity the *right half of the diagram shows them taking place over two strides* after one out of three positions has been eliminated in order to display more clearly the maxima (h) and the minima (lo).
- Finally in the **horizontal plane** (Fig. 26) the picture is much clearer, since the oscillations are as frequent. The pelvis is shown in half three positions: right stride **r**, left stride **le**, right stride **r**.

These diagrams do not represent the sum total of the movements of the pelvis since it undergoes horizontal and vertical translations as well as two types of rotation, one around a vertical axis and the other around an anteroposterior axis, as will be discussed later.

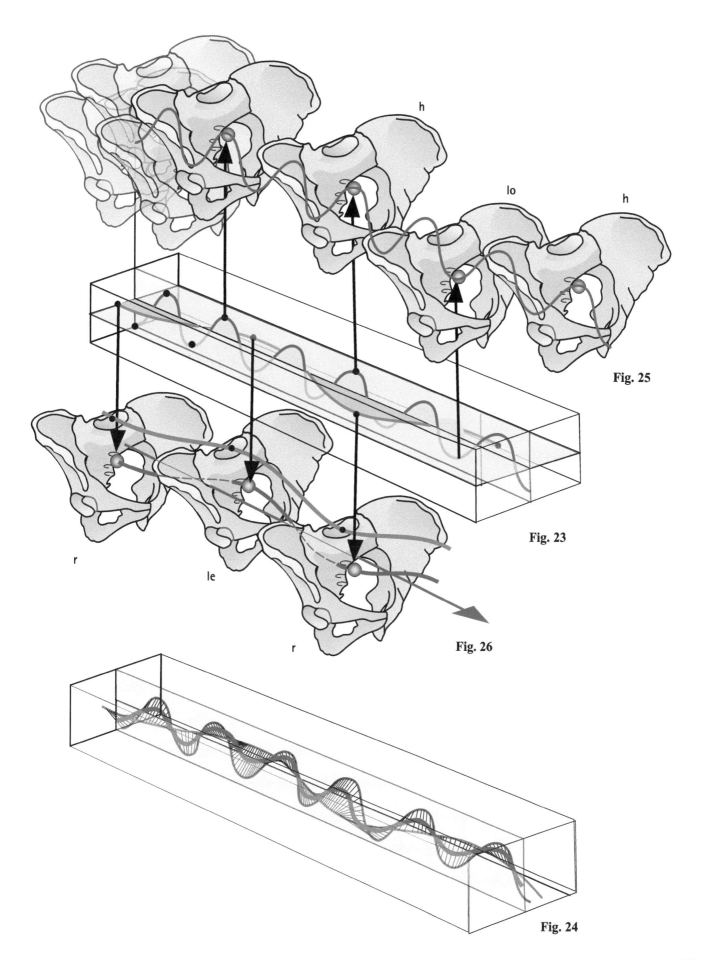

h

lo   h

Fig. 25

Fig. 23

r

le

r

Fig. 26

Fig. 24

277

Tilting of the pelvis

The side-to-side and vertical translations of the pelvis are coupled with rotations, one around a vertical axis and the other around an anteroposterior axis.

The rotation around the anteroposterior axis causes the pelvis to tilt in a movement similar to the rolling movement of a ship (Fig. 27: sequence of steps viewed from the back).

During the single-limb support, the opposite side of the pelvis is depressed, despite the checking action of the gluteus minimus and gluteus medius on the supporting side. This rolling movement is indicated by the inclination of the line joining the two sacral articular facets and corresponding to the **short axis of the lozenge of Michaelis** (see Volume 3, p. 83, Figs 76 and 78). This inclination of the sacrum towards the non-supporting limb **causes the lumbar spine to bend** on the same side and impact the thoracic and even the cervical spine in such a way

that the **scapular girdle is bent in the opposite direction**, as evidenced by a lowering of the intershoulder line towards the supporting side.

In summary, the intershoulder line and the pelvic line, which are horizontal and thus parallel in the symmetrical upright position, become **inversely oblique to each other** and **converge on the side of single-limb support.**

During a normal sequence of steps, the pelvic line and the intershoulder line undergo inverse displacements in conjunction with sinusoidal movements of the spine.

This phenomenon is recaptured in the diagram (Fig. 28), which illustrates the **movements in space of the pelvic line** in the shape of a wavy ribbon formed by the successive tilts of the pelvis. Similarly, the **inter-shoulder line** describes in space a similar wavy ribbon but with inverse inclinations.

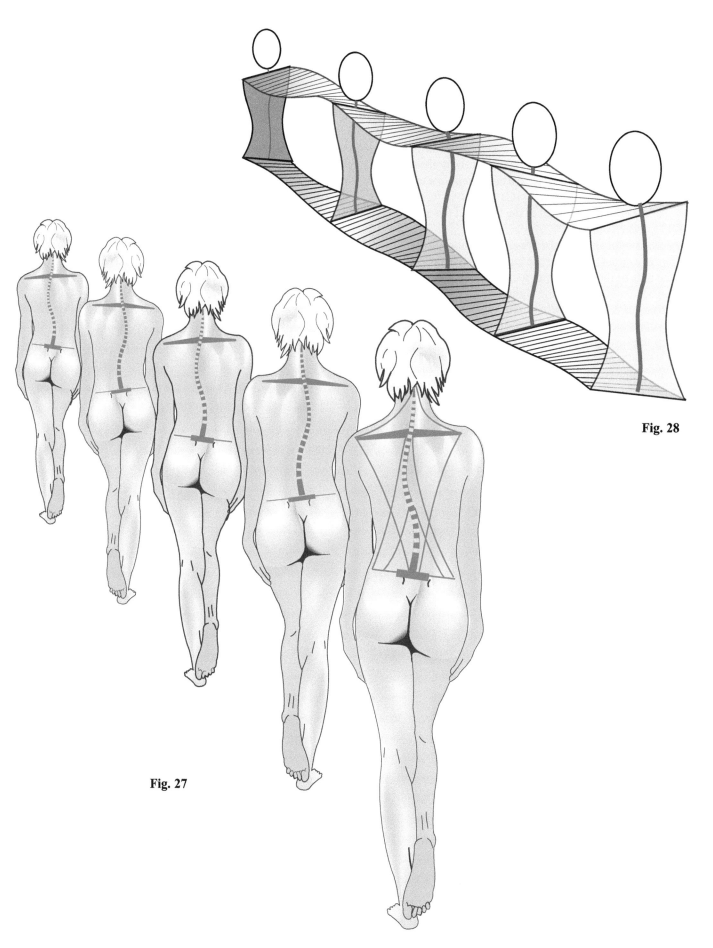

Fig. 27

Fig. 28

Torsion of the trunk

The tilt of the pelvis around an anteroposterior axis is associated with **rotation around a vertical axis** induced by the **forward movement of the swing limb** relative to the supporting limb. As the swing limb moves forward, it pulls the pelvis forward. This rotation takes place on the **head of the femur of the supporting limb (Fig. 29) as follows:**

- The starting position is the symmetrical upright position I, where the common axis of the hips (in red) is perpendicular to the axis of the direction of locomotion.
- If the advancing limb is the **right**, the pelvis (II) *rotates on the femoral head medially at the left hip joint on the left femoral head, and laterally on the right femoral head.*
- When the next step is taken (III), the opposite occurs: the pelvis rotates laterally on the right femoral head belonging to the now supporting limb, and the swinging left limb causes the *pelvis to rotate laterally on the left femoral head.*

At the same time, because of the **automatic swinging of the upper limbs** (see next page), the advance of the upper limb opposite to the leading limb (Fig. 30) causes the scapular girdle and the intershoulder line **to run obliquely in the opposite direction:**

- In position A, the intershoulder line crosses obliquely the interhip line in space since the *left upper limb is in the forward position, while the right lower limb is the swing limb.*
- In the next positions, B, C and D, these two lines cross each other with alternating obliquity.

This **torsion of the trunk** can be represented diagrammatically (Fig. 31) with the help of a **warped sail-like plane** twisted on itself. It is reminiscent of a caravel sail[*], and it connects the intershoulder and interhip lines.

Thus, walking calls into action the entire body. Only the head stays stable because the gaze is fixed in the direction of the goal and elicits compensatory rotations in the cervical spine. The head undergoes only **vertical oscillations** parallel to those of the pelvis, but with some dampening, although not enough to take stable photographs while moving forward.

---

[*] The square sail is hung from the mast by a horizontal yard, which can be likened to the scapular girdle. Its lower edge is kept stretched by another horizontal structure, the boom, which is jointed to the base of the mast and corresponds to the pelvis **(Figs. 30 and 31).**

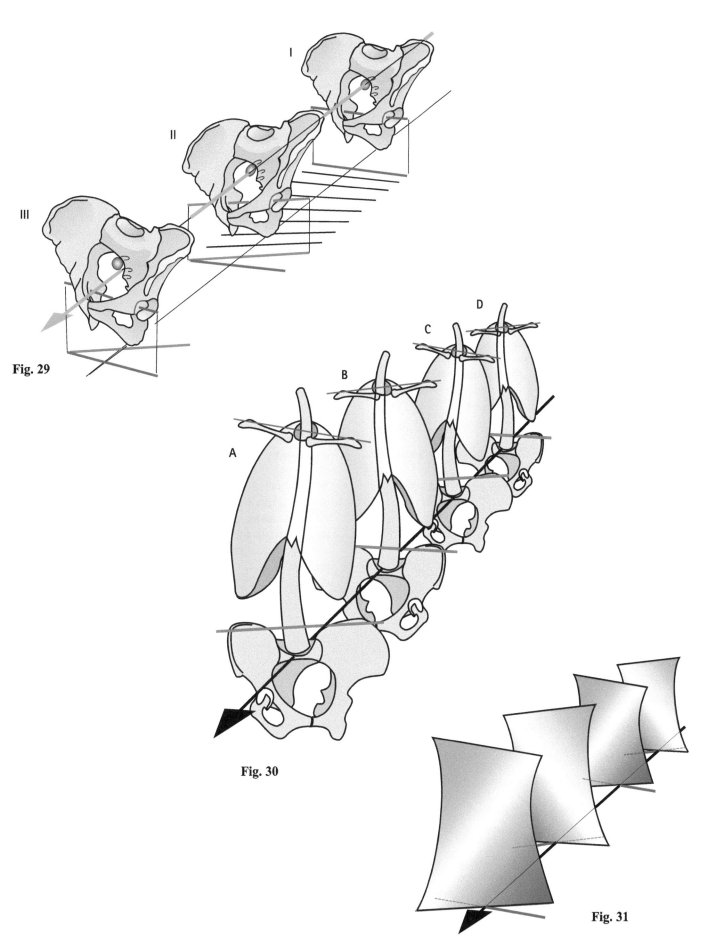

Fig. 29

Fig. 30

Fig. 31

281

Swinging of the upper limbs

As part of their genetic heritage, human beings have retained the diagonal-sequence gait of their quadruped ancestors. Among the land animals **(Fig. 30)** only the reptiles, such as lizards or crocodiles, move like our tetrapod ancestor, the ichthyosega, i.e., by keeping their limbs spread laterally in the transverse plane a and moving by pushing their shoulders and hips forwards and backwards. Mammals move their limbs in a parasagittal plane, i.e., parallel to the long axis of the body b. All quadrupeds, such as the horse, **(Fig. 32bis)** move their diagonally opposite feet simultaneously, since their supporting feet provide greater stability for their bodies b. The only animals that amble are the giraffe **(Fig. 33)**, the camel, the elephant, the llama, the bear and the okapi, i.e., they move their ipsilateral feet forward simultaneously. The horse can also amble, but only after dressage.

The human gait **(Fig. 34)** includes flexion of the upper limb on the side opposite to the swinging lower limb, as illustrated in the diagram showing the three successive events: the left upper limb in phase with the right leg and the inverse in the second step of the stride.

This movement occurs automatically without thinking, and usually the elbow is more flexed during shoulder extension. In some neurological diseases, as in Parkinson's disease, the automatic swinging of the limbs is lost. Military marches will be discussed later.

One can question the value of this swinging movement.

The forward propulsion of the upper limb **(Fig. 36)** displaces forward a and b, the common barycentres of the upper limbs (blue circle), followed by (see inset) displacement of the common barycentre of the four limbs (red circle), which then provides an additional impetus to the trunk by projecting its barycentre forward from the position of the pink rose to that of the red rose. The forward torsion of the trunk during the first step **(Fig. 35)** is well seen in a superior view, which illustrates the diagonal way the limbs swing: at the start of the first step a, the right arm is propelled forward, while the left leg trails posteriorly, and during midstance c, the limbs lie in an inverse position.

During fast walking, as in competitions, the swinging of the upper limbs takes place with flexed elbows. This arrangement of the upper limbs provides a greater impetus, as shown by drawing the barycentres viewed from above **(Fig. 36)**:

- after the position of the partial barycentre C **(Fig. a)** has been calculated
- the location of the partial barycentre C' **(Fig. b)** of the upper limb appears displaced forward with respect to its position with "the elbows slightly flexed," which then provides a greater impetus to the general barycentre of the body, as the partial barycentre moves forward from position C to position C'.
- thus simply flexing the elbows significantly increases the efficiency of the swinging of the upper limbs.
- for this reason, it is a fact that walking is far less easy when the two upper limbs are not used and cannot swing, This is why prisoners are handcuffed behind their backs, since it is more difficult for them to escape by running away. It is the same with carrying a child, which could perhaps explain why mothers of certain ethnic groups prefer to carry their children on their backs.

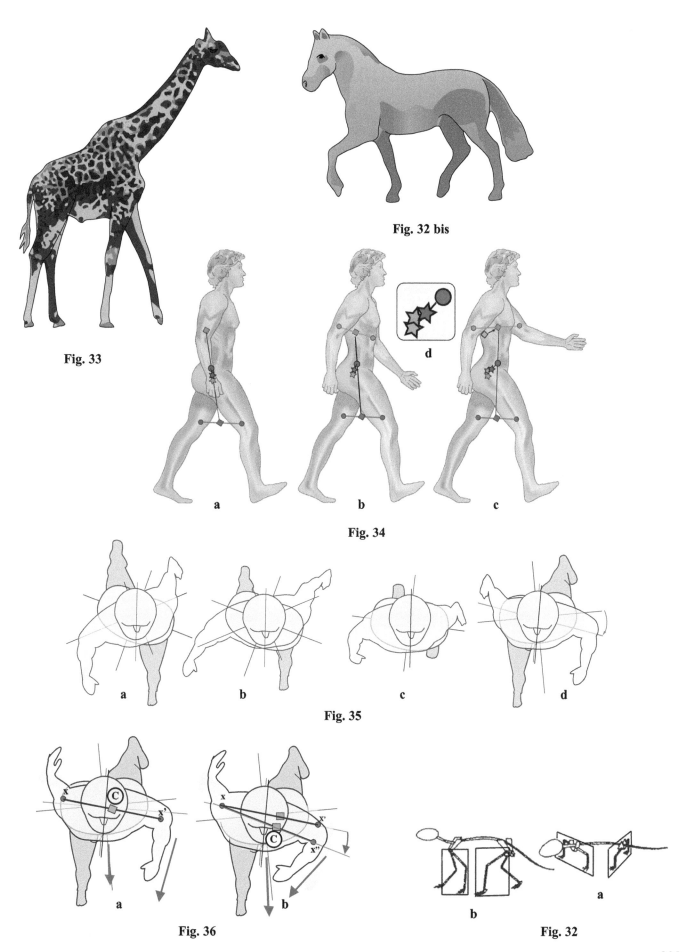

Fig. 32 bis

Fig. 33

Fig. 34

Fig. 35

Fig. 36

Fig. 32

Muscles involved in walking

All the muscles of the lower limbs are important during walking, so that deficiency of a single muscle can disturb walking more or less severely.

The nine diagrams on the next page illustrate the activation of the muscles of the right lower limb with the left limb included for reference. They show a complete gait cycle with the movements alternating from side to side:

1. **Early advance of the leading limb** (Fig. 37)
   - hip flexion by iliopsoas **1**
   - knee flexion by the hamstrings and the biceps femoris **2**
   - ankle flexion by the ankle flexors **3**, i.e. tibialis anterior, fibularis tertius
   - toe extension by the extensors digitorum longus and brevis and the extensor hallucis **4**.

2. **Initial heel contact with the ground** (Fig. 38)
   - end of hip flexion by the iliopsoas **1**
   - knee extension by the quadriceps **5**
   - end of ankle flexion by the ankle flexors **3** and the toe extensors **4**.

3. **The vertical single-limb support (the foot-flat or loading response**, Fig. 39)
   - continuing activity of the quadriceps **5**
   - early contraction of the gluteus maximus **6**.

4. **The mid-stance with fall forward** (Fig. 40):
   - hip extension by the gluteus maximus **6** with the help of the hamstrings **7** and in antagonism-synergism with the quadriceps **5**

   - ankle flexion by the flexors **3** in synergy with the gluteus maximus **6**.

5. **The first propulsive motion (the heel-off stage before the end of double support**, Fig. 41)
   - continuing hip extension by **6** and **7**
   - continuing knee extension by **5**
   - ankle extension by the triceps **8** and the toe flexors **9**.

6. **The second propulsive motion (the pre-swing phase**, Fig. 42)
   - the supporting limb is fully extended as the swing limb is about to land on the ground
   - increased activity of **5**, **6**, **7**, **8**, and **9**, particularly of the flexor hallucis longus **9**.

7. **The early swing with the other foot in single support** (Fig. 43)
   - posterior displacement of the swing leg by contraction of the hamstrings **7** and ankle flexors **3**
   - hip flexion by the iliopsoas **1**.

8. **The mid-swing with forward movement of the swing limb** (Fig. 44)
   - increased contraction of **1** and **5** and relaxation of **3**
   - knee extension by quadriceps contraction **5**
   - elevation of the toes by the toe extensors **10**.

9. **Terminal contact of the swing limb with the ground** (Fig. 45)
   - start of a new cycle **1**, **5** and **3**.

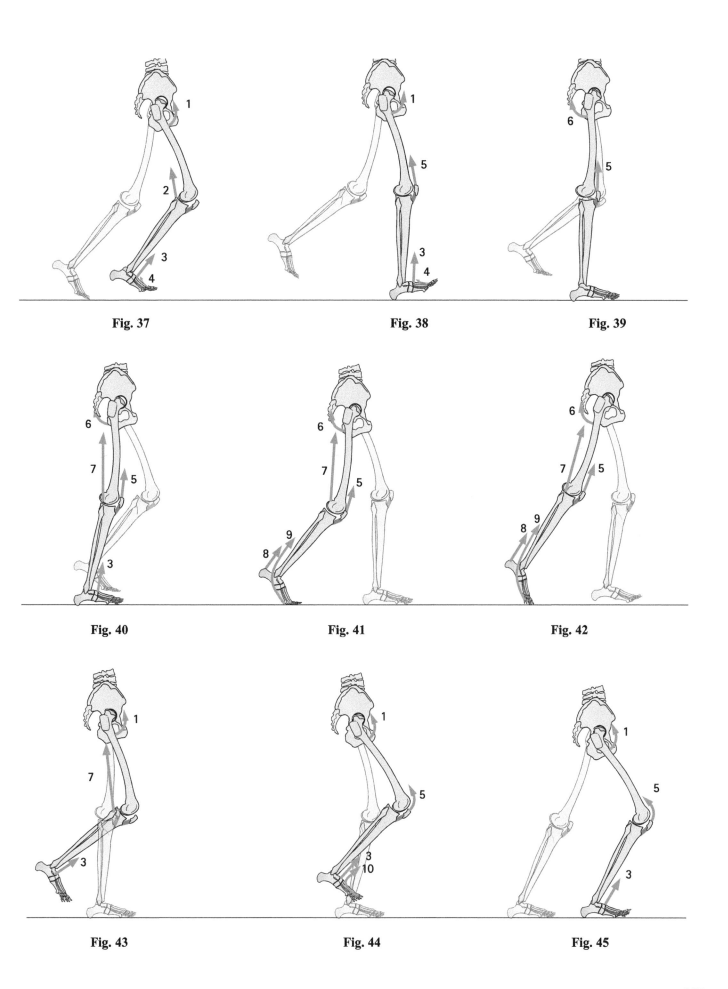

Fig. 37

Fig. 38

Fig. 39

Fig. 40

Fig. 41

Fig. 42

Fig. 43

Fig. 44

Fig. 45

Muscular chains during running

It would be wrong to believe that all these muscles work by themselves and without coordination. In fact they work in accordance with very precise **motion blueprints**, which are under the control of the nervous system, particularly of the cerebellum (the coordinating centre), and which combine examples of **antagonism-synergism** and **synergism** to form **muscular chains.**

These muscular chains are very important functionally, e.g. the chain controlling **extension of the lower limb** (Fig. 46: start of the race) *during the propulsive phase.* This chain highlights the usefulness of biarticular muscles, i.e. the rectus femoris R and the triceps surae T. *Their action on the distal joint depends on the position of the proximal joint*, which determines their state of pre-tension. In the case shown here, as the gluteus maximus G extends the hip, it stretches the rectus femoris and thus enhances its action as a knee extensor. In its turn, as the rectus femoris extends the knee, it stretches the gastrocnemius and thus enhances the power of the triceps surae in extending the ankle and maximizing the propulsive force.

In sum, **part of the power of the gluteus maximus is transferred first to the rectus femoris and then to the triceps via the rectus femoris.** This system has a *high mechanical advantage*, since, in accordance with the principle of muscle power = muscle weight, the gluteus maximus, the most powerful muscle in the body, is located at the root of the limb, i.e. **near the centre of gravity of the body.** The advantage of placing muscle masses near the root of the lower limb is to *bring its segmental barycentre closer to the root and to decrease the global moment of force of the lower limb*, thus increasing the efficiency of the muscles.

Walking is not always as described on the previous page, and peculiar and artificial modes of walking, e.g. goose-stepping (Fig. 47) are used during the parades of some armies. It requires very strong hip flexors at considerable physical cost and therefore cannot be used for long periods.

Finally, there is running (Fig. 48), which is a derivative of walking; it is characterized by the **loss of the period of double-limb support** (note how the shadows of the supports are separated), and its replacement by **the double-float period**, which is also the initial phase of jumping.

This chapter, due to space constraints, has not fully covered the characteristics of walking and of its derivatives. This will be covered in the next few pages.

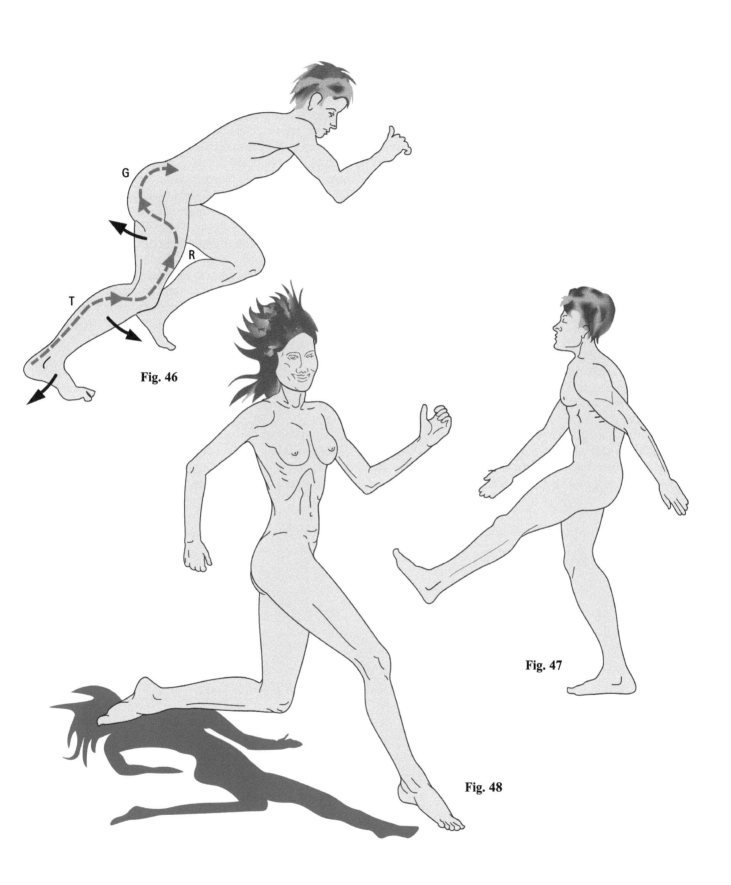

G

R

T

Fig. 46

Fig. 47

Fig. 48

The different types of walking and jumping

There are many ways of walking, to the point that one can be recognized by one's gait. The diagonal swinging of the upper limbs is an invaluable aid to normal walking, but, excluding neurological diseases that deprive us of this aid (as in Parkinson's disease), there are occasions when the upper limbs are not available to participate, as, for example, when one carries a suitcase in each hand **(Fig. 49)**. Walking then becomes doubly difficult because of the weight to be carried and the loss of the swinging upper limbs. Men and women have managed to find many ways to recover the use of their hands while walking: for example, by carrying their loads on their heads **(Fig. 50)** – a very common practice in Africa – which requires a great sense of balance and also bestows a queenly bearing. In any case, this practice produces an excellent cervical musculature.

One can carry a bundle on one's head but certainly not a child. To avoid carrying children in their arms, mothers of small children can carry them in a harness attached to the front of the chest **(Fig. 51)**; this allows the upper limbs to swing free but does not help in performing work. While working, mothers can carry their children on their backs with the help of a different type of harness or even with the use of a piece of cloth properly draped and tied, as in the case of African women who can thus work in the fields while their babies benefit from being rocked by the swinging movements of their mothers' bodies.

Normal walking can be turned into race-walking **(Fig. 53**: long-distance race-walker). It must retain the double-limb support phase to avoid disqualification because its absence signifies running. The double-limb support phase disappears when one runs and is replaced by a period of non-support with both feet off the ground. This is well seen in the picture, where a runner is seen landing on his swinging limb.

This movement of non-support is required during jumping, and the picture **(Fig. 55)** shows a high jumper using the Forsbury flop, which has become the standard technique, since it allows the barycentre of the body to move above the bar while the feet are raised in time to avoid catching on the bar.

To clear the even higher bar in the pole vault the athlete must not only run quickly with his pole to gather momentum but also use his upper limbs to lift himself upside down on his pole in order to allow his barycentre to be raised above the bar.

The upper limbs are also useful in the long jump **(Fig. 56)**. As they are raised rapidly, their momentum increases the upward thrust, which is combined with the forward thrust to produce the longest possible parabolic trajectory. On landing, when the four limbs are thrust forward to lower the jumper's barycentre and ensure a landing on the buttocks with the body bent forward to indicate the length of the jump on the sandpit. Thus, the hands must not trail behind the jumper.

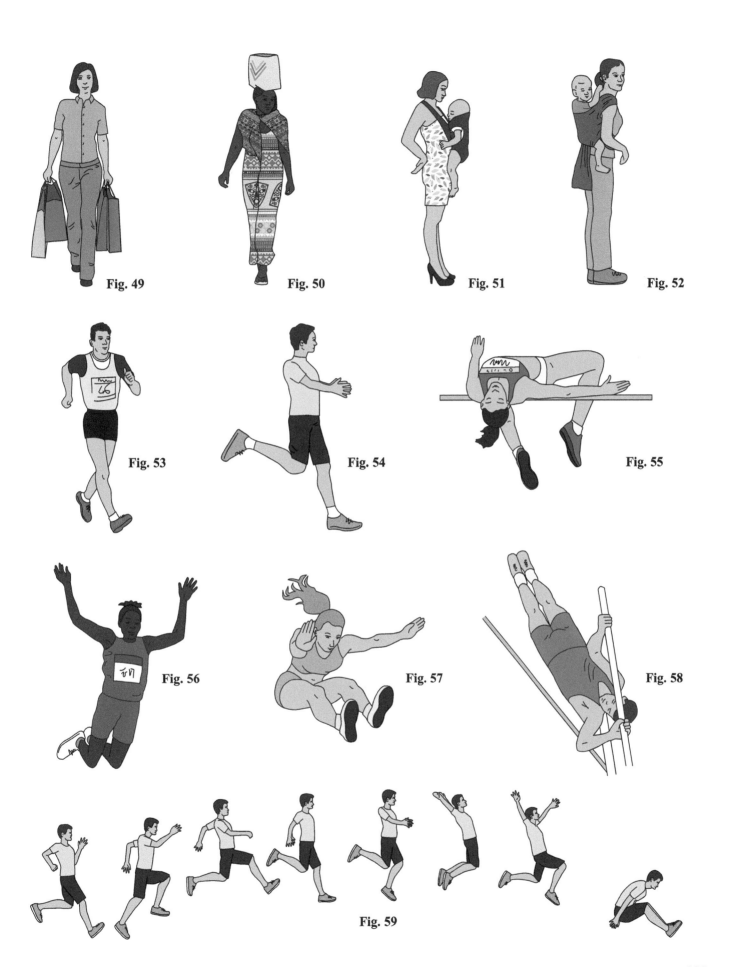

Fig. 49

Fig. 50

Fig. 51

Fig. 52

Fig. 53

Fig. 54

Fig. 55

Fig. 56

Fig. 57

Fig. 58

Fig. 59

Military marches and dancing

There is a big difference between the way an ordinary citizen walks and the way soldiers walk when they march past in public. These many modes of walking depend above all on two factors:

- the rhythm, more or less rapid, which typifies certain army units, e.g., the fast march of the "Mountain Infantry" or the slow march, as with the "Consular March" of the Napoleonic Guard or the "emphatically" slow "March of the Janissaries" so popular in the old Ottoman Empire

- the synchronisation of the basic movements of all the soldiers during a parade. For a perfect show the movements in each row must be synchronised so that anyone watching one row must see all the soldiers of that row "disappear" after the first soldier. This synchronisation must work for all the rows in the parade. Some countries are known for the precision and coordination of their military parades.

It must be recognized that the fulfilment of these two imperatives is made much easier by the military music, whose rousing duple-time rhythm acts as a metronome.

The normal walk **(Fig. 60)**, with the usual swinging of the upper limbs, is certainly the most often used in parades and is the least tiring. It can be used by a soldier on patrol duty **(Fig. 61)**, who nonetheless uses his hands to hold his gun. In some more war-like parades the gun can be held at the ready, which precludes swinging of the arms and thus makes the walk more tiring. In parades of soldiers going off to war **(Fig. 63)** each soldier carries his gear in a backpack and his gun slung across his shoulder, thus allowing his upper arms to swing freely and making the walk much easier.

There are also official parades of certain units **(Fig. 64)**, where the gun is carried in front of the trunk by the right hand with only the left arm able to swing. In some countries the swing of the arms can be intensified (**Fig. 65**: very elegant female Chinese soldier) or exaggerated, which gives it an aggressive look. Finally in the so-called "authoritarian" countries the troops goose-step with the swinging leg kept rigid and flexed at 80° at least. This walk acquires a lot of effort on the part of the soldier and cannot be unduly prolonged.

In contrast to animals, apart from language, poetry, mathematics and music (laughter must not be included, according to Rabelais) humans are the only species able to do something with their feet other than walking, i.e. dancing. So-called civilized human beings are familiar with social dancing, which in a playful way is really a display of seduction. Quite different is classical dance **(Fig. 69)**, which, with its complex and graceful movements and attitudes, could be described as the poetry of human biomechanics or the language of the heart expressed by the body. It is indeed a great privilege given to us by the "Great Spirit of the Universe" (to use ecumenical language).

But to end the story let us come back to Earth with the so-called normal walk, which for some of us can regress to quadrupedalism, as in the Nordic walk **(Fig. 70)**. It comes from cross-country skiing and is practised using long poles that provide an extra thrust forward. This walk, which remains a diagonal-sequence gait, is now very fashionable and, according to its fans, represents the most complete form of sports thanks to the use of the shoulder girdle. Its only fault is to make obsolete the riddle of the Sphinx, in which the mythological animal walks on "three feet in the evening."

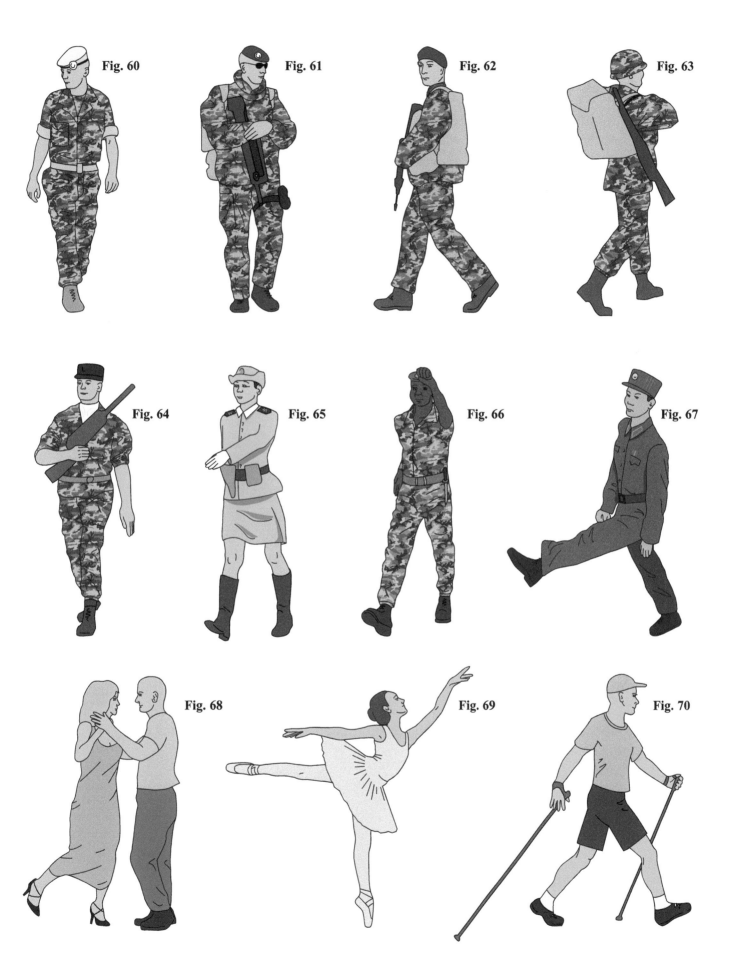

Fig. 60

Fig. 61

Fig. 62

Fig. 63

Fig. 64

Fig. 65

Fig. 66

Fig. 67

Fig. 68

Fig. 69

Fig. 70

Walking is freedom

Walking is the first of our freedoms and is essential for our **independence**: we can thus escape danger, go to whoever gives us food and drink, climb mountains, travel over the vastness of the world and approach other people.

This freedom, acquired at a heavy cost, can be lost during life as a result of nervous system lesions, loss of elementary coordinated movements, interruption of neural conductivity, spinal cord lesions, myopathic muscular insufficiency, decreases in or loss of articular mobility due to inflammatory or degenerative arthritis or simply after a severe trauma.

Sometimes after a prolonged and difficult rehabilitation, we can learn again how to walk. In other cases, the loss is final, but we can walk after a fashion with a stick, an external prosthesis that can temporarily restore balance in walking, i.e. a third leg (see the riddle of the Sphinx, p. 262). Often, however, the stick implies the definitive loss of our autonomy.

Once the freedom to walk is compromised, one can be condemned to an armchair, a wheelchair or, even worse, to bed before the end.

People who walk without difficulty should be at least conscious of this freedom, which allows them to run, jump, dance – in short to enjoy life to the fullest!

The diagram corresponding to this page is based on a drawing by Michelangelo.

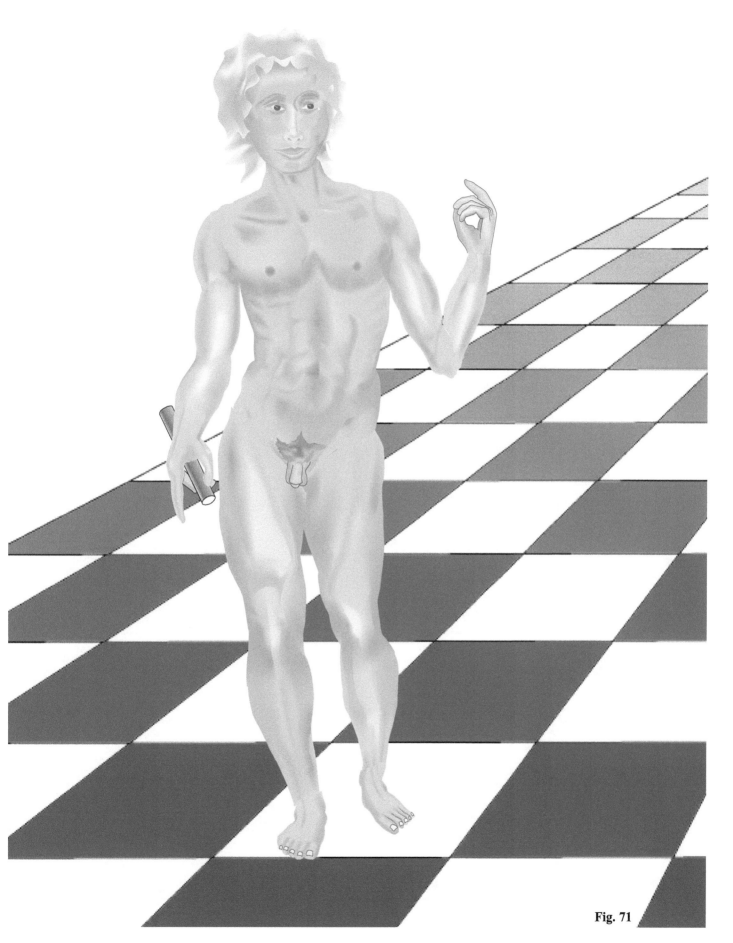

Fig. 71

APPENDICES

The nerves of the lower limb

The nerves of the lumbar and sacral plexuses and their branches supplying the lower limb are shown in detail in the 'Synoptic Table of the Nerves of the Lower Limb' (Fig. 1), which can be read easily. Each muscle is named in accordance with the International Anatomical Terminology. The origins of these nerves and their communications are numerous, but on the whole it is very easy to recognize the functions and supply territories of each of the major nerve trunks.

The lumbar plexus
It supplies the motor nerves to the muscles at the root of the lower limb. Three of its roots (L2-L4) give rise to two main nerve trunks: the femoral and obturator nerves.

1. The femoral nerve
It innervates almost all of the pelvic muscles and in particular the muscles of the anterior compartment of the thigh, i.e. the quadriceps, the sartorius and one of the adductors, i.e. the adductor longus. It is thus the nerve for **knee extension**. It also gives rise to a very long sensory nerve, the **saphenous nerve**, which supplies the anteromedial surface of the lower limb right down to the foot.

2. The obturator nerve
It innervates a single pelvic muscle, i.e. the obturator externus, but is the major motor nerve to the adductor muscles, it is therefore the nerve for **adduction**. It also contains the sensory nerves for the medial surface of the thigh.

The sacral plexus
It consists of the three upper sacral roots and receives an important contribution from the lumbar plexus, i.e. the lumbosacral trunk (formed by the roots of L4 and L5). It sends motor nerves to the pelvic muscles, especially the glutei. It forms two large nerve trunks on the posterior surface of the thigh: the posterior cutaneous nerve of the thigh and the sciatic nerve:

1. The posterior cutaneous nerve of the thigh
It contributes to the motor innervation of the pelvic muscles, in particular the gluteus maximus; hence it is the nerve for **thigh extension**. It also contains sensory fibres from the posterior surface of the thigh and the upper half of the leg.

2. The sciatic nerve
It innervates the muscles of the posterior surface of the thigh; hence it is the nerve for **knee flexion**. It also sends out nerves to the anterior compartment of the thigh, making it a contributor to **adduction**. It divides distally into two large branches, the tibial nerve and the common fibular nerve.

- The **tibial nerve** sends motor branches to the muscles of the posterior compartment of the leg and is thus the nerve for **ankle extension** and **toe flexion**. It then divides into two terminal branches, the **medial plantar nerve** and the **lateral plantar nerve**, which together innervate the plantar flexor and adductor-abductor muscles of the toes and carry sensory nerves from the sole of the foot. It also gives rise to the **sural nerve**, which supples sensory fibres to the posterior aspect of the leg and to the sole of the foot.
- The **common fibular nerve** sends motor branches to the muscles of the anterior and lateral compartments of the leg, i.e. the fibularis muscles. It is thus responsible for **flexion** and **side-to-side movements of the ankle** and also for **toe extension**. It terminates in the extensor digitorum brevis, which is the only muscle in the dorsum of the foot. It carries sensory nerves from the anterior and lateral surfaces of the leg and the dorsum of the foot.

SYNOPTIC TABLE OF NERVES OF THE LOWER LIMB

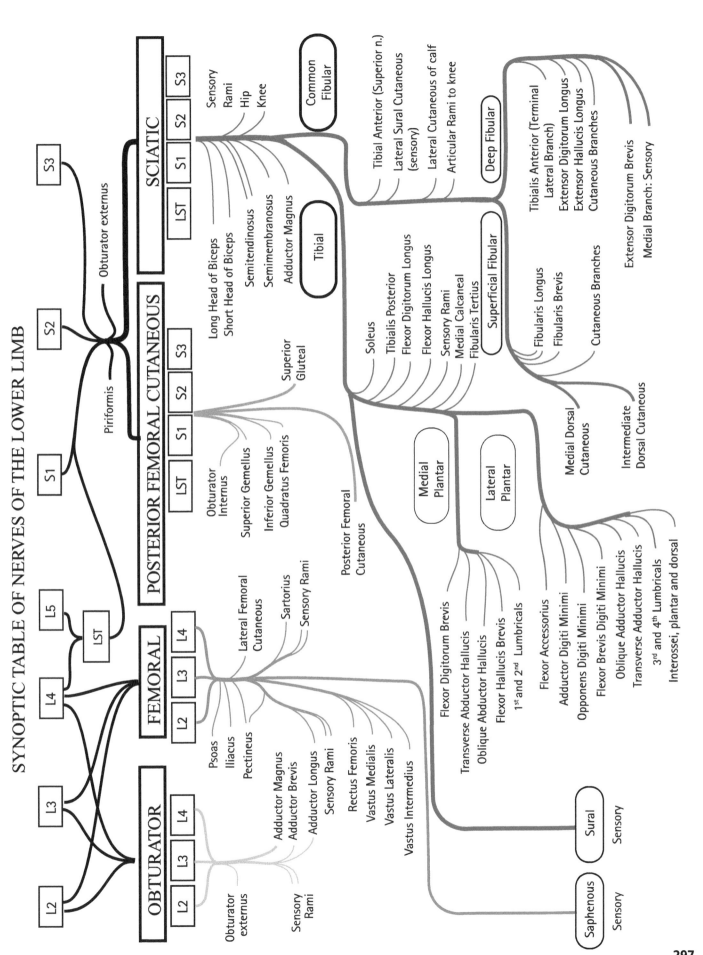

Sensory compartments of the lower limb

The sensory compartments form irregular patches that run along the entire lower limb and are clearly visible on (Fig. 2) an anterior (left) and a posterior view (right).

The lateral cutaneous nerve of the thigh **1** a branch of the femoral nerve, innervates the lateral surface of the thigh.

The iliohypogastric nerve, a collateral branch of the lumbar plexus (L1), supplies sensory nerves to a small patch of skin **2** near the anterior superior iliac spine; the ilio-inguinal nerve supplies the upper part of the medial aspect of the thigh close to the genital organs.

The buttocks **3** are innervated by the inferior clunial branches of the posterior cutaneous nerve of the thigh.

The anterior surface of the thigh **4** is innervated by the intermediate cutaneous femoral nerve.

The genitofemoral **5** nerve supplies the femoral triangle.

The medial surface of the thigh **6** is supplied by the medial cutaneous nerve of the thigh, which is a branch of the femoral nerve.

The lateral surface of the thigh **1** is supplied by the lateral cutaneous femoral nerve, a branch of the lumbar plexus.

The medial surface of the knee **7** receives sensory fibres from the obturator nerve and the infrapatellar branch of the saphenous nerve, a branch of the femoral nerve.

The lateral surface of the leg **8** receives sensory fibres from the lateral sural cutaneous nerve and from the sural communicating nerve, which are branches of the common fibular nerve.

The anteromedial surfaces of the thigh **9** and of the knee and the medial surface of the leg are innervated by the saphenous nerve, a branch of the femoral nerve.

The dorsal surface of the foot **10** receives sensory fibres from the musculocutaneous nerve (a branch of the common fibular nerve); its lateral border **11** from the terminal branch of the sural nerve and the sole of the foot as well as the distal phalanges of the toes **12** from the plantar nerves (terminal branches of the tibial nerve). It is a very interesting clinical observation that the dorsal aspect of the interspace between the big toe and the second toe **1** is innervated by the terminal fibres of the deep fibular nerve and therefore a sensory loss in this very limited area indicates a lesion of this nerve, due, for example, to compression in the anterior compartment of the thigh.

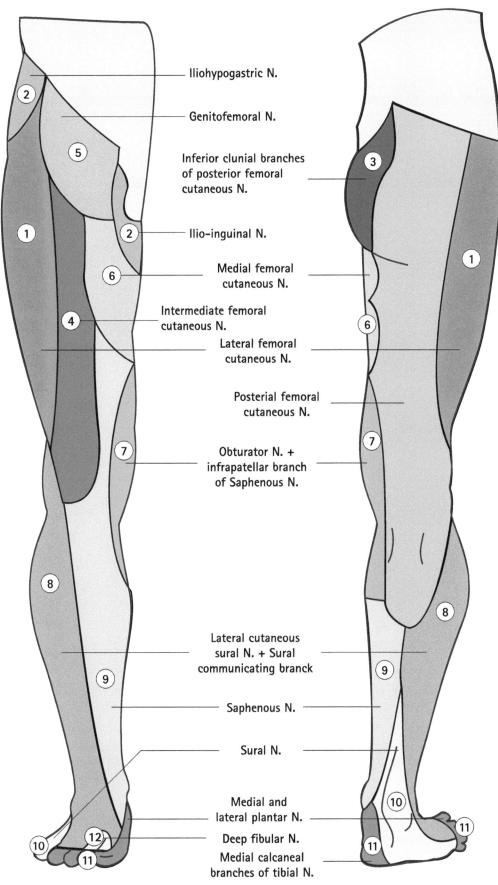

Iliohypogastric N.

Genitofemoral N.

Inferior clunial branches of posterior femoral cutaneous N.

Ilio-inguinal N.

Medial femoral cutaneous N.

Intermediate femoral cutaneous N.

Lateral femoral cutaneous N.

Posterial femoral cutaneous N.

Obturator N. + infrapatellar branch of Saphenous N.

Lateral cutaneous sural N. + Sural communicating branck

Saphenous N.

Sural N.

Medial and lateral plantar N.

Deep fibular N.

Medial calcaneal branches of tibial N.

Fig. 1

Fig. 2

Bibliography

Barnett CH, **Davies DV**, **MacConaill MA** 1961 *Synovial joints. Their structure and mechanics*. CC Thomas, Springfield

Barnier L 1950 *L'analyse des mouvements*. PUF, Paris

Basmajian JV 1962 *Muscles alive. Their function revealed by electromyography*. Williams and Wilkins, Baltimore

Biesalski K, **Mayer L** 1916 *Die physiologische Sehnenverpflanzung*. Springer, Berlin

Boehler L 1944 Traitement des fractures de la colonne dorsale inférieure et lombaire sans paralysie. In: *Technique du traitement des fractures*. Paris: éditions médicales de France: 285-322

Bonnel F 2002 *Abrégé d'anatomie fonctionnelle et biomécanique*, tome III: Membre Inférieur. Sauramps Medical Ed., Montpellier

Bousquet G, **Le Beguec P**, **Girardin Ph** 1991 *Les laxités chroniques du genou: physiologie, physiopathologie, étude clinique et traitement*. Ed Medsi/McGraw-Hill

Bridgeman GB 1939 *The human machine. The anatomical structure and mechanism of the human body*. Vol 1. Dover, New York

Bunnell S 1970 *Surgery of the hand*, ed 3. Revised by Boyes. Lippincott, Philadelphia

Cardano, Gerolamo (Italian mathematician 1501-1576) on the universal joint: see the Internet.

De Doncker E, **Kowalski C** 1979 *Kinésiologie et rééducation du pied*. Masson, Paris

De Doncker E, **Kowalski C** 1970 Le pied normal et pathologique. *Acta Orthop Belg* 36:386-559.

Descamps L 1950 *Le jeu de la hanche*. Thèse, Paris

Duchenne (de Boulogne) GBA 1867 *Physiologie des mouvements*. Vol 1. J-B. Baillière, Paris (out of print; edited facsimile published by Annales de Médecine Physique, 1967)

Duchenne (de Boulogne) GBA 1949 *Physiology of motion*. Translated by EB Kaplan. WB Saunders, Philadelphia

Farabeuf LH 1893 *Précis de manuel operatoire* Masson, Paris 4e édition

Fick R 1904 *Handbuch der Anatomie und Mechanik der Gelenke, unter Berücksichtigung der bewegenden Muskeln*. Gustav Fishcer, Iena

Fick R 1911 *Handbuch der Anatomie und Mechanik der Gelenke*. Gustav Fischer, Iena

Fischer O 1907 *Kinematik organischer Gelenke*. F. Vierweg und Sohn, Braunschweig

Frain P 1980 Facteurs géométriques et cinétiques liant le condyle fémoral interne et le ligament interne du genou. *Rev Chir Orthop Réparatrice Appar Mot* 66(4):285-295

Frain P, **Fontaine C**, **D'Hondt D** 1984 Contraintes du genou par dérangement ménisco-ligamentaire. Etude de l'Articulation Condylo-Tibiale Interne. *Rev Chir Orthop Réparatrice Appar Mot* 70(5):361-369

Gauss, Karl Friedrich German mathematician (1777-1855): *La géométrie non-euclidienne* (on Codman's paradox). See the Internet.

Ghyka Matila C 1978 *Le Nombre d'Or*. Vol. 1, p. 190. Gallimard, Paris

Hauser EDW 1950 *Diseases of the Foot*. WB Saunders Co, Philadelphia, London

Henke J 1859 *Die Bewegungen der Handwurzel*. Zeitschrift für rationelle Medizine, Zürich

Henke W 1863 *Handbuch der Anatomie und Mechanik der Gelenke*. CF Wintersche Verlaghandlung, Heidelberg

Hilgenreiner H 1935 Zur Frühdiagnose der angeborenen Hüftgelenksverrenkung. *Med Klin* 21:1385-1388, 1425-1429.

Hohmann G 1950 (quoted in *McGlamy's Comprehensive Textbook of Foot and Ankle Surgery*. Banks AS, Downey MB, Martin DE, Miller SJ Lippincott Williams & Wilkins, 3rd ed. 2001)

Kapandji AI 1987 La Biomécanique 'Patate'. *Ann Chir Main* 5:260-263

Kapandji AI 1997 Vous avez dit Biomécanique? La Mécanique 'Floue' ou 'Patate'. *Maîtrise Orthopédique* 64:1, 4-11.

Kapandji AI 2011 *Qu'est-ce que la biomécanique?*, 1 vol., Sauramps Medical Ed., Montpellier.

Lapidus PW 1963 Kinesiology and mechanical anatomy of the tarsal joints. *Clin Orthop* 30:30-34

Le Cœur P 1938 *La pince malléolaire: physiologie et pathologie du péroné*. Louis Arnette, Paris

MacConaill MA, **Barnett CH**, **Davis DV** 1962 *Synovial joints*. Longmans, London

MacConaill MA 1953 Movements of bones and joints. Significance of shape. *J Bone Joint Surg* 35B:290

MacConaill MA 1946 Studies in the mechanics of synovial joints: displacement on articular surfaces and significance of saddle joints. *Irish J M Sci* 21(7):223-225

MacConaill MA 1946 Studies in the mechanics of synovial joints; hinge joints and nature of intra-articular displacements. *Irish M Sci* 21(9):620-626

MacConaill MA 1966 *Studies on the anatomy and function of bones and joints* F. Gaynor Evans, New York

MacConaill MA 1966 The geometry and algebra of articular kinematics. *Bio Med Eng* 1:205-212

MacConaill MA, **Basmadjian JV** 1969 *Muscle and movements: a basis for human kinesiology*. Williams & Wilkins, Baltimore

Maquet PGJ 1976 *Biomechanics of the knee*. Springer, Berlin

Maquet PGJ 1972 Biomécanique de la gonarthrose. *Acta Orthop Belg* 38:33-54

Maquet P 1963 Un traitement biomécanique de l'arthrose fémoro-patellaire: l'avancement du tendon rotulien. *Rev Rhum Mal Osteoartic* 30:779

Marey EJ. 1882 Emploi de la chronophotographie pour déterminer la trajectoire des corps en mouvement avec leur vitesse à chaque instant et leurs positions relatives. Application à la mécanique animale. *Comptes Rendus à l'Académie des Sciences* 7 Aug: 267-270

Marey EJ, **Demeny G** 1885 Locomotion humaine: mécanisme du saut. *Comptes Rendus à l'Académie des Sciences* 7 Aug:489-494

Marey EJ, **Pagès C** 1887 La locomotion comparée: mouvements du membre pelvien chez l'homme, l'éléphant et le cheval: mécanisme du saut. *Comptes Rendus à l'Académie des Sciences* 24 Aug: 149-156

Marey EJ 1873 *La machine animale*. Vol I. Alcan, Paris

Menschik A 1974 Mechanik des Kniegelenkes. *Z Orthop* 112:481-495

Menschik A 1975 Mechanik des Kniegelenkes. *Z Orthop* 113:388-400

Menschik A 1987 *Biometrie. Das Konstruktionsprinzip des Kniegelenks, des Hüftgelenks, der Beinlänge und der Körpergrösse*. Springer, Berlin

Merkel FS 1913 *Die Anatomie des Menschen*. Editions PLUS, Berlin

Moreaux A 1959 *Anatomie artistique de l'Homme*. Vol 1. Maloine, Paris

Morton DJ 1935 *The Human Foot*. Columbia Univ. Press, NY 1935

Ockham, William of: English Franciscan monk, scholastic philosopher (1280-1349) *The Principle of Universal Economy*. See the Internet

Ombredanne L, Mathieu P 1937 *Traité de chirurgie orthopédique*. Masson, Paris

Poirier P, Charpy A 1926 *Traité d'anatomie humaine*, ed 4. Masson, Paris

Rasch PJ, Burke RK 1971 *Kinesiology and Applied Anatomy; the science of human movement*. Vol. 1. Lea & Febiger, Philadelphia

Riemann, Georg Friedrich Bernhard, German mathematician (1826-1866) *Non-Euclidian geometry* (on Codman's paradox). See the Internet

Roud A 1913 *Mécanique des articulations et des muscles de l'homme*. Rouge & Cie, Librairie de l'Université de Lausanne

Rouvière H 1948 *Anatomie humaine descriptive et topographique*, ed 4. Masson, Paris

Seitz WH 1997 quoted in Daentzer D, Wilkes, Zimmermann. Observations concerning the transverse metatarsal arch. *Foot and Ankle Surgery* 3(1): 1-48

Slocum DB, Larson RL 2007 Rotatory instability of the knee: its pathogenesis and a clinical test to demonstrate its presence. *Clin Orthop Relat Res* 454:5-13

Soeur R 1958 Flat-foot contracture and synosteosis of the tarsus. *Bull Acad R Med Belg* 23(7):551-582

Steindler A 1964 *Kinesiology of the human body*. Vol I, p. 708. CC Thomas, Springfield

Strasser H 1917 *Lehrbuch der Muskel und Gelenkemechanik*. Vol IV. Springer, Berlin

Testut L 1893 *Traité d'anatomie humaine*. Doin, Paris

Trendelenburg GF 1895 *Deutsche Med. Woch.*, St Petersburg

Vandervael F 1956 *Analyse des mouvements du corps humain*. Maloine, Paris

Von Recklinghausen H 1920 *Gliedermechanik und Lähmungsprostesen*. Vol I. Springer, Berlin

Weber W, Weber E 1836 *Mechanik der menschlichen Gehwerkzeuge*. Dietrich, Göttingen

Weber W, Weber E 1837 Ueber die Mechanik der menschlichen Gehwerkzeuge nebst der Beschreibung eines Versuches über das Herausfallen des Schenkelkopfes in luftverdünnren Raum. *Annals Physics Chem* 40:1-13.

Welker H 1876 Ueber das Hüftgelenk, nebst Bemerkungen über Gelenke überhaupt. *Zeitschrift für Anatomie und Entwicklungsgeschichte, Leipzig*

Wiberg G 1941 Rœntgenographic and anatomic studies on the patellar joint. *Acta Orthop Scand* 12:319-410

Index

Models of joint biomechanics

Recommendations

Why do we need models of joint biomechanics? It is because these **hand-made models**, requiring careful attention from readers with enough patience to build them, are veritable **three-dimensional diagrams** providing an intuitive understanding of how joints work. Moreover, they are devices that can be used for teaching, either by having the students assemble them or for the purpose of demonstration. They constitute an original contribution to these volumes devoted to the functional anatomy of the locomotor system.

If you wish to assemble one of these models, you must first transfer the drawing on to a sheet of cardboard **1 mm thick** or, failing that, on to a thick Bristol board. The easy solution is to glue directly to the cardboard each sheet of the model removed from the book, but this should be avoided since it will destroy your book and, if you make a mistake you will not be able to make up for it. It is better therefore to glue on to the cardboard a *photocopy of the page in question*. The best solution is *to trace on to the cardboard a carbon copy of the diagram*, which has the advantage of avoiding the problem of having to use glued sheets of paper later. Finally, a useful solution is to obtain an enlarged photocopy (A3 format), which allows you to make larger models. Assembling these models is easy if you *strictly follow the directions* which are provided with the plates and are illustrated with mounting instructions. *Do not ever start cutting out before reading all the instructions.* If you make a mistake, you can always transfer the piece on to another sheet of cardboard of the same thickness and start again.

The **folding lines** are sharp and regular when the cardboard has first been lightly incised to a depth of one-quarter of its thickness on the outer aspect of the fold with a razor blade, a craft knife or a scalpel. Be careful, therefore, to notice *which way the cardboard will be folded*, as indicated below:

*   The folding lines marked by broken lines must be *cut on the front of the cardboard and folded on the back* (for reference, the front is the side with the printed sheet, and the back is the blank side).
*   The folding lines marked by lines of alternating dots and dashes must be *cut on the back* and *folded towards the front* of the board. To mark these lines on the front, it is useful to *place a fine needle at each end of the folding line.*

Use a fast-acting cellulose glue for **gluing the pieces together.** The *shaded surfaces*, demarcated by dotted lines (not to be confused with the lines indicating the folds) correspond to the spots *on the front of the cardboard for gluing.* Whenever possible, the two surfaces to be glued together have been marked with the same letter. Glue the pieces one by one and *wait until two glued spots on the same piece are quite dry before gluing other spots on the same piece.*

Meanwhile, go on gluing the spots on the other pieces. While the glue is drying, keep the pieces tied to a wooden plank by elastic bands, or use the needles for marking the folds to steady the piece.

Exceptionally in model 5, the folds representing the articular hinges must be made without any incisions (or with only shallow incisions) in order to prevent the wear and tear of usage.

You will also need the **following materials:**

*   A thick cardboard (1 mm thick) to strengthen some of the pieces or to serve as bases (for Models 1 and 3)
*   The smallest available paper fasteners (for Model 3), which can be obtained from a stationery shop
*   Fine elastic threads used in the welts of socks; these can be obtained from a haberdashery
*   Thick threads or fine strings or, even better, braided cords to represent the tendons.

Building the models

Model 1: to illustrate the role of the cruciates and of the collateral ligaments of the knee

This model allows you to illustrate how the cruciates and the collateral ligaments are selectively stretched during certain movements (see p. 125) and to explain, in particular, how the femoral condyle is 'pulled back' on the tibial articular surfaces during movements of flexion-extension.

Assembly (Plate I)

Before you cut out any piece at all it is preferable to transfer the two pieces of this model (Fig. 1), i.e. the femoral cross-section A and tibial cross-section B, on to a thick cardboard (1 mm thick). Then follow the assembly instructions and position the elastic bands, of different colours if possible, to correspond to the two cruciates and the medial collateral ligament. To do this, take three rubber bands and cut each to make a strand. Make a knot at one end of these strands, and then thread them through the holes in the tibial cross-section from back to front so that the knot comes to lie at the back. Next, glue the tibial cross-section on to a rectangular piece of strong cardboard (see assembly instructions, Fig. 2). If the knots interfere with the gluing, hollow out the cardboard slightly to receive them.

Then thread each elastic band through the corresponding hole in the femoral cross-section from front to back so that:

*   the anterior cruciate runs from a to b
*   the posterior cruciate runs from c to d
*   the medial collateral ligament runs from e to f.

Mobilization

The anterior cruciate is elongated during flexion (red arrow), felt as tension in the elastic band. For this ligament to maintain the same length, the condyle must be pulled back anteriorly. This movement corresponds to the *condylar pull-back effected by the anterior cruciate.*

Likewise, starting from the position of flexion, the posterior cruciate is elongated during extension (blue arrow). To regain its initial length, the condyle must be pulled back posteriorly. This corresponds to the *pullback movement of the posterior cruciate.* By making the femoral condyle *roll and slide* on the tibial articular surface, you can see the *ligament being stretched farther during extension than during flexion.*

Model 2: articulated plates illustrating the anteroposterior stability of the knee

(see Fig. 185, p. 125)

This model (Fig. 3) allows you to understand how the cruciates preclude any antero-posterior sliding without preventing flexion-extension of the knee.

Assembly (Plate I)

1. Cut out the two rectangles A and B (Plate I).

2. From a piece of stronger cardboard, cut out two other rectangles of exactly the same dimensions as A and B

3. From a piece of ordinary paper, cut out three strips one centimetre wide along the full length of the paper (A4 format).

4. As per **assembly instructions** (Fig. 4), glue one end of each paper strip on to the shaded areas a, b and c, making sure that the strips remain strictly parallel to the longer sides of the rectangles (**step a**).

5. On top of the rectangle A and of the ends of the three paper strips already glued down, glue one of the rectangles from the strong cardboard, which must cover exactly the rectangle **A**.

6. Place this combination on the table (**step b**) with the strong cardboard rectangle at the bottom and then fold over the rectangle A, ensuring that the three paper strips remain parallel to one another and to the long side of the rectangle A.

7. Then place rectangle B on top, with its front facing upwards and the shaded area **a'** overlying the free end of the middle paper strip.

8. Fold the free ends of the three paper strips over rectangle B so that they can be glued to areas a', b' and c'. These three rectangles must be pressed against one another.

9. On top of rectangle B glue the second rectangle of strong cardboard (**step c**), pull hard on the three paper strips, place a weight on top of this assembly and wait till the glue is quite dry.

10. Finally, cut off (**step d**) any paper strips that stick out.

Inside this assembly the paper strips, which correspond to the cruciates, cross one another in space in such a way that the rectangles cannot be pulled apart vertically because of the tension developed in these strips.

Mobilization

With this model you can verify (Fig. 5) that it is impossible to make any one of the rectangles slide past another lengthwise (a).

On the other hand, if you pick up only the upper rectangle and swing it over to one side or the other, *it will rotate about the hinge located at one of the short sides of the assembly* (b) and also at the other short side of the assembly (c). The two rectangles do not appear to be stuck to each other, and *yet they are articulated at their extremities.*

The femoral condyles and the tibial articular surfaces are similarly arranged except that the paper strips corresponding to the cruciates are not equal in length and are not fixed to a base of similar length. As a result, rotation takes place, not only around two axes, but also around *a succession of axes aligned along the curves of the condyles,* as demonstrated in the next model.

Model 3: Experimental demonstration of the determinants of trochlear and condylar contours

With this model (see Figs 54 and 55, p. 87) you can yourself trace the contours of the condyles and of the trochlea and thus illustrate the **role of the ligaments in determining the shapes of the articular surfaces.**

Assembly (Plate II)

1. Cut out the different pieces of this model:
- the tibial plateau A
- the piece called the femoral *Base* B, which will come to lie on top of the deck C
- the rectangular platform on which the contours will be drawn. Already drawn are two thick lines corresponding to the sites of junction between the articular contour and the femoral diaphysis, which will be drawn later
- the patella prolonged downwards by the ligamentum patellae
- one patellar retinaculum (PR).
- the anterior cruciate ligament (ACL)
- the posterior cruciate ligament (PCL)
- three thick strips for the production of three thick discs needed for the assembly.

2. Accordion-pleat these strips to produce the 'washers' and then make a hole through all six layers in one step (not easy!).

3. At each end of the PCL, make two folding lines before piercing the holes 3 and 4.

4. Make the holes on the other pieces exactly in the positions indicated.

Assembly (Plate III)

Use the smallest paper fastener available at the stationer's to assemble the model (Fig. 6).

The holes on each of the pieces are numbered to correspond to each other. Match these holes in numerical order, remembering to insert washers between holes 5, 6 and 7. Finally, fix the femoral base **B** to the shaded deck **C** at holes 8 and 9. You will notice that, for the model to work properly, you must make a dent (arrow p) in the washer 4 without denting the PCL itself.

Mobilization

This model is now ready to use (Fig. 7).

From the position of extension, where the tibial plateau is pulled as far as possible to the left because of the dent in the washer of hole 4, move it progressively to the right (red arrow), and at each position pencil in the posterior contour of the patella and the superior contour of the tibial plateau.

As the tibial plateau moves to the right, you can see its *superior surface tracing the curvature of the condyle*, while at the same time the *posterior surface and the posterosuperior angle of the patella trace the contour of the trochlea* (Fig. 8). If the model has been well assembled, these two curves join the two thick lines already drawn on the platform, and the curve of the trochlea links up with that of the condyle.

This experiment also demonstrates that the contours of the condyles and of the trochlea correspond respectively to the **enveloping curves of the successive positions** of the tibial plateau and of the patella, within a **mechanical system** defined by the *relative lengths and arrangement of the cruciates as well as the ligamentous connections of the patella.* You could easily generate other contours by changing one or more of the components of this mechanical assembly.

Model 4: Model of the foot

This model is a simplified version of the model presented in the first editions of this work. It is much easier to build and allows you to perform virtually the same experiments.

Building Model 4 (Plate IV)

1. Cut out the following pieces of the model:
- the leg **A**, with its articulated segments at the bottom end corresponding to the universal joint of the ankle; you must make the two slits carefully using a scalpel or a craft knife
- the intermediate piece **B** corresponding to the anterior tarsus
- **C** corresponding to the calcaneus
- **D** corresponding to the stabilizer of the calcaneus
- the five rays of the foot, numbered I-V.

2. To increase the rigidity of the leg component of piece **A** you can glue two similar bands of cardboard parallel to each other along its two edges.

Assembly (Plate V)

A blown-up view (Fig. 9) shows the arrangement and the interlocking of the various pieces:
- The leg piece **A** has three folds running in opposite directions x, y and z (Fig. 10); these folds will in the assembled model correspond to the 'heterokinetic universal joint' of the ankle in conjunction with the axis of the ankle x and Henke's axis z.
- Make the assembly *rigid* by inserting the calcaneal piece **C**, i.e. by slipping the two tongue-like projections into the appropriate slits and securing them with *split pins* pushed through the holes in the projections. For split pins you can use toothpicks or matchsticks.

- Complete the calcaneal piece **C** with the calcaneal stabilizer **D**, whose slit is made to slide into the corresponding calcaneal slit so that the edge of **D** is flush with that of **C**.
- Make the five rays of the foot by making shallow incisions into each piece on its top side, folding the flaps towards each other and gluing them together (Fig. 11). Wait until the glue is secure before proceeding.
- Glue each ray to the corresponding projection of the intermediate piece **B** representing the anterior tarsus, making sure that they are set at the proper distance apart and at the proper inclination, as indicated on piece **B.** The front of this piece will already have an incision made at the base of each projection to correspond to the flexion-extension axes of the metatarsals.
- When the assembly made up of piece **B** and the five rays is solid, you can glue it to the superior surface of the part **T** of the leg piece to link the tarsus to the metatarsals.

The model is now complete, but *you have not yet stabilized the assembly* with the help of tighteners, which are essential to ensure at least that the foot is stable when placed on a horizontal plane.

The **elastic tighteners** are best represented by elastic threads used in sewing. You can easily fix them on to the cardboard plates by jamming them into tiny slits made in the cardboard with a scalpel or a craft knife.

On the model (Fig. 9) these five slits are flagged by small red arrows.

On an **antero-medial view** (Fig. 12), a **medial view** (Fig. 13) or a **lateral view** (Fig. 14) you can see how these elastic threads are arranged to simulate the *balanced tonus of the muscles*:
- The *blue thread*, between the first ray and the calcaneus, simulates the muscles forming the *chord of the anterior arch.* You can easily control its tension at the level of its attachment to the calcaneus.
- The *red thread* forms a *triangle* as it runs from the tarsus to the calcaneal tuberosity via the leg piece. It simulates the *balance between the ankle flexors and extensors*. You can control the balance of tensions in this thread at the level of the slit in the leg piece.

After *patiently* making repeated attempts to find the right degree of tension for these threads, you will have a model that stays in balance on a horizontal surface; it is the miracle long awaited! You can then make the model take up all the positions of the foot relative to the leg, in particular those of eversion (Fig. 15) and inversion (Fig. 16) of the sole of the foot, which can easily be seen to occur preferentially in certain directions because of the **heterokinetic nature of the universal joint of the ankle.** You can also simulate the pes cavus (Fig. 17) by verticalizing the calcaneus, and the pes planus (Fig. 18) by causing collapse of the medial arch combined with a valgus of the calcaneus.

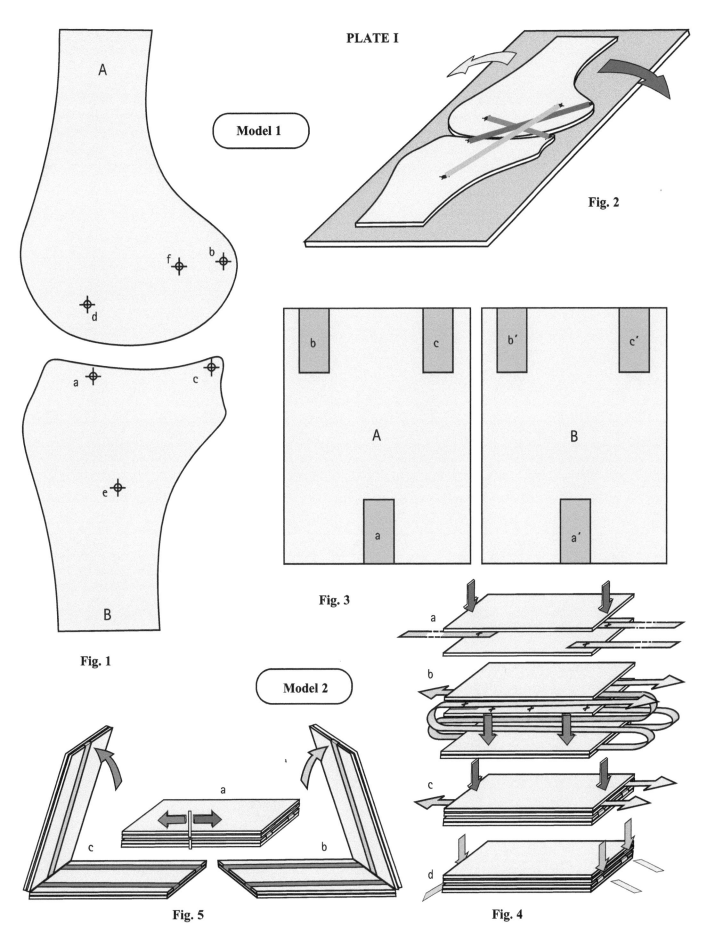

PLATE I

Model 1

Fig. 1

Fig. 2

Fig. 3

Model 2

Fig. 4

Fig. 5

313

PLATE II

Model 3

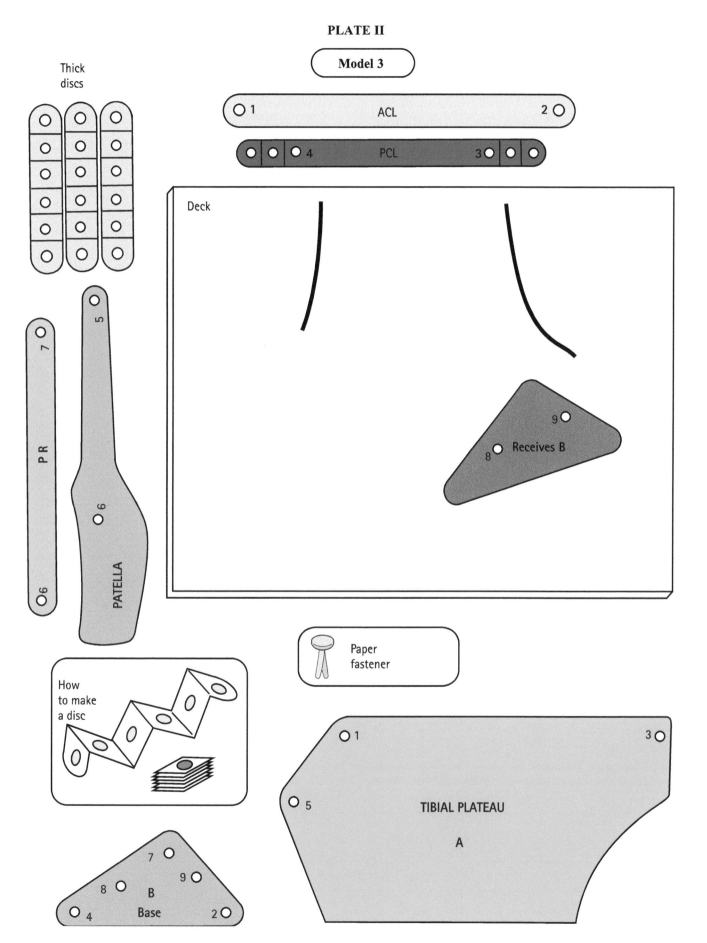

Thick discs

1 ACL 2

4 PCL 3

Deck

9

8 Receives B

P R

7

5

6

PATELLA

6

How to make a disc

Paper fastener

1 3

5 TIBIAL PLATEAU

A

7

9

8 B

Base

4 2

PLATE III

Model 3

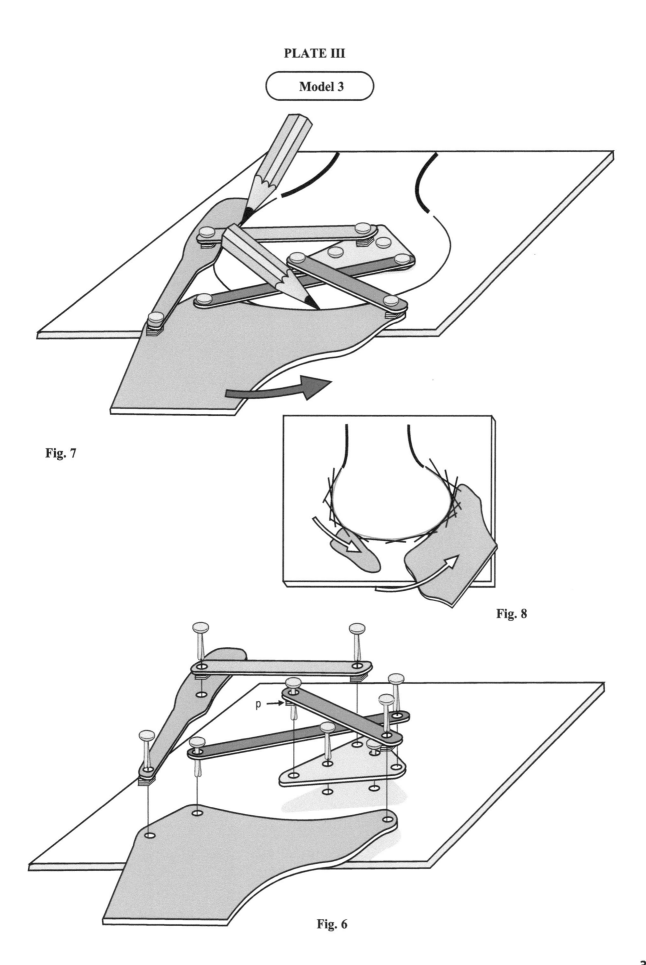

Fig. 7

Fig. 8

Fig. 6

PLATE IV

Model 4

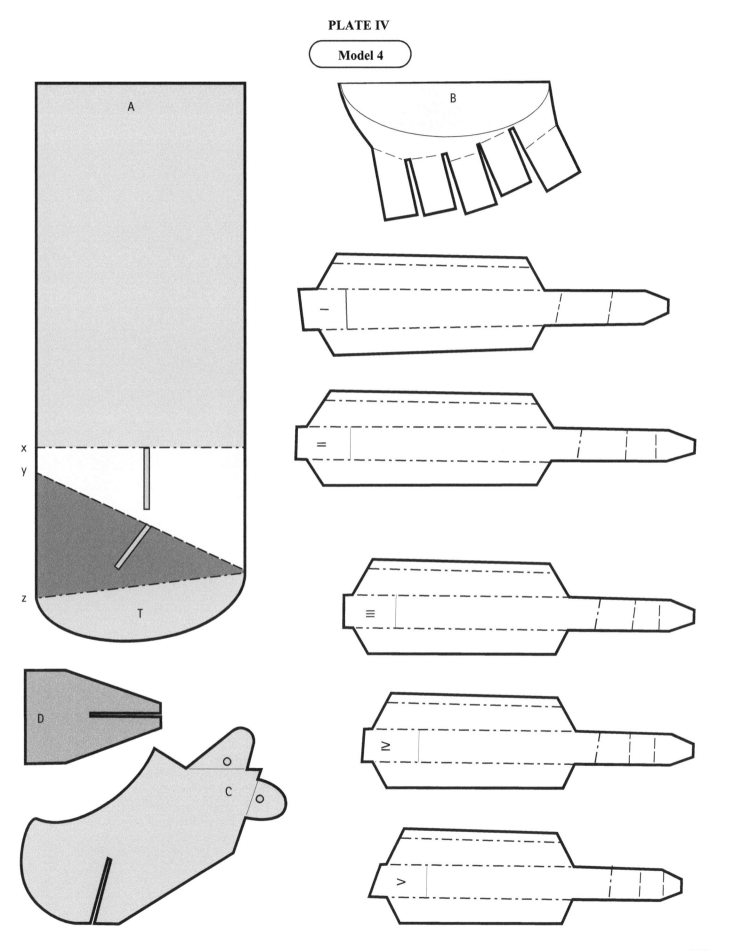

PLATE V

Model 4

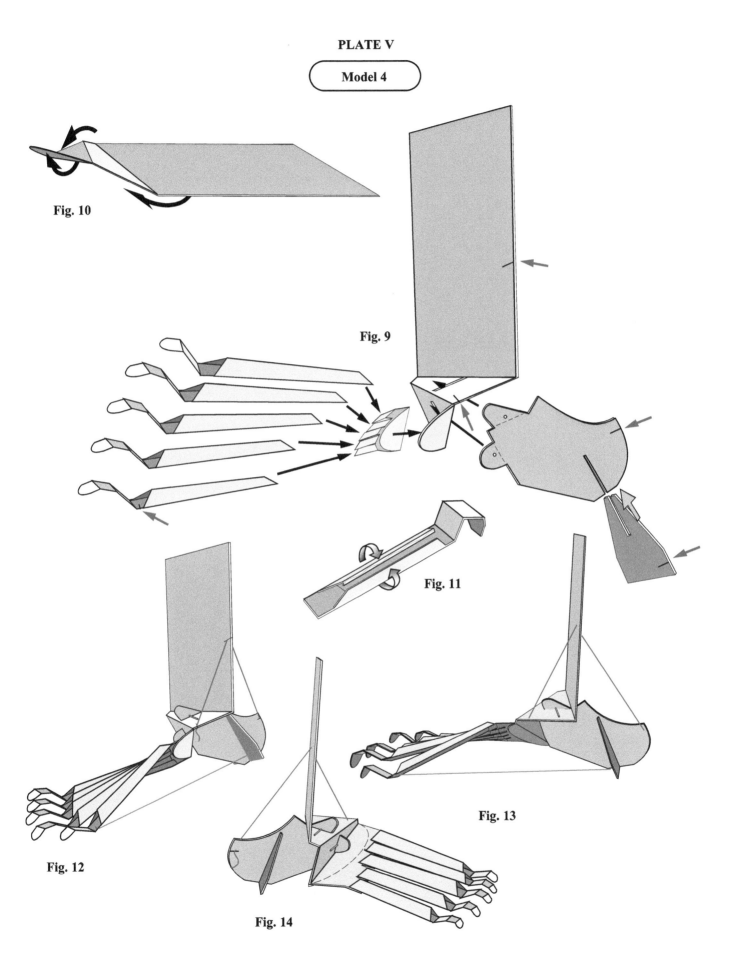

Fig. 10

Fig. 9

Fig. 11

Fig. 12

Fig. 14

Fig. 13

PLATE VI

Model 4

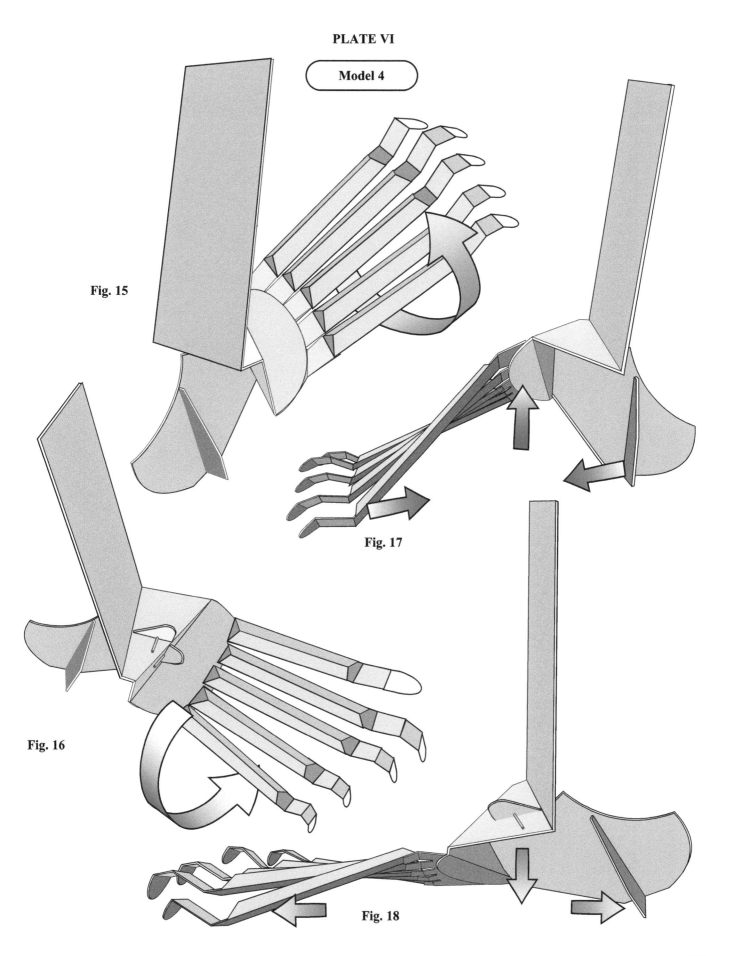

Fig. 15

Fig. 16

Fig. 17

Fig. 18